Hepatocellular Cancer

CURRENT CLINICAL ONCOLOGY

Maurie Markman, MD, SERIES EDITOR

Hepatocellular Cancer: *Diagnosis and Treatment,* edited by *BRIAN I. CARR,* 2005

Squamous Cell Head and Neck Cancer, edited by *DAVID J. ADELSTEIN,* 2005

Biology and Management of Multiple Myeloma, edited by *JAMES R. BERENSON,* 2004

Cancer Immunotherapy at the Crossroads: *How Tumors Evade Immunity and What Can Be Done,* edited by *JAMES H. FINKE AND RONALD M. BUKOWSKI,* 2004

Treatment of Acute Leukemias: *New Directions for Clinical Research,* edited by *CHING-HON PUI,* 2003

Allogeneic Stem Cell Transplantation: *Clinical Research and Practice,* edited by *MARY J. LAUGHLIN AND HILLARD M. LAZARUN,* 2003

Chronic Leukemias and Lymphomas: *Biology, Pathophysiology, and Clinical Management,* edited by *GARY J. SCHILLER,* 2003

Colorectal Cancer: *Multimodality Management,* edited by *LEONARD SALTZ,* 2002

Breast Cancer: *A Guide to Detection and Multidisciplinary Therapy,* edited by *MICHAEL H. TOROSIAN,* 2002

Melanoma: *Biologically Targeted Therapeutics,* edited by *ERNEST C. BORDEN,* 2002

Cancer of the Lung: *From Molecular Biology to Treatment Guidelines,* edited by *ALAN B. WEITBERG,* 2001

Renal Cell Carcinoma: *Molecular Biology, Immunology, and Clinical Management,* edited by *RONALD M. BUKOWSKI AND ANDREW NOVICK,* 2000

Current Controversies in Bone Marrow Transplantation, edited by *BRIAN J. BOLWELL,* 2000

Regional Chemotherapy: *Clinical Research and Practice,* edtied by *MAURIE MARKMAN,* 2000

Intraoperative Irradiation: *Techniques and Results,* edited by *L. L. GUNDERSON, C. G. WILLETT, L. B. HARRISON, AND F. A. CALVO,* 1999

Hepatocellular Cancer

Diagnosis and Treatment

Edited by

Brian I. Carr, MD, FRCP, PhD
University of Pittsburgh Medical Center,
Pittsburgh, PA

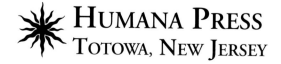

Humana Press
Totowa, New Jersey

999 Riverview Drive, Suite 208
Totowa, New Jersey 07512
humanapress.com

For additional copies, pricing for bulk purchases, and/or information about other Humana titles, contact Humana at the above address or at any of the following numbers: Tel.: 973-256-1699; Fax: 973-256-8341, E-mail: humana@humanapr.com; or visit our Website: http://humanapress.com

Cover design by Patricia F. Cleary

Cover illustrations from Figs. 1A and 2A in Chapter 11, "Interventional Radiology Techniques for Intra-Arterial Chemo-Embolization" by Nikhil B. Amesur, Albert B. Zajko, and Philip D. Orons; Fig. 8 in Chapter 4, "Pathologic Aspects of Hepatocellular Tumors," by Hale Kirimlioglu, Anthony J.Demetris, and Michael A. Nalesnik; and Fig. 1A (left side) in Chapter 12, "Medical Therapy of Hepatocellular Carcinoma," by Brian I. Carr.

This publication is printed on acid-free paper. ∞
ANSI Z39.48-1984 (American National Standards Institute) Permanence of Paper for Printed Library Materials.

Printed in the United States of America. 10 9 8 7 6 5 4 3 2 1
e-ISBN: 1-59259-844-7
Library of Congress Cataloging-in-Publication Data

Hepatocellular cancer : diagnosis and treatment / edited by Brian I. Carr.
p. ; cm. -- (Current clinical oncology)
Includes bibliographical references and index.
ISBN 1-58829-125-1 (alk. paper)
1. Liver--Cancer.
[DNLM: 1. Carcinoma, Hepatocellular--therapy. 2. Carcinoma, Hepatocellular--diagnosis.
WI 735 H5289 2005] I. Carr, Brian I. II. Series.
RC280.L5H4555 2005
616.99'436--dc22 2004006683

Dedication

To my daughters, Ophira and Feridey

Preface

You are not obliged to complete the task,
nor are you free to desist from trying.
—Talmud, Avot

Hepatocellular carcinoma (HCC) used to be regarded as a rare disease. The increasing numbers of chronic hepatitis C virus carriers in the United States and subsequent increased incidence of HCC seen in most large medical centers means that it is no longer an uncommon disease for most gastroenterologists or oncologists to encounter.

During the times when liver resection or systemic chemotherapy were the only real therapeutic modalities available, the outcomes were generally dismal, especially because most patients presented with advanced-stage tumors. Several recent factors seem to have changed this. They include the more frequent use of aggressive surveillance by ultrasound and computed tomography (CT) scanning in patients who have chronic hepatitis or cirrhosis from any cause (and thus are known to be at risk for subsequent development of HCC) to detect tumors at an earlier and therefore more treatable stage. Advances in CT scanning, particularly the introduction of multihead fast helical scans, mean that this vascular tumor can often be detected at an earlier stage, or multiple lesions can be diagnosed when only large single lesions were formerly seen, so that unnecessary resections are not performed.

Liver transplantation has had a profound effect on the therapeutic landscape. There have always been two hopes for this modality: namely, to eliminate cirrhosis as a limiting factor for surgical resection and also to extend the ability of the surgeon to remove ever-larger tumors confined to the liver. Regional chemotherapy and hepatic artery chemoembolization have been around for a long time and have been practiced mainly in the Far East and Europe.

There has not been a consensus for which drug or drug combination is best or whether embolization is important and, if so, what type and size of particle are optimal. Although there is still no consensus on these matters, it has recently become clear from two randomized controlled clinical trials that hepatic artery chemoembolization for unresectable nonmetastatic HCC seems to bestow a survival advantage compared to no treatment. The high recurrence rates after resection have led numerous investigators to evaluate preresection and postresection chemotherapy in the hope of decreasing recurrence rates. Only recently have clinical trials begun to provide evidence of enhanced survival for multimodality therapy involving resection and either chemotherapy or ^{131}I-lipiodol. The introduction of ^{90}Yttrium microspheres, which appear to offer the promise of relatively nontoxic tumoricidal therapy to the liver, appears to be a major therapeutic addition to our treatment choices, and its role alone or in combination with other therapies is just beginning to be explored.

In addition, we are beginning to enter the phase in which proteomics is applied to many tumor types, including HCC. This raises the possibility of being able to categorize patients into prognostic subsets, prior to any therapy. We are also just at the beginning of the age of cell cycle modulating factors including hormones, growth factors, and growth factor receptor antagonists and agents that specifically alter defined aspects of the cell cycle.

For these reasons, it seemed reasonable to produce a book that represents much of the current therapy and thinking on HCC. Admittedly, there is a bias toward expressing the experience of one center, the Liver Cancer Center at the University of Pittsburgh Starzl Transplant Institute, in which over 250 new cases of HCC have been seen each year for the last 15 years. This is an exciting time to be in the field of HCC basic science as well as clinical management because so many changes are simultaneously occurring at multiple levels of our understanding and management of the disease.

Brian I. Carr, *MD, FRCP, PhD*

Contents

Contributors

JAWAD AHMAD MD, MRCP (UK) • *Division of Gastroenterology, Hepatology, and Nutrition, Department of Medicine, University of Pittsburgh School of Medicine, Pittsburgh, PA*

NIKHIL B. AMESUR, MD • *Department of Radiology, University of Pittsburgh School of Medicine, Pittsburgh, PA*

C. ANDREW BONHAM, MD • *Department of Transplantation Surgery, University of Pittsburgh Medical Center, Pittsburgh, PA*

BRIAN I. CARR, MD, FRCP, PhD • *Liver Cancer Center, Thomas E. Starzl Transplantation Institute, Department of Surgery, University of Pittsburgh Medical Center, Pittsburgh, PA*

KAPIL B. CHOPRA, MD, DM, FACP • *Department of Medicine, University of Pittsburgh School of Medicine, Pittsburgh, PA*

MARIE C. DEFRANCES, MD, PhD • *Department of Pathology, University of Pittsburgh School of Medicine, Pittsburgh, PA*

ANTHONY J. DEMETRIS, MD • *Division of Transplantation and Hepatic Pathology, Department of Pathology, Thomas E. Starzl Transplantation Institute, University of Pittsburgh Medical Center, Pittsburgh, PA*

IGOR DVORCHIK, PhD • *Department of Transplantation Surgery, University of Pittsburgh Medical Center; Department of Biostatistics, Graduate School of Public Health, University of Pittsburgh, Pittsburgh, PA*

MICHAEL P. FEDERLE, MD • *Department of Radiology, University of Pittsburgh School of Medicine, Pittsburgh, PA*

SYDNEY D. FINKELSTEIN, MD • *Department of Pathology and Laboratory Medicine, University of Pittsburgh Medical Center, Pittsburgh, PA*

DAVID A. GELLER, MD • *Liver Cancer Center, Thomas E. Starzl Transplantation Institute, University of Pittsburgh School of Medicine, Pittsburgh, PA*

MARTIN GOODMAN, MD • *Thomas E. Starzl Transplantation Institute, University of Pittsburgh School of Medicine, Pittsburgh, PA*

TAKASHI KANEMATSU, MD, PhD • *Department of Surgery II, Nagasaki University School of Medicine, Nagasaki, Japan*

VIBHU KAPOOR, MD • *Department of Radiology, University of Pittsburgh School of Medicine, Pittsburgh, PA*

ANDREW S. KENNEDY, MD • *Radiation Oncology, Wake Radiology Oncology, Cary, NC*

HALE KIRIMLIOGLU, MD • *Pathology Department, Inonu University, Malatya, Turkey*

J. WALLIS MARSH, MD, MBA • *Department of Surgery, University of Pittsburgh School of Medicine, Pittsburgh, PA*

GEORGE K. MICHALOPOULOS, MD, PhD • *Department of Pathology, University of Pittsburgh School of Medicine, Pittsburgh, PA*

MICHAEL A. NALESNIK, MD • *Division of Transplantation and Hepatic Pathology, Department of Pathology, Thomas E. Starzl Transplantation Institute, University of Pittsburgh Medical Center, Pittsburgh, PA*

SADAYUKI OKUDAIRA, MD, PhD • *Department of Transplantation and Digestive Surgery, Nagasaki University Graduate School of Biomedical Sciences, Nagasaki, Japan*

PHILIP D. ORONS, DO • *Departments of Radiology and Surgery, University of Pittsburgh School of Medicine, Pittsburgh, PA*

MICHAEL J. PAYNE, MD • *Department of Radiology, University of Pittsburgh School of Medicine, Pittsburgh, PA*

MORDECHAI RABINOVITZ, MD • *Division of Gastroenterology, Hepatology, and Nutrition, Department of Medicine, University of Pittsburgh School of Medicine, Pittsburgh, PA*

DAVID A. SASS, MD • *Division of Gastroenterology, Hepatology, and Nutrition, Department of Surgery, University of Pittsburgh School of Medicine, Pittsburgh, PA*

F. LELAND THAETE, MD • *Department of Radiology, University of Pittsburgh School of Medicine, Pittsburgh, PA*

KATSUHIKO YANAGA, MD, PhD • *Department of Surgery, The Jikei University School of Medicine, Tokyo, Japan*

ALBERT B. ZAJKO, MD • *Departments of Radiology and Surgery, University of Pittsburgh School of Medicine, Pittsburgh, PA*

Value-Added eBook/PDA

This book is accompanied by a value-added CD-ROM that contains an eBook version of the volume you have just purchased. This eBook can be viewed on your computer, and you can synchronize it to your PDA for viewing on your handheld device. The eBook enables you to view this volume on only one computer and PDA. Once the eBook is installed on your computer, you cannot download, install, or e-mail it to another computer; it resides solely with the computer to which it is installed. The license provided is for only one computer. The eBook can only be read using Adobe® Reader® 6.0 software, which is available free from Adobe Systems Incorporated at www.Adobe.com. You may also view the eBook on your PDA using the Adobe® PDA Reader® software that is also available free from Adobe.com.

You must follow a simple procedure when you install the eBook/PDA that will require you to connect to the Humana Press website in order to receive your license. Please read and follow the instructions below:

1. Download and install Adobe® Reader® 6.0 software

You can obtain a free copy of the Adobe® Reader® 6.0 software at www.adobe.com

*Note: If you already have the Adobe® Reader® 6.0 software installed, you do not need to reinstall it.

2. Launch Adobe® Reader® 6.0 software

3. Install eBook: Insert your eBook CD into your CD-ROM drive

PC: Click on the "Start" button, then click on "Run"

At the prompt, type "d:\ebookinstall.pdf" and click "OK"

*Note: If your CD-ROM drive letter is something other than d: change the above command accordingly.

MAC: Double click on the "eBook CD" that you will see mounted on your desktop.

Double click "ebookinstall.pdf"

4. Adobe® Reader® 6.0 software will open and you will receive the message:

"This document is protected by Adobe DRM" Click "OK"

*Note: If you have not already activated the Adobe® Reader® 6.0 software, you will be prompted to do so. Simply follow the directions to activate and continue installation.

Your web browser will open and you will be taken to the Humana Press eBook registration page. Follow the instructions on that page to complete installation. You will need the serial number located on the sticker sealing the envelope containing the CD-ROM.

If you require assistance during the installation, or you would like more information regarding your eBook and PDA installation, please refer to the eBookManual.pdf located on your CD. If you need further assistance, contact Humana Press eBook Support by e-mail at ebooksupport@humanapr.com or by phone at 973-256-1699.

*Adobe and Reader are either registered trademarks or trademarks of Adobe Systems Incorporated in the United States and/or other countries.

Color Plates

Color Plates 1–8 appear as an insert following page 210.

PLATE 1 Two mass lesions arising in a noncirrhotic liver. (*See* Fig. 1, Chapter 4.)

PLATE 2 Focal nodular hyperplasia. (*See* Fig. 3, Chapter 4.)

PLATE 3 Hepatocelular carcinoma. (*See* Fig. 4, Chapter 4.)

PLATE 4 Hepatocelular carcinoma with portal vein invasion. (*See* Fig. 4, Chapter 4.)

PLATE 5 Hepatocelular carcinoma. (*See* Fig. 8, Chapter 4.)

PLATE 6 Hepatocelular carcinoma, fibrolamellar subtype. (*See* Fig. 10, Chapter 4.)

PLATE 7 Electron micrograph of glass microspheres adjacent to a human hair for perspective and CT-based reconstruction from radiation treatment planning software of a predominantly right-sided tumor with transparent liver volume. (*See* Fig. 1A,B, Chapter 13.)

PLATE 8 Glass microspheres in clusters within a tumor nodule of HCC. (*See* Fig. 2, Chapter 13.)

1 Etiology and Epidemiology of Hepatocellular Carcinoma

Jawad Ahmad, MD
and Mordechai Rabinovitz, MD

Contents

1. INTRODUCTION

Hepatocellular carcinoma (HCC) is one of the leading causes of worldwide cancer mortality, with an estimated 1 million deaths annually and a 5-year survival rate of less than 5% *(1)*. Cirrhosis of the liver is the main risk factor for the development of HCC, but the incidence of HCC varies considerably depending on, among other factors, geographical location and the cause of liver disease. HCC incidence of 4 to 15 per 100,000 has been reported in Western countries, compared with 120 per 100,000 in Asia and Africa *(2)*. Similarly, higher incidences of HCC have been reported in chronic liver disease related to viral hepatitis B and C compared with alcoholic liver disease. Tables 1 and 2 list some of the causes and possible mechanisms of HCC development.

2. RISK FACTORS FOR HCC

2.1. Hepatitis B Virus

Several case-control studies in the 1970s demonstrated that hepatitis B surface antigen (HBsAg) was present in the serum of patients with HCC substantially more frequently than in controls *(3–5)*. This was contrary to earlier reports that doubted such an association *(6,7)*. The issue was resolved by the landmark cohort

From: *Current Clinical Oncology: Hepatocellular Cancer: Diagnosis and Treatment*
Edited by: B. I. Carr © Humana Press Inc., Totowa, NJ

Table 1
Risk Factors for the Development of HCC

Hepatitis B
Hepatitis C
Cirrhosis
Aflatoxin β1
Hereditary hemochromatosis
α-1-antitrypsin deficiency
Hereditary tyrosinemia
Alcohol
Male gender
Age
Tobacco smoking
Radiation exposure
Inorganic arsenic
Radioactive thorium dioxide
Oral contraceptive use
Glycogen storage disease
Membranous obstruction of the vena cava
Safrole oil

Table 2
Possible Pathogenic Mechanisms in the Development of HCC

Risk factor	*Possible mechanism*
Hepatitis B	Integration into host genome
	HBx protein and p53 suppression
Hepatitis C	Persistent inflammation and cirrhosis
	HCV capsid induced genetic modulation
Aflatoxin	Genetic polymorphism, p53 tumor suppression
Male gender	Androgenic stimulation of transforming growth factor α

study by Beasley et al. *(8)*, who followed up almost 23,000 Chinese subjects in Taiwan for an average of 3.3 years, 15% of whom were HBsAg positive. Of the 41 people who died of HCC, all but one was HBsAg positive, a relative risk of 223 compared with HBsAg-negative controls. A similar increased risk of HCC was seen in a prospective study of 1400 Alaskan natives with chronic hepatitis B *(9)*.

The precise mechanism for HCC development in chronic hepatitis B virus (HBV) is unclear, but integration of the viral genome into cellular DNA has been found in almost all HBV-induced HCC cases *(10)*. The X gene of the viral genome codes for functionally active transactivator proteins, including the X protein (HBx), which is oncogenic in transgenic mice *(11)*. The HBx protein interacts directly with promoter-bound transcription factors, or proto-oncogene promoters such as NFκB and also stimulates cellular second messenger systems, including the *ras* mitogen-activated protein-kinase signaling cascade and the protein kinase C pathway *(12)*. The pivotal role of HBx protein in initiating carcinogenesis is given further credence by the demonstration that it binds to the p53 tumor-suppressor protein and may inhibit p53-mediated apoptosis, leading to a clonally selected population of hepatocytes that expresses the incorporated viral genome *(13,14)*.

The strong association between hepatitis B infection and HCC is demonstrated further by examining the effect of interferon (IFN)-α therapy. IFN-α leads to loss of serological markers, including hepatitis B DNA and hepatitis B e antigen, appearance of hepatitis B e antibody (seroconversion), and can even result in the loss of HBsAg. This, in turn, would be expected to reduce the risk of HCC. Indeed, a recent meta-analysis of nine randomized controlled trials suggested that IFN-α therapy may reduce the absolute cumulative lifetime incidence of HCC by 4% *(15)*. It is unclear whether this is related to the direct anticarcinogenic effect of IFN-α or its antiviral effect. This argument is supported further by the striking decline in HCC incidence after the introduction of hepatitis B vaccine. Chang et al. *(16)* examined the effect on the incidence of HCC of a nationwide hepatitis B vaccination program begun in Taiwan in 1984. There was a stepwise decline in the annual incidence of HCC in children age 6 to 14 years from 0.7 per 100,000 between 1981 and 1986, to 0.57 per 100,000 between 1986 and 1990, to 0.36 per 100,000 between 1990 and 1994. Similarly, the incidence in children age 6 to 9 years declined from 0.52 per 100,000 in those born between 1974 and 1984 to 0.13 per 100,000 for those born between 1984 and 1986. The same group also suggested that the reduction in HCC attributed to hepatitis B vaccination is significant only in male children, with no decline witnessed in female children vaccinated over the same time period *(17)*. However, a recent study in the same population demonstrated that HBV vaccination decreased childhood HCC by up to 70% in boys and by up to 62% in girls *(18)*.

Previous infection with hepatitis B also may confer a risk for carcinogenesis. Matsuzaki et al. *(19)* recently demonstrated an increased incidence of hepatitis B DNA integration into the host genome in some Japanese patients with HCC who had no serological evidence of hepatitis B or hepatitis C infections. This suggests that prior hepatitis B infection may play a role in neoplastic progression.

2.2. Hepatitis C Virus

Hepatitis C virus (HCV) is an RNA virus and does not integrate into the host genome as seen with HBV *(20)*. Despite this, numerous series from throughout the world have demonstrated the high incidence of serum antibodies to hepatitis C (anti-HCV) in patients with HCC *(21–33)* and also have detected HCV RNA in liver and tumor tissue *(34–36)*. Most of the HCC cases develop in patients with underlying cirrhosis several decades after the initial infection, at a rate of 1–7% per year *(37,38)*. Tong et al. *(39)* reported a cohort of 131 patients with chronic posttransfusion hepatitis seen over a 14-year period and followed up for 4 years. Of these, 5% had evidence of HCC at presentation, and a further 5% developed HCC during the follow-up period.

Although cirrhosis greatly increases the risk of HCC, it can also develop in patients without cirrhosis. In patients with chronic hepatitis without cirrhosis, the incidence of HCC over a 3-year cumulative period was 4%, compared with almost 13% in those with established cirrhosis *(40)*. Indeed, HCV RNA can be found in patients with HCC in the absence of cirrhosis or fibrosis *(41)*.

The rate of liver cell proliferation also may play a role in the development of HCC. Persistent regeneration and proliferation of liver cells is a key feature of the hepatitis process, and products of the HCV genome may be involved in regulating liver cell proliferation. The HCV capsid can modulate the effect of several cellular genes, such as the human c-*myc* promoter gene *(42)*, and can transform rat embryo fibroblasts into a malignant phenotype when transfected with the *ras* oncogene *(43)*. Both in vitro and in vivo studies have underscored the capacity of viral proteins to induce tumorigenesis *(44)*. Some investigators have demonstrated clinical correlation of these models with higher rates of HCC in patients with chronic HCV or cirrhosis who expressed markers of liver cell dysplasia or periportal hepatocyte regeneration *(45–47)*. Recently, a retrospective study of 115 patients with chronic viral hepatitis identified large liver cell dysplasia as an independent risk factor for the development of HCC *(48)*. This may be related to the association of HCV replication with overexpression of transforming growth factor (TGF)-α and insulin-like growth factor II, both of which are related to hepatocyte transformation *(49)*.

The effect of hepatitis C treatment further emphasizes the role of HCV in the development of HCC. IFN-α with or without ribavirin is effective in reducing hepatic inflammation, in clearing HCV RNA in some patients with chronic HCV infection, or both *(50,51)*. Nishiguchi et al. conducted a randomized trial of IFN-α in patients with chronic HCV infection and cirrhosis *(52)*. Ninety patients were randomized to IFN-α or placebo and were followed up for 2–7 years. HCC developed in only 4% of the IFN-α groupcompared with 38% of the placebo group, although most patients in this study had HCV genotype 2. Another study analyzed the effect of IFN-α on more than 1500 patients with chronic HCV, most of whom had genotype 1. The risk of HCC was decreased in treated patients, but this effect was seen mostly in those patients who cleared HCV RNA during treatment or normalized their serum transaminases *(53)*. Other studies also demonstrated the effect of treatment on HCC. In patients with a sustained response, relapse, or nonresponse to IFN therapy, the relative risk of developing HCC compared with historical controls was 0.06, 0.51, and 0.95, respectively *(54)*. Further analysis of these findings suggested that age of 50 years or older, male gender, and advanced fibrotic stage were associated with an increased risk of HCC.

Liver fibrosis seems to be a crucial factor in determining carcinogenesis. A recent retrospective study of 2890 patients in Japan demonstrated a strong correlation between the annual incidence of HCC and the degree of liver fibrosis. IFN therapy was associated with a reduced risk of HCC, again most significantly in those who had a virological or biochemical response *(55)*.

In patients with chronic hepatitis C, several other factors seem to affect the progression to HCC. Coinfection with the human immunodeficiency virus (HIV), which is a frequent problem because of its common mode of acquisition, has been made increasingly relevant by the improved life expectancy of HIV-infected persons with the introduction of highly effective antiretroviral therapies. Although data are limited, there is some evidence that HCC may occur earlier and after a shorter period of HCV infection in patients coinfected with HIV *(56)*.

The role of alcohol in persons with hepatitis C also has received some attention. Yamauchi et al. *(57)* retrospectively studied 133 patients with either alcohol- or HCV-induced cirrhosis and determined that the 10-year cumulative occurrence rate of HCC was 18.5% in anti-HCV-negative alcoholic cirrhosis, 56.5% in nonalcoholic HCV-induced cirrhosis, and 80.7% in patients with alcoholic cirrhosis who were positive for anti-HCV. Similarly, diabetes mellitus may have a synergistic effect on progression to HCC in chronic hepatitis C *(58)*. A recent study from Japan indicated that genetic polymorphisms in proinflammatory cytokines such as the interleukin-1 family also may increase the risk of HCC in HCV patients *(59)*.

2.3. Hepatitis B and Hepatitis C Coinfection

The common modes of acquisition of hepatitis B and C infection may result in coinfection. Several investigators have hypothesized a possible synergistic effect on the development of HCC. Donato et al. *(60)* carried out a meta-analysis of 32 case-control studies looking at the impact of HBV and HCV infection on HCC development. Although the odds ratio for developing HCC in anti-HCV-positive persons was 17.3 and was 22.5 for HBsAg-positive subjects, the odds ratio for those with combined infection was 165. Similarly, a recent Italian study of 259 cirrhotic patients followed over 5 years suggested that patients positive for both anti-HCV and HbsAg were twice as likely to experience HCC compared with patients with hepatitis C infection alone and four times as likely compared with those with just hepatitis B infection *(61)*. However, data from a prospective Taiwanese cohort of more than 12,000 men contradict these earlier reports and suggest that HCV and HBV act independently in the pathogenesis of HCC, with a similar relative risk of developing HCC in patients who were HBsAg positive, anti-HCV positive, or positive for both *(62)*.

The mechanisms for HCC development in coinfection are unclear but probably occur through common and different pathways, because the data suggest a less than multiplicative effect of the two viruses. One simple model would involve HBV acting as an initiator by integrating into the host genome, and both HBV and HCV may then promote carcinogenesis by stimulating repeated cycles of inflammation, necrosis, and regeneration.

2.4. Hereditary Hemochromatosis

Hereditary hemochromatosis (HH) is an autosomal recessive disorder with homozygous frequency estimates of 1 in 220 to 1 in 400 in some populations *(63)*. Niederau et al. *(64)* followed 163 patients with HH for more than 10 years and found that in patients with cirrhosis, the frequency of HCC was more than 200 times that of an age- and gender-matched population. The same study demonstrated that venesection before the development of cirrhosis is associated with a normal life expectancy. The importance of cirrhosis as a risk factor in HH has been shown in a similar cohort of homozygous Italian patients who were followed prospectively for up to 229 months. Of the 97 patients who had cirrhosis, HCC developed in 28 during follow-up, whereas there were no cases of HCC observed in the 55 noncirrhotic patients *(65)*. However, the presence of cirrhosis is not an absolute prerequisite for the development of HCC, as some investigators have shown *(66,67)*. Interestingly, the development of HCC in HH, although associated with cirrhosis in most cases, is not usually associated with markers of hepatitis B or C infection or with the degree of iron deposition *(68)*.

2.5. α-1 Antitrypsin Deficiency

α-1 antitrypsin (A1AT) deficiency is an autosomal recessive disorder that is a common cause of liver disease and liver transplantation in children and may cause cirrhosis and HCC in adults *(69)*. The homozygous PiZZ phenotype is associated with liver injury, presumably because of the accumulation of the abnormally folded A1AT deficiency mutant in the endoplasmic reticulum of liver cells. Transgenic mice carrying the mutant Z allele develop severe liver disease and HCC with intrahepatocytic globules of A1AT *(70)*.

As seen with HCV infection, liver cell dysplasia often is found in patients with A1AT deficiency *(71)*. In a retrospective Swedish study *(72)*, homozygous PiZZ type was found more frequently in patients with cirrhosis and HCC compared with age- and gender-matched controls. Also in that study, HCC developed even in patients without evidence of cirrhosis and in those who had the heterozygous PiZ state *(73)*. However, other investigators found no correlation with an increased HCC risk *(74,75)*. The exact mechanism of carcinogenesis is unclear but may follow a stepwise model of preneoplastic nodules, adenomas, and HCC over several years *(76)*.

2.6. Aflatoxin Exposure

Aspergillus flavus is an ubiquitous fungus that produces hepatotoxins called aflatoxins, which contaminate staple foodstuffs in several tropical and subtropical regions. Exposure to aflatoxins, particularly aflatoxin β1, is associated with HCC as proved by several ecological and molecular epidemiological studies *(77–79)*. The magnitude of risk of HCC may be related to genetic polymorphism of hepatic metabolizing enzymes, particularly microsomal epoxide hydrolase *(80)*. There is a close association between aflatoxin exposure and mutation in the p53 tumor suppressor gene, one of the most frequently mutated genes in human cancers. Aflatoxin β1 induces a G to T transversion at the third position of codon 249 of p53 in human HCC cells *(81)*, and the same mutation has been observed in patients with HCC in areas of the world with high levels of aflatoxin exposure *(82,83)*. Results of a recent cohort study of some 6500 subjects in the Penghu Islets of Taiwan suggested that in patients with HCC, there was an adjusted odds ratio of 5.5 for heavy exposure to aflatoxins *(84)*. Although the vast majority of these HCC patients were HBsAg positive, the earlier onset of HCC in these patients compared with the rest of Taiwan suggests a synergistic effect of aflatoxin exposure and hepatitis B infection.

2.7. Other Risk Factors

Porphyria cutanea tarda is the most common and readily treated of the porphyrias and is characterized by chronic, blistering lesions of sun-exposed skin. Reports suggest that the prevalence of HCC is up to 16% in these patients, although this may be related to the presence of underlying hepatic fibrosis and the 80–90% incidence of HCV infection in these patients *(85,86)*. Similarly, acute intermittent porphyria is associated with HCC (87), particularly in women *(88)*.

Primary sclerosing cholangitis is well known to increase the risk of cholangiocarcinoma, but also may increase the risk of HCC *(89)*. Primary biliary cirrhosis also recently has been shown to result in a similar incidence of HCC as other causes of cirrhosis *(90,91)*.

Older age is another possible risk factor, but likely reflects the several decades required for cirrhosis to develop in patients with viral hepatitis. A recent European study examined this more closely by using birth order as a surrogate marker for age at infection with hepatitis B *(92)*. First- or second-born children tend to acquire common infections at school, whereas later-born children are exposed earlier through their older siblings. Compared with HBsAg-positive controls, those with HCC who were HBsAg-positive were twice as likely to have been later-born children, reflecting a longer period of infection. This was true even allowing for the confounding effect of an increased carrier state in patients infected at a younger age. The same relationship was not seen with hepatitis C-related HCC, reflecting the later onset of infection.

Tobacco smoke and alcohol have been implicated in the cause of many cancers and may play a role in the causation of HCC in patients with underlying liver disease. A recent European study of 333 patients with HCC indicated a dose–response association between smoking and HCC risk and a supermultiplicative effect of heavy smoking and heavy drinking. Interestingly, the effect was more noticeable in patients without evidence of HBV or HCV infection *(93)*. However, in a Chinese cohort of almost 90,000 people followed for 8 years, HCC did not seem to be associated with alcohol consumption. In males, there was no association with smoking, although a positive association between HCC and smoking was seen in females *(94)*. Alcohol itself has some carcinogenic potential through its metabolism to acetaldehyde, which inhibits nuclear repair enzymes, and also because of the generation of oxygen free radicals induced by cytochrome P450 2E1. This enzyme is involved in activating several compounds, including nitrosamines, to carcinogens. In addition, chronic alcohol use depletes liver retinoic acid, which is associated with increased expression of *AP1* genes (c-*fos* and c-*jun*), leading to cellular hyperproliferation. This effect can be reversed in experimental animals by adding retinoic acid and subsequent normalization of *AP1* gene expression and cellular regeneration *(95)*.

There are case reports of plant products associated with HCC. Safrole is an oil found in high concentration in *Piper betle*, a leafy plant used in betel quid that is chewed in many countries. Safrole is a rodent hepatocarcinogen and has been found in the livers of patients with HCC in the form of safrole DNA adducts, in the absence of other causes of tumor *(96)*.

Membranous obstruction of the inferior vena cava (MOVC) is an uncommon disorder of unclear origin leading to blockage of hepatic outflow, similar to Budd–Chiari syndrome (BCS). However, unlike BCS, MOVC is associated with the development of HCC in up to 40% of cases, in the absence of hepatitis viral markers *(97)*.

Male gender is associated with a two- to fourfold increase in HCC, even when the higher rates of confounding factors, such as viral hepatitis and alcoholic liver disease in men, are adjusted for *(98,99)*. The reasons for this discrepancy are unclear but may be related to androgenic stimulation. Studies in a transgenic mouse model in which overexpression of TGF-α leads to spontaneous development of liver tumors in 75% of male mice in 12 months, found that castration of male mice led to a decrease in liver tumors, which could be reversed by the addition of dihydrotestosterone *(100)*. Similarly, oophorectomy can increase the incidence of tumor formation to levels seen in male mice *(101)*.

Cirrhosis of any cause predisposes to HCC, although the risk varies according to the cause of cirrhosis. For example, hemochromatosis and viral liver disease are associated with higher rates of HCC than alcoholic liver disease. Nonetheless, the duration of cirrhosis seems to be the most important factor, regardless of cause *(102)*. Cirrhosis resulting from multiple risk factors present at one time may be associated with an increased incidence of HCC, and indeed, a recent study suggested that multinodular HCC is more prevalent in this group of patients *(103)*.

Cryptogenic cirrhosis or cirrhosis thought to be associated with nonalcoholic fatty liver disease (NAFLD) also may increase the risk of HCC. A recent study indicated that obesity was an independent predictor for HCC in patients with alcoholic cirrhosis or cryptogenic cirrhosis *(104)*. There also seems to be an increased incidence of NAFLD in patients with HCC, with one report from the United States suggesting that, although hepatitis C was still the predominant cause, NAFLD contributed to at least 13% of cases *(105)*.

Greater hepatocyte turnover in patients with cirrhosis may lead to an increased incidence of HCC as seen with HCV infection. One method of assessing cell turnover is liver cell proliferative activity measured by immunostaining of liver tissue for proliferating cell nuclear antigen (PCNA). In a cohort of 208 well-compensated cirrhotic patients, Donato et al. *(106)* were able to demonstrate a relative risk of almost 5 for the development of HCC in patients with a high level of PCNA compared with those with lower levels. This relative risk extended to patient survival. Cirrhotic patients with spontaneous bacterial peritonitis are also at increased risk of developing HCC *(107)*.

The presence of cirrhosis is not a prerequisite for HCC formation. However, even in cases of HCC in noncirrhotic livers, abnormal histological results, including fibrosis and iron overload, often are seen in the nontumorous liver, underscoring the importance of hepatocyte dysplasia or regeneration in the cause of HCC *(108,109)*.

Oral contraceptive pills (OCPs) are associated with the development of hepatic adenomas *(110)*. Several studies and case reports have demonstrated that prolonged use (particularly longer than 8 years) of OCPs and higher synthetic estrogen content, increases the relative risk of hepatic adenoma and HCC *(111–116)*. The occurrence of neoplastic change may be related to the propensity of estrogen to promote hepatocyte proliferation *(117)*. The effect on adenoma formation may be reversible with discontinuation of the OCPs *(118)*, but HCC still can occur after resolution of the adenoma *(119)*. The absolute risk of HCC is small, but the relative risk of 2.6 reported in case-control studies could have implications in societies where OCP use is prevalent and other risk factors are uncommon, especially because the risk of HCC does not decrease for at least 10 years after prolonged OCP use *(120)*.

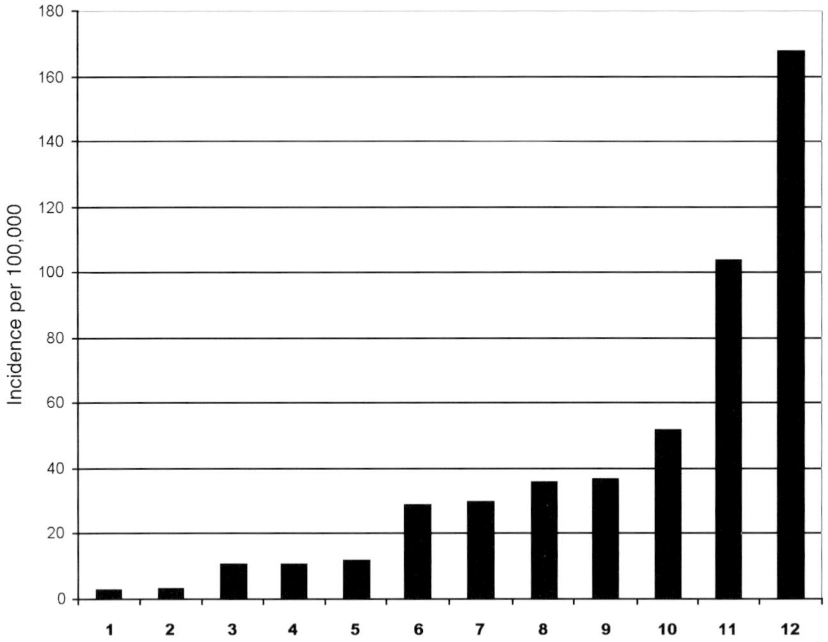

Fig. 1. Age-adjusted incidence of HCC in men according to geographical location. Data from refs. *1,132,133,*and *144* and from *Cancer Incidence in Five Continents*, Vol VII. IARC Scientific Publication No. 143. Cancer Base no. 2, 1997. Key: 1, United States; 2, U.K.; 3, Italy; 4, France; 5, Nigeria; 6, South Africa; 7, Zimbabwe; 8, Hong Kong; 9, Japan; 10, Thailand; 11, Mozambique; 12, Haimen City, China.

Hereditary tyrosinemia is an autosomal recessive disorder of tyrosine metabolism that results in liver disease and HCC in childhood. There is evidence of hepatocellular dysplasia before the development of HCC and DNA ploidy *(121)*. Therefore, it has been suggested that liver transplantation should be considered at younger than 2 years, because the risks of dysplasia and HCC increase substantially after this age *(122)*. Also, radiation exposure, inorganic arsenic ingestion, and radioactive thorium dioxide all may increase HCC risk *(123,124)*.

3. WORLDWIDE DISTRIBUTION OF HCC

The global distribution of HCC varies widely (Fig. 1), with two-thirds of the estimated 350,000 new cases per year occurring in the Far East, only several thousand occurring annually in the United States, and some 30,000 cases being diagnosed per year in Europe *(125)*. Even within these locations, HCC incidence differs according to age, gender, and cause. The situation becomes complex by the effect of immigration, particularly in the United States, where Chinese Americans have rates of HCC much higher than the indigenous population, and

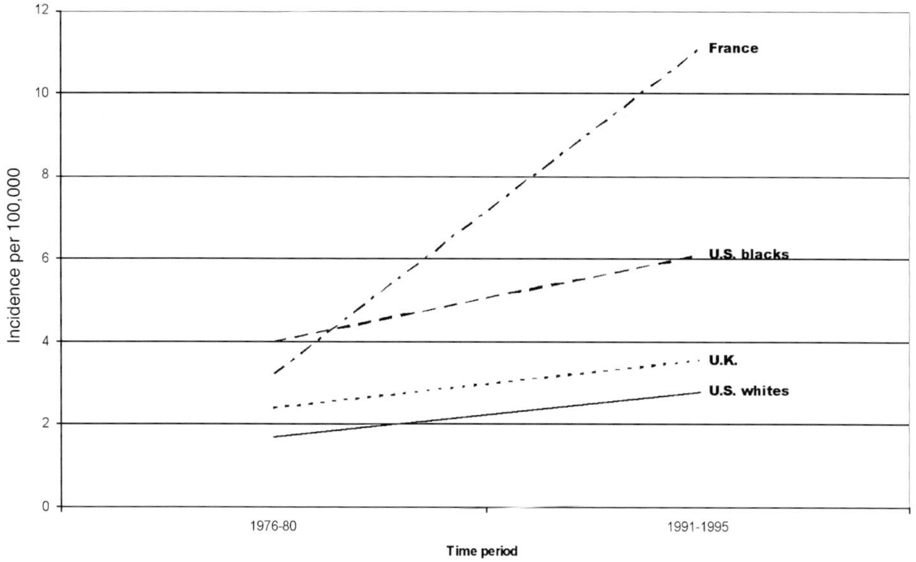

Fig. 2. Rising age-adjusted incidence of HCC among males in the West from 1976 through 1995. The data for 1976 through 1980 and for 1991 through 1995 from France and the UK refer to data from 1979 and 1994, respectively. Data from refs. *1*, *132*, and *133*.

rates may take several generations to fall *(126)*. In the Western world overall, HCC incidence is rising (Fig. 2).

3.1. HCC in the United States

The lower incidence of HCC in the United States (approx 2.5 per 100,000) is likely a result of lower rates of chronic HBV infection. A recent report demonstrated that in patients with HBV, rates of HCC are as high as 1000 per 100,000, very similar to those seen in high-incidence countries *(127)*. The emergence of chronic HCV infection over the last 30 years is likely to impact on the HCC incidence in the United States as the population ages.

Viral hepatitis accounts for most cases of HCC worldwide, as in the United States. Liang et al. *(128)* studied 91 American patients with HBsAg-negative HCC. Using sensitive polymerase chain reaction and three sets of primers for both HBV DNA and HCV RNA to optimize the detection of the viral genomes, they were able to demonstrate that 71% of these patients had evidence of either or both viruses in serum or liver tissue. Almost half the cases had evidence of HCV infection, which seems to be the most common cause of HCC in the United States.

The incidence of HCC cases in the United States has risen over the last two decades *(1)*. El-Serag and Mason *(129)* examined three national databases and found a 41% increase in the mortality rate from HCC and a 46% increase in hospitalizations resulting from HCC from the late 1970s to the early 1990s. It has been attributed to a rise in the overall age-adjusted incidence of HCC from 1.4 per 100,000 during the period from 1976 through 1980 to 2.4 per 100,000 from 1991 through 1995. The incidence of HCC increased particularly in younger persons age 40–60 years, and there were a disproportionate number of males and nonwhites affected. The authors hypothesized that HBV and HCV infections acquired during the 1960s and 1970s were responsible, at least in part, for the increase in the incidence in males and blacks, who are at greater risk of HBV and HCV infection. Further investigation revealed that HCV infection accounted for most of the increase in HCC cases, whereas the rates for HCC associated with HBV, alcohol, and other risk factors were unchanged. These findings were confirmed by the same group controlling for differences in age, gender, race, and geographic region. The increase in incidence of HCC rose the fastest in white males age 45–54 years, perhaps explained by the consequences of HCV infection acquired during the 1960s and 1970s *(130)*. Even within the United States, significant geographic variation exists in the incidence of HCC that cannot be explained by differences in race, age, or gender, with age-adjusted incidence rates as high as 4.6 per 100,000 in Hawaii, compared with 1.1 per 100,000 in Iowa and 1.0 per 100,000 in Utah *(131)*.

3.2. HCC in Europe

As in the United States, there has been a rise in the incidence of HCC in the United Kingdom *(132)*. Age-adjusted mortality rates increased from 2.39 to 3.56 per 100,000 in the male population between 1979 and 1994. An even greater rise was seen in women. The authors hypothesized that HCV infection was responsible for this trend and warned that HCC incident rates would continue to increase as those infected in the 1960s and 1970s from intravenous drugs experienced cirrhosis, and subsequently HCC, at an annual rate of 5%. Similar trends have been seen in France *(133)*. A recent case-control study in southern Italy, an area where HCV infection is hyperendemic, demonstrated a high incidence of HCC *(134)*. National statistics in Italy have shown that the age-standardized mortality rate from HCC rose from 4.8 to 10.9 per 100,000 over a 25-year period (1969–1994). Hepatitis C infection again would seem to be chiefly responsible, because more than 70% of cases of HCC diagnosed from 1996 through 1997 were anti-HCV-positive and only 11.5% were HBsAg-positive *(135)*. Closer analysis of these data revealed that HCC in older patients was more likely to be HCV-related, and the discrepancy in the incidence of HCC between males and females was more marked in HBsAg-positive patients. More than 90% of all patients had underlying cirrhosis. These results are in contrast to the one-third of cirrhotic patients who were HBsAg-positive in the early 1970s *(136)*. The use of reusable glass syringes in the 1950s and 1960s may have led to an increase in HCV infection rates.

In Greece, where the prevalence of chronic HBV infection is 10 times higher than that of chronic HCV infection, almost 60% of HCC cases are attributed to HBV and only 12% to HCV *(137)*. Even in Germany, which has a lower incidence of HCC, most cases are related to viral infection *(2)*.

The impact of viral hepatitis on HCC actually may be underestimated. Most studies have used the presence of HBsAg and anti-HCV to document the presence of HBV or HCV infection. A European cooperative group reported that HBsAg was present in 19% of HCC cases and anti-HCV was present in 40%. However, HBV DNA was detected in 33% of HBsAg-negative patients, and HCV RNA was detected in 7% of anti-HCV-negative cases of HCC. These findings emphasize the importance of HBV and HCV in the etiology of HCC and also stress the importance of using viral genome detection methods in epidemiological studies of HCC *(138)*.

3.3. HCC in Asia

In areas of the world with the highest rates of HCC, HBV infection is the most common etiological agent. In parts of China and Taiwan, almost one-fifth of the population are carriers of HBV, and the vast majority of persons with HCC are HBsAg-positive *(139)*. Although HCV infection is the main risk factor in HBsAg-negative HCC, HCV prevalence is low, with only 0.9% of healthy blood donors positive for anti-HCV *(140)*. The positive impact of HBV vaccination programs as detailed above may alter the cause of HCC in the Far East in the future.

A similar situation exists in India *(141)* , where a recent study showed that 53 of 74 HCC cases had evidence of HBV infection, compared with only 3 patients with HCV infection alone and 6 patients with dual infection with both HBV and HCV.

In contrast to the rest of Asia, cases of HCC in Japan are mainly related to HCV infection, and its incidence, as in the West, is rising but on a larger scale *(99)*. The reasons underlying this difference are likely related to the wide transmission of HCV to young people in Japan from contaminated blood and needles after the Second World War. It also seems that in Japanese patients with chronic viral hepatitis, the progression to HCC occurs at an accelerated rate in HCV infection compared with HBV infection. Takano et al. followed a cohort of 251 patients for a mean of 6 years and demonstrated that HCC was 2.7 times more common in patients with HCV than in patients with HBV *(142)*. Similarly, in a prospective study of 2215 patients followed for 10 years, HCC developed in 13.6% of the patients who were anti-HCV-positive. In contrast, HCC developed in only 4.9% of HBsAg-positive patients during that period *(143)*.

4. SUMMARY

The cause of HCC varies according to geographical location, but viral hepatitis is involved in most cases. Hepatitis B remains the most common cause in the developing world, and integration of the viral genome into the host is an important step in carcinogenesis. Mass vaccination programs are likely to dramatically alter the incidence of HCC in Asia. Hepatocellular carcinoma related to HCV is becoming an increasing problem in the developed world, but the factors leading to tumor formation are not yet well-understood. More effective treatments of HCV infection will be required to impact on the predicted increase in HCC in the coming decades.

REFERENCES

1. El-Serag HB, Mason AC. Rising incidence of hepatocellular carcinoma in the United States. *N Engl J Med* 1999;340:745–750.
2. Kubicka S, Rudolph KL, Hanke M, Tietze MK, Tillmann HL, Trautwein C, et al. Hepatocellular carcinoma in Germany: a retrospective epidemiological study from a low-endemic area. *Liver* 2000;20:312–318.
3. Prince AM, Szmuness WM, Michon J, Demaille J, Diebolt G, Linhard J, et al. A case/control study of the association between primary liver cancer and hepatitis B in Senegal. *Int J Cancer* 1975;16:376–383.
4. Simons MJ, Yap EH, Yu M, Shanmugaratnam K. Australia antigen in Chinese patients with hepatocellular carcinoma and comparison groups: influence of technique sensitivity on differential frequencies. *Int J Cancer* 1972;10:320–325.
5. Nishioka K, Hirayama T, Sekine T, Okouchi K, Mayumi M. Australia antigen and hepatocellular carcinoma. *GANN Mono Cancer Res* 1973;14:167–175.
6. Smith JB, Blumberg BS. Viral hepatitis, post-necrotic cirrhosis, and hepatocellular carcinoma. *Lancet* 1969;ii:953.
7. Simons MJ, Yu M, Chew BK, Tan AY, Yap EH, Seah CS, et al. Australia antigen in Singapore Chinese patients with hepatocellular carcinoma. *Lancet* 1971;i:1149–1151.
8. Beasley RP, Hwang L-Y, Lin C-C, Chien C-S. Hepatocellular carcinoma and hepatitis B virus. *Lancet* 1981;2:1129–1133.
9. McMahon BJ, Alberts SR, Wainwright RB, Bulkow L, Lanier AP. Hepatitis B related sequelae. Prospective study in 1400 Hepatitis B surface antigen positive Alaska Native carriers. *Arch Intern Med* 1990;150:1051–1054.
10. Kew MC. Hepatitis B and C viruses and hepatocellular carcinoma. *Clin Lab Med* 1996;16:395–406.
11. Kim CM, Koike K, Saito I, Miyamura T, Jay G. HBx gene of hepatitis B virus induces liver cancer in transgenic mice. *Nature* 1991;351:317–320.
12. Henkler FF, Koshy R. Hepatitis B virus transcriptional activators: mechanisms and possible role in oncogenesis. *J Viral Hepatitis* 1996;3:109–121.
13. Truant R, Antunovic J, Greenblatt J, Prives C, Cromlish JA. Direct interaction of the hepatitis B virus HBx protein with p53 leads to inhibition by HBx of p53 response element-directed transactivation. *J Virol* 1995;69:1851–1859.
14. Wang XW, Gibson MK, Vermeulen W, Yeh H, Forrester K, Sturzbecher HW, et al. Abrogation of p53-induced apoptosis by the hepatitis B virus X gene. Cancer Res 1995;55:6012–6016.

15. Wong JB, Koff RS, Tine F, Pauker SG. Cost-effectiveness of interferon-α2b treatment for hepatitis B e antigen-positive chronic hepatitis B. *Ann Intern Med* 1995;122:664–675.
16. Chang M-H, Chen C-J, Lai M-S, Wu T-C, Kong M-S, Liang D-C, et al. Universal hepatitis B vaccination in Taiwan and the incidence of hepatocellular carcinoma in children. *N Engl J Med* 1997;336:1855–1859.
17. Chang M-H, Shau W-Y, Chen C-J, Wu T-C, Kong M-S, Liang D-C, et al. Hepatitis B vaccination and hepatocellular carcinoma rates in boys and girls. *JAMA* 2000;284: 3040–3042.
18. Lee CL, Hsieh KS, Ko YC. Trends in the incidence of hepatocellular carcinoma in boys and girls in Taiwan after large-scale hepatitis B vaccination. *Cancer Epidemiol Biomarkers Prev* 2003;12:57–59.
19. Matsuzaki Y, Sato M, Saito Y, Karube M, Doy M, Shoda J, et al. The role of previous infection of hepatitis B virus in Hbs antigen negative and anti-HCV negative Japanese patients with hepatocellular carcinoma: etiological and molecular biological study. *J Exp Clin Cancer Res* 1999;18:379–389.
20. Sherlock S. Viruses and hepatocellular carcinoma. *Gut* 1994;35:828–832.
21. Nishioka K, Watanabe J, Furuta S, Tanaka E, Iino S, Suzuki S, et al. A high prevalence of antibody to the hepatitis C virus in patients with hepatocellular carcinoma in Japan. *Cancer* 1991;67:429–433.
22. Bruix J, Barrera JM, Calvet X, Ercilla G, Costa J, Sanchez-Tapias JM, et al. Prevalence of antibodies to hepatitis C virus in Spanish patients with hepatocellular carcinoma and hepatic cirrhosis. *Lancet* 1989;2:1004–1006.
23. Colombo M, Kuo G, Choo QL, Donato MF, Del Ninno E, Tommasini MA, et al. Prevalence of antibodies to hepatitis C virus in Italian patients with hepatocellular carcinoma. *Lancet* 1989;2:1006–1008.
24. Hasan F, Jeffers LJ, De Medina M, Reddy KR, Parker T, Schiff ER, et al. Hepatitis C-associated hepatocellular carcinoma. *Hepatology* 1990;12:589–591.
25. Yu MC, Yuan JM, Ross RK, Govindarajan S. Presence of antibodies to the hepatitis B surface antigen is associated with an excess risk for hepatocellular carcinoma among non-Asians in Los Angeles County, California. *Hepatology* 1997;25:226–228.
26. Jeng JE, Tsai JF. Hepatitis C virus antibody in hepatocellular carcinoma in Taiwan. *J Med Virol* 1991;34:74–77.
27. Hadziyannis S, Tabor E, Kaklamani E, Tzonou A, Stuver S, Tassopoulos N, et al. A case-control study of hepatitis B and C virus infections in the etiology of hepatocellular carcinoma. *Int J Cancer* 1995;60:627–631
28. Baur M, Hay U, Novacek G, Dittrich C, Ferenci P. Prevalence of antibodies to hepatitis C virus in patients with hepatocellular carcinoma in Austria. *Arch Virol* 1992;4:76–80.
29. Coursaget P, Leboulleux D, Le Cann P, Bao O, Coll-Seck AM. Hepatitis C virus infection in cirrhosis and primary hepatocellular carcinoma in Senegal. *Trans R Soc Trop Med Hyg* 1992;86:552–553.
30. Al Karawi MA, Shariq S, El Shiekh Mohamed AR, Saeed AA, Ahmed AM. Hepatitis C virus infection in chronic liver disease and hepatocellular carcinoma in Saudi Arabia. *J Gastroenterol Hepatol* 1992;7:237–239.
31. Ramesh R, Munshi A, Panda SK. Prevalence of hepatitis C virus antibodies in chronic liver disease and hepatocellular carcinoma patients in India. *J Gastroenterol Hepatol* 1992;7:393–395.
32. Di Bisceglie AM, Order SE, Klein JL, Waggoner JG, Sjogren MH, Kuo G, et al. The role of chronic viral hepatitis in hepatocellular carcinoma in the United States. *Am J Gastroenterol* 1991;86:335–338.
33. Bukh J, Miller RH, Kew MC, Purcell RH. Hepatitis C virus RNA in southern African blacks with hepatocellular carcinoma. *Proc Natl Acad Sci U S A* 1993;90:1848–1851.

34. Mangia A, Vallari DS, Di Bisceglie AM. Use of confirmatory assays for diagnosis of hepatitis C viral infection in patients with hepatocellular carcinoma. *J Med Virol* 1994;43: 125–128.
35. Gerber MA, Shieh YS, Shim KS, Thung SN, Demetris AJ, Schwartz M, et al. Detection of replicative hepatitis C virus sequences in hepatocellular carcinoma. *Am J Pathol* 1992;141:1271–1277.
36. Takeda S, Shibata M, Morishima T, Harada A, Nakao A, Takagi H, et al. Hepatitis C virus infection in hepatocellular carcinoma. Detection of plus-strand and minus-strand viral RNA. *Cancer* 1992;70:2255–2259.
37. Di Bisceglie AM. Hepatitis C and hepatocellular carcinoma. *Hepatology* 1997;26(suppl 1):34S–38S.
38. Colombo M, De Franchis R, Del Ninno E, Sangiovanni A, De Fazio C, Tommasini M, et al. Hepatocellular carcinoma in Italian patients with cirrhosis. *N Engl J Med* 1991;325: 675–680.
39. Tong MJ, El-Farra NS, Reikes AR, Co RL. Clinical outcomes after transfusion-associated hepatitis C. *N Engl J Med* 1995;332:1463–1466.
40. Tsukuma H, Hiyama T, Tanaka S, Nakao M, Yabuuchi T, Kitamura T, et al. Risk factors for hepatocellular carcinoma among patients with chronic liver disease. *N Engl J Med* 1993;328:1797–1801.
41. De Mitri MS, Poussin K, Baccarini P, Pontisso P, D'Errico A, Simon N, et al. HCV-associated liver cancer without cirrhosis. *Lancet* 1995;345:413–415.
42. Ray RB, Lagging LM, Meyer K, Steele R, Ray R. Transcriptional regulation of cellular and viral promoters by the hepatitis C virus core protein. *Virus Res* 1995;37:209–220.
43. Ray RB, Lagging LM, Meyer K, Ray R. Hepatitis C virus core protein cooperates with ras and transforms primary rat embryo fibroblasts to tumorigenic phenotype. *J Virol* 1996;70: 4438–4443.
44. Colombo M. Natural history and pathogenesis of hepatitis C related hepatocellular carcinoma. *J Hepatol* 1999;31(suppl 1):25–30.
45. Borzio M, Bruno S, Roncalli M, Mels GC, Ramella G, Borzio F, et al. Liver cell dysplasia is a major risk for hepatocellular carcinoma in cirrhosis: A prospective study. *Gastroenterology* 1995;108:812–817.
46. Shibata M, Morizane T, Uchida T, Yamagami T, Onozuka Y, Nakano M, et al. Irregular regeneration of hepatocytes and risk of hepatocellular carcinoma in chronic hepatitis and cirrhosis with hepatitis C virus infection. *Lancet* 1998;351:1773–1777.
47. Makino Y, Shiraki K, Sugimoto K, Ito T, Yamanaka T, Fujikawa K, et al. Histological features of cirrhosis with hepatitis C virus for prediction of hepatocellular carcinoma development: a prospective study. *Anticancer Res* 2000;20:3709–3715.
48. Libbrecht L, Craninx M, Nevens F, Desmet V, Roskams T. Predictive value of liver cell dysplasia for development of hepatocellular carcinoma in patients with non-cirrhotic and cirrhotic chronic viral hepatitis. *Histopathology* 2001;39:66–73.
49. Tanaka S, Takenaka K, Matsumata T, Mori R, Sugimachi K. Hepatitis C virus replication is associated with expression of transforming growth factor-alpha and insulin-like growth factor-II in cirrhotic livers. *Dig Dis Sci* 1996;41:208–215.
50. Davis GL, Esteban-Mur R, Rustgi V, Hoefs J, Gordon SC, Trepo C, et al. Interferon alfa-2b alone or in combination with ribavirin for the treatment of relapse of chronic hepatitis C. International Hepatitis Interventional Therapy Group. *N Engl J Med* 1998;339:1493–1499.
51. McHutchison JG, Gordon SC, Schiff ER, Shiffman ML, Lee WM, Rustgi VK, et al. Interferon alfa-2b alone or in combination with ribavirin as initial treatment for chronic hepatitis C. Hepatitis Interventional Therapy Group. *N Engl J Med* 1998;339:1485–1492.
52. Nishiguchi S, Kuroki T, Nakatani S, Morimoto H, Takeda T, Nakajima S, et al. Randomised trial of effects of interferon-α on incidence of hepatocellular carcinoma in chronic active hepatitis C with cirrhosis. *Lancet* 1995;346:1051–1055.

53. Ikeda K, Saitoh S, Arase Y, Chayama K, Suzuki Y, Kobayashi M, et al. Effect of interferon therapy on hepatocellular carcinogenesis in patients with chronic hepatitis type C: a long-term observation study of 1,643 patients using statistical bias correction with proportional hazard analysis. *Hepatology* 1999;29:1124–1130.
54. Imai Y, Kawata S, Tamura S, Yabuuchi I, Noda S, Inada M, et al. Relation of interferon therapy and hepatocellular carcinoma in patients with chronic hepatitis C. *Ann Intern Med* 1998;129:94–99.
55. Yoshida H, Shiratori Y, Moriyama M, Arakawa Y, Ide T, Sata M, et al. Interferon therapy reduces the risk for hepatocellular carcinoma: national surveillance program of cirrhotic and noncirrhotic patients with chronic hepatitis C in Japan. *Ann Intern Med* 1999;131:174–181.
56. Garcia-Samaniego J, Rodriguez M, Berenguer J, Rodriguez-Rosado R, Carbo J, Asensi V, et al. Hepatocellular carcinoma in HIV-infected patients with chronic hepatitis C. *Am J Gastroenterol* 2001;96:179–183.
57. Yamauchi M, Nakahara M, Maezawa Y, Satoh S, Nishikawa F, Ohata M, et al. Prevalence of hepatocellular carcinoma in patients with alcoholic cirrhosis and prior exposure to hepatitis C. *Am J Gastroenterol* 1993;88:39–43.
58. Cimino L, Oriani G, D'Arienzo A, Manguso F, Loguercio C, Ascione A, et al. Interactions between metabolic disorders (diabetes, gallstones and dyslipidemia) and the progression of chronic hepatitis C virus infection to cirrhosis and hepatocellular carcinoma. A cross-sectional multicentre survey. *Dig Liver Dis* 2001;33:240–246.
59. Wang Y, Kato N, Hoshida Y, Yoshida H, Taniguchi H, Goto T, et al. Interleukin-1 beta gene polymorphisms associated with hepatocellular carcinoma in hepatitis C virus infection. *Hepatology* 2003;37:65–71.
60. Donato F, Boffetta P, Puoti M. A meta-analysis of epidemiological studies on the combined effect of hepatitis B and C virus infections in causing hepatocellular carcinoma. *Int J Cancer* 1998;75:347–354.
61. Chiaramonte M, Stroffolini T, Vian A, Stazi MA, Floreani A, Lorenzoni U, et al. Rate of incidence of hepatocellular carcinoma in patients with compensated viral cirrhosis. *Cancer* 1999;85:2132–2137.
62. Sun CA, Wu DM, Lin CC, Lu SN, You SL, Wang LY, et al. Incidence and cofactors of hepatitis C virus-related hepatocellular carcinoma: a prospective study of 12,008 men in Taiwan. *Am J Epidemiol* 2003;157:674–682.
63. Edwards CQ, Griffin LM, Goldgar DE, Drummond C, Skolnick MH, Kushner JP. Prevalence of hemochromatosis among 11,065 presumably healthy blood donors. *N Engl J Med* 1988;318:1355–1362.
64. Niederau C, Fischer R, Sonnenberg A, Stremmel W, Trampisch HJ, Strohmeyer G. Survival and causes of death in cirrhotic and in noncirrhotic patients with primary hemochromatosis. *N Engl J Med* 1985;313:1256–1262.
65. Fargion S, Fracanzani AL, Piperno A, Braga M, D'Alba R, Ronchi G, et al. Prognostic factors for hepatocellular carcinoma in genetic hemochromatosis. *Hepatology* 1994;20:1426–1431.
66. Fellow IW, Stewart M, Jeffcoate WJ, Smith PG, Toghill PJ. Hepatocellular carcinoma in primary hemochromatosis in the absence of cirrhosis. *Gut* 1988;29:1603–1606.
67. Blumberg RS, Chopra S, Ibrahim R, Crawford J, Farraye FA, Zeldis JB, et al. Priamry hepatocellular carcinoma in idiopathic hemochromatosis after reversal of cirrhosis. *Gastroenterology* 1988;95:1399–1402.
68. Niederau C, Fischer R, Purschel A, Stremmel W, Haussinger D, Strohmeyer G. Longterm survival in patients with hereditary hemochromatosis. *Gastroenterology* 1996;110:1107–1119.
69. Qu D, Teckman JH, Perlmutter DH. Review: α1-antitrypsin deficiency associated liver disease. *J Gastroenterol Hepatol* 1997;12:404–416.
70. Geller SA, Nichols WS, Dycaico MJ, Felts KA, Sorge JA. Histopathology of α1-antitrypsin liver disease in a transgenic mouse model. *Hepatology* 1990;12:40–47.

71. Cohen C, Derose PB. Liver cell dysplasia in alpha-1-antitrypsin deficiency. *Mod Pathol* 1994;7:31–36.
72. Elzouki AN, Eriksson S. Risk of hepatobiliary disease in adults with severe alpha-1-antitrypsin deficiency (PiZZ): is chronic viral hepatitis B or C an additional risk factor for cirrhosis and hepatocellular carcinoma? *Eur J Gastroenterol Hepatol* 1996;8:989–994.
73. Zhou H, Fischer H-P. Liver carcinoma in PiZ alpha-1-antitrypsin deficiency. *Am J Surg Pathol* 1998;22:742–748.
74. Rabinovitz M, Gavaler JS, Kelly RH, Prieto M, Van Thiel D. Lack of increase in heterozygous alpha-1-antitrypsin deficiency phenotypes among patients with hepatocellular and bile duct carcinoma. *Hepatology* 1992;15:407–410.
75. Propst T, Propst A, Dietze O, Judmaier G, Braunsteiner H, Vogel W. Prevalence of hepatocellular carcinoma in alpha-1-antitrypsin deficiency. *J Hepatol* 1994;21:1006–1011.
76. Geller SA, Nichols WS, Kim SS, Tolmachoff T, Lee S, Dycaico MJ, et al. Hepatocarcinogenesis is the sequel to hepatitis in Z#2 alpha-1-antitrypsin transgenic mice: histopathological and DNA ploidy studies. *Hepatology* 1994;19:389–397.
77. Ross RK, Yuan JM, Yu MC, Wogan GN, Qian GS, Tu JT, et al. Urinary aflatoxin biomarkers and risk of hepatocellular carcinoma. *Lancet* 1992;339:943–946.
78. Qian GS, Ross RK, Yu MC, Yuan JM, Gao YT, Henderson BE, et al. A follow-up study of urinary markers of aflatoxin exposure and liver cancer risk in Shanghai, People's Republic of China. *Cancer Epidemiol Biomarker Prev* 1994;3:3–10.
79. Allen SJ, Wild CP, Riley EM, Montesano R, Bennett S, Whittle HC, et al. Aflatoxin exposure, malaria and hepatitis B infection in rural Gambian children. *Trans R Soc Trop Med Hyg* 1992;58:426–430.
80. Tiemersma EW, Omer RE, Bunschoten A, van't Veer P, Kok FJ, Idris MO, et al. Role of genetic polymorphism of glutathione-S-transferase T1 and microsomal epoxide hydrolase in aflatoxin-associated hepatocellular carcinoma. *Cancer Epidemiol Biomarkers Prev* 2001;10:785–791.
81. Aguilar F, Hussain SP, Cerutti P. Aflaoxin B1 induces the transversion of G to T in codon 249 of the p53 tumor suppressor gene in human hepatocytes. *Proc Natl Acad Sci USA* 1993; 90:8586–8590.
82. Ozturk M. P53 mutation in hepatocellular carcinoma after aflatoxin exposure. *Lancet* 1991;338:1356–1359.
83. Scorsone KA, Zhou YZ, Butel JS, Slagle BL. P53 mutations cluster at codon 249 in hepatitis B virus positive hepatocellular carcinomas from China. *Cancer Res* 1992;52:1635–1638.
84. Chen C-J, Wang L-Y, Lu S-N, Wu M-H, You S-L, Zhang Y-J, et al. Elevated aflatoxin exposure and increased risk of hepatocellular carcinoma. *Hepatology* 1996;24:38–42.
85. Salata H, Cortes JM, Enriquez de Salamanca R, Oliva H, Castro A, Kusak E, et al. Porphyria cutanea tarda and hepatocellular carcinoma. Frequency of occurrence and related factors. *J Hepatol* 1985;1:477–487.
86. Tsukazaki N, Watanabe M, Irifune H. Porphyria cutanea tarda and hepatitis C virus infection. *Br J Dermatol* 1998;138:1015–1017.
87. Andersson C, Bjersing L, Lithner F. The epidemiology of hepatocellular carcinoma in patients with acute intermittent porphyria. *J Intern Med* 1996;240:195–201.
88. Andant C, Puy H, Faivre J, Deybach J-C. Acute hepatic porphyrias and primary liver cancer. *N Engl J Med* 1998;338:1853–1854.
89. Harnois DM, Gores GJ, Ludwig J, Steers JL, LaRusso NF, Wiesner RH. Are patients with cirrhotic stage primary sclerosing cholangitis at risk for the development of hepatocellular cancer? *J Hepatol* 1997;27:512–516.
90. Caballeria L, Pares A, Castells A, Gines A, Bru C, Rodes J. Hepatocellular carcinoma in primary biliary cirrhosis: similar incidence to that in hepatitis C virus-related cirrhosis. *Am J Gastroenterol* 2000;96:1160–1163.

91. Floreani A, Baragiotta A, Baldo V, Menegon T, Farinati F, Naccarato R. Hepatic and extra-hepatic malignancies in primary biliary cirrhosis. *Hepatology* 1999;29:1425–1428.
92. Kuper H, Hsieh C-C, Stuver SO, Mucci LA, Tzonou A, Zavitsanos X, et al. Birth order, as a proxy for age at infection, in the etiology of hepatocellular carcinoma. *Epidemiology* 2000;11:680–683.
93. Kuper H, Tzonou A, Kaklamani E, Hsieh CC, Lagiou P, Adami HO, et al. Tobacco smoking, alcohol consumption and their interaction in the causation of hepatocellular carcinoma. *Int J Cancer* 2000;85:498–502.
94. Evans AA, Chen G, Ross EA, Shen FM, Lin WY, Lodon WT. Eight-year follow-up of the 90,000-person Haimen City cohort: I. Hepatocellular carcinoma mortality, risk factors, and gender differences. *Cancer Epidemiol Biomarkers Prev* 2002;11:369–376.
95. Inoue H, Seitz HK. Viruses and alcohol in the pathogenesis of primary hepatic carcinoma. *Eur J Cancer Prev* 2001;10:107–110.
96. Liu C-J, Chen C-L, Chang K-W, Chu C-H, Liu T-Y. Safrole in betel quid may be a risk factor for hepatocellular carcinoma: case report. *Can Med Assoc J* 2000;162:359–360.
97. Matsui S, Ichida T, Watanabe M, Sugitani S, Suda T, Takahashi T, et al. Clinical features and etiology of hepatocellular carcinoma arising in patients with membranous obstruction of the inferior vena cava: In reference to hepatitis viral infection. *J Gastroenterol Hepatol* 2000;15:1205–1211.
98. Ikeda K, Saitoh S, Koida I, Arase Y, Tsubota A, Chayama K, et al. A multivariate analysis of risk factors for hepatocellular carcinogenesis: a prospective observation of 795 patients with viral and alcoholic cirrhosis. *Hepatology* 1993;18:47–53.
99. El-Serag HB. Epidemiology of hepatocellular carcinoma. *Clin Liver Dis* 2001;5:87–107.
100. Matsumoto T, Takagi H, Mori M. Androgen dependency of hepatocarcinogenesis in TGFα transgenic mice. *Liver* 2000;20:228–233.
101. Takagi H, Sharp R, Hammermeister C, Goodrow T, Bradley MO, Fausto N, et al. Molecular and genetic analysis of liver oncogenesis in TGFα transgenic mice. *Cancer Res* 1992;52:5171–5177.
102. Del Olmo JA, Serra MA, Rodriguez F, Escudero A, Gilabert S, Rodrigo JM. Incidence and risk factors for hepatocellular carcinoma in 967 patients with cirrhosis. *J Cancer Res Clin Oncol* 1998;124:560–564.
103. Fasani P, Sangiovanni A, De Fazio C, Borzio M, Bruno S, Ronchi G, et al. High prevalence of multinodular hepatocellular carcinoma in patients with cirrhosis attributable to multiple risk factors. *Hepatology* 1999;29:1704–1707.
104. Nair S, Mason A, Eason J, Loss G, Perrillo RP. Is obesity an independent risk factor for hepatocellular carcinoma in cirrhosis? *Hepatology* 2002;36:150–155.
105. Marrero JA, Fontana RJ, Su GL, Conjeevaram HS, Emick DM, Lok AS. NAFLD may be a common underlying liver disease in patients with hepatocellular carcinoma in the United States. *Hepatology* 2002;36:1349–1354.
106. Donato MF, Arosio E, Del Ninno E, Ronchi G, Lampertico P, Morabito A, et al. High rates of hepatocellular carcinoma in cirrhotic patients with high liver cell proliferative activity. *Hepatology* 2001;34:523–528.
107. Llovet JM, Moitinho E, Sala M, Bataller R, Rodriguez-Iglesias P, Castells A, et al. Prevalence and prognostic value of hepatocellular carcinoma in cirrhotic patients presenting with spontaneous bacterial peritonitis. *J Hepatol* 2000;33:423–429.
108. Grando-Lemaire V, Guettier C, Chevret S, Beaugrand M, Trinchet J-C. Hepatocellular carcinoma without cirrhosis in the West: epidemiological factors and histopathology of the non-tumorous liver. *J Hepatol* 1999;31:508–513.
109. Bralet MP, Regimbeau JM, Pineau P, Dubois S, Loas G, Degos F, et al. Hepatocellular carcinoma occurring in nonfibrotic liver: epidemiologic and histopathologic analysis of 80 French cases. *Hepatology* 2000;32:200–204.

110. Baum JK, Holtz F, Bookstein JJ. Possible association between benign hepatomas and oral contraceptives. *Lancet* 1973;2:926–929.
111. Rooks JB, Ory HW, Ishak KG, et al. Epidemiology of hepatocellular adenoma. The role of oral contraceptive use. *JAMA* 1979;242:644–648.
112. Edmondson HA, Henderson BE, Benton B. Liver cell adenomas associated with the use of oral contraceptives. *N Engl J Med* 1976;294:470–472.
113. Henderson BE, Preston-Martin S, Edmondson HA, Peters RL, Pike MC. Hepatocellular carcinoma and oral contraceptives. *Br J Cancer* 1983;48:437–440.
114. Neuberger J, Forman D, Doll R, Williams R. Oral contraceptives and hepatocellular carcinoma. *BMJ* 1986;292:1355–1357.
115. Forman D, Vincent TJ, Doll R. Cancer of the liver and the use of oral contraceptives. *BMJ* 1986;292:1357–1361.
116. Mant JWF, Vessey MP. Trends in mortality from primary liver cancer in England and Wales 1975–1992: influence of oral contraceptives. *Br J Cancer* 1995;72:800–803.
117. Thung SN, Gerber MA. Precursor stage of hepatocellular neoplasm following long exposure to orally administered contraceptives. Hum Pathol 1981;12:472–475.
118. Edmondson HA, Reynolds TB, Henderson B, Benton B. Regression of liver cell adenomas associated with oral contraceptives. *Ann Intern Med* 1977;86:180–182.
119. Gordon SC, Reddy R, Livingstone AS, Jeffers LJ, Schiff ER. Resolution of a contraceptive-steroid-induced hepatic adenoma with subsequent evolution into hepatocellular carcinoma. *Ann Intern Med* 1986;105:547–549.
120. Tavani A, Negri E, Parazzini F, Franceschi S, La Vecchia C. Female hormone utilisation and risk of hepatocellular carcinoma. *Br J Cancer* 1993;67:635–637.
121. Zerbini C, Weinberg DS, Hollister KA, Perez-Atayde AR. DNA ploidy abnormalities in the liver of children with hereditary tyrosinemia type I. Correlation with histopathologic features. *Am J Pathol* 1992;140:1111–1119.
122. Mieles LA, Esquivel CO, Van Thiel DH, Koneru B, Makowka L, Tzakis AG, Starzl TE. Liver transplantation for tyrosinemia. A review of 10 cases from the University of Pittsburgh. *Dig Dis Sci* 1990;35:153–157.
123. Gilbert ES, Koshurnikova NA, Sokolnikov M, Khokhryakov VF, Miller S, Preston DL, et al. Liver cancers in Mayak workers. *Radiat Res* 2000;154:246–252.
124. Chen C-J, Yu M-W, Liaw Y-F. Epidemiological characteristics and risk factors of hepatocellular carcinoma. *J Gastroenterol Hepatol* 1997;12:S294–S308.
125. Schafer DF, Sorrell MF. Hepatocellular carcinoma. *Lancet* 1999;353:1253–1257.
126. Hanley AJG, Choi BCK, Holoway EJ. Cancer mortality among Chinese migrants: a review. *Int J Epidemiol* 1995;24:255–265.
127. Di Bisceglie AM, Carithers RL, Gores GJ. Hepatocellular carcinoma. *Hepatology* 1998;28:1161–1165.
128. Liang TJ, Jeffers LJ, Reddy KR, De Medina M, Parker IT, Cheinquer H, et al. Viral pathogenesis of hepatocellular carcinoma in the United States. *Hepatology* 1993;18:1326–1333.
129. El-Serag HB, Mason AC. Risk factors for the rising rates of primary liver cancer in the United States. *Arch Intern Med* 2000;160:3227–3230.
130. El-Serag HB, Davila JA, Petersen NJ, McGlynn KA. The continuing increase in the incidence of hepatocellular carcinoma in the United States: an update. *Ann Intern Med* 2003;139:817–823.
131. Davila JA, Petersena NJ, Nelson HA, El-Serag HB. Geographic variation within the United States in the incidence of hepatocellular carcinoma. *J Clin Epidemiol* 2003;56:487–493.
132. Taylor-Robinson SD, Foster GR, Arora S, Hargreaves S, Thomas HC. Increase in primary liver cancer in the UK, 1979–94. *Lancet* 1997;350:1142–1143.
133. Deuffic S, Poynard T, Buffat L, Valleron A-J. Trends in primary liver cancer. *Lancet* 1998;351:214–215.

134. Montella M, Crispo A, Izzo F, Ronga D, Tamburini M, De Marco M, et al. HCV and hepatocellular carcinoma: a case-control study in an area of hyperendemicity. *Int J Mol Med* 2000;6:571–574.
135. Stroffolini T, Andreone P, Andriulli A, Ascione A, Craxi A, Chiaramonte M, et al. Characteristics of hepatocellular carcinoma in Italy. *J Hepatol* 1998;29:944–952.
136. Bianchi P, Bianchi-Porro G, Coltorti M, Dardanoni L, Del Vecchio Blanco C, Fagiolo V, et al. Occurrence of Australia antigen in chronic hepatitis in Italy. *Gastroenterology* 1972;63:482–485.
137. Kuper HE, Tzonou A, Kaklamani E, Hadziyannis S, Tasopoulos N, Lagiou P, et al. Hepatitis B and C viruses in the etiology of hepatocellular carcinoma: a study in Greece using third-generation assays. *Cancer Causes Control* 2000;11:171–175.
138. Brechot C, Jaffredo F, Lagorce D, Gerken G, zum Buschenfelde KM, Papakonstontinou A, et al. Impact of HBV, HCV and GBV-C/HGV on hepatocellular carcinomas in Europe: results of a European concerted action. *J Hepatol* 1998;29:173–183.
139. Yuan JM, Govindarajan S, Henderson BE, Yu MC. Low prevalence of hepatitis C infection in hepatocellular carcinoma (HCC) cases and population controls in Guangxi, a hyperendemic region for HCC in the People's Republic of China. *Br J Cancer* 1996;74:491–493.
140. Chen DS, Kuo GC, Sung JL, Lai MY, Sheu JC, Chen PJ, et al. Hepatitis C virus infection in an area hyperendemic for hepatitis B and chronic liver disease: the Taiwan experience. *J Infect Dis* 1990;161:817–822.
141. Sarin SK, Thakur V, Guptan RC, Saigal S, Malhotra V, Thyagarajan SP, et al. Profile of hepatocellular carcinoma in India: an insight into the possible etiologic associations. *J Gastroenterol Hepatol* 2001;16:666–673.
142. Takano S, Yokosuka O, Imazeki F, Tagawa M, Omata M. Incidence of hepatocellular carcinoma in chronic hepatitis B and C: a prospective study of 251 patients. *Hepatology* 1995;21:650–655.
143. Ikeda K, Saitoh S, Suzuki Y, Kobayashi M, Tsubota A, Koida I, et al. Disease progression and hepatocellular carcinogenesis in patients with chronic viral hepatitis: a prospective observation of 2215 patients. *J Hepatol* 1998;28:930–938.
144. Hussain SA, Ferry DR, El-Gazzaz G, Mirza DF, James ND, McMaster P, et al. Hepatocellular carcinoma. *Ann Oncol* 2001;12:161–172.

2 Molecular Mechanisms of Hepatocellular Carcinoma

Insights to Therapy

Marie C. DeFrances, MD, PhD
and George K. Michalopoulos, MD, PhD

Contents

1. INTRODUCTION

The incidence of hepatocellular carcinoma (HCC) is increasing in the United States *(1)* and elsewhere *(2)*. Because of its late presentation, its aggressiveness, and its limited response to therapy, HCC is a major cause of cancer death with possibly up to 1 million deaths yearly attributed to HCC worldwide *(3)*. Current treatment modalities for HCC are only modestly successful with orthotopic liver

From: *Current Clinical Oncology: Hepatocellular Cancer: Diagnosis and Treatment*
Edited by: B. I. Carr © Humana Press Inc., Totowa, NJ

transplantation or resection offering the best hope for long-term survival in select patients *(3)*.

Human HCC is commonly associated with underlying chronic liver disease and cirrhosis caused by persistent infection with hepatitis B virus (HBV) and/or hepatitis C virus (HCV), alcohol abuse, or certain metabolic diseases including hereditary hemochromatosis or α-1-antitrypsin deficiency *(4)*. Although each of these disease processes appears to increase the risk of subsequent HCC development, neither the exact causative insult(s) nor the overall risk posed by these diseases is clearly defined. In general terms, increased hepatocyte replication accompanied by DNA damage and outgrowth of clonal cell populations appears to underlie hepatocarcinogenesis caused by known HCC risk factors. However, it is unclear whether the DNA damage that accompanies the increased mitotic rate is the result of replication errors imparted by abnormal and rapid progression through the cell cycle and/or owing to mutagenesis of the hepatocyte genome directly by toxins or through oxidative stress induced by inflammation or other mechanisms *(5)*. The question of whether similar mechanisms of hepatocyte transformation are shared among the various predisposing conditions or whether unique pathways are employed is under intense scrutiny.

To this end, substantial efforts have been made to understand the genetic basis of HCC, and multiple avenues of research are now converging to offer insight into the molecular mechanisms of liver cancer. It is proposed that five to six separate genetic events are necessary for transformation of a normal hepatocyte into a malignant cell *(6)*, and the use of animal models of HCC, as well as analysis of human HCC tissue samples, has yielded important clues about the molecular steps that lead to the development of HCC. Although mismatch repair mechanisms may play a role in some human HCCs *(7)*, genomic instability characterized by repeated losses and gains of particular chromosomal regions in HCC cells occurs more frequently. Nonrandom losses of heterozygosity (LOH) have been noted on chromosomes 1p, 4q, 6q, 8p, 9p, 10q, 13q, 16p, 16q, and 17p in HCCs, whereas gains of genomic material were identified on chromosomes 1q, 6p, 8q, and 17q *(8)*. The regions of loss or gain are thought to harbor tumor suppressor genes and oncogenes, respectively, and in some instances, these changes correlate with underlying disease condition, tumor differentiation, or patient outcome. Identification of the potential genes lying within the regions has been the focus of many studies, and from them and other experimental evidence such as that obtained from gene expression profiling using cDNA/oligonucleotide microarrays or serial analysis of gene expression (SAGE), some recurrent themes are emerging that may direct the development of novel therapies. Aberrant signaling via cell surface receptors and intracellular effector molecules, deregulation of the cell cycle and apoptosis, extracellular matrix remodeling, and induction of vascular remodeling and growth all appear to contribute to the neoplastic transformation, growth, and/or subsequent invasion of hepatocellular carcinoma. These pathways in human HCC are highlighted here.

2. HEPATIC MITOGENS IN HCC

Most peptide growth factors bind to and activate cell growth, motility. and survival pathways through cell surface tyrosine kinase-bearing receptors. Their importance to hepatic homeostasis has been a focus of study over the last quarter century, and several growth factors such as hepatocyte growth factor (HGF), epidermal growth factor (EGF), and the EGF-related protein, transforming growth factor (TGF)-α are likely to be important in vivo regulators of hepatocyte growth *(9)*. Other modulators such as insulin-like growth factor (IGF)-I and IGF-II have been demonstrated to stimulate hepatocyte DNA synthesis in vitro *(10)*.

2.1. Hepatocyte Growth Factor

In cultured hepatocytes, HGF induces motility *(11)*, causes the adoption of complex hepatic architecture *(12)*, and acts as an anti-apoptotic agent *(13,14)*. It is also the most potent known mitogen for hepatocytes in culture and is thought to be one of the key stimulants of hepatocyte replication in vivo following surgical removal of the liver *(9)*. The biological actions of HGF are mediated through the receptor tyrosine kinase, Met *(15)*. The importance of HGF and Met in liver biology is highlighted by the fact that animals null for HGF or Met die *in utero* with liver, placental, and other abnormalities *(16–18)*.

Several studies show that Met expression is upregulated in human HCC tissues *(19–21)* and, when abundantly overexpressed, may correlate with the presence of intrahepatic metastases and poor patient outcome *(20)*. Activating mutations of the *met* gene *(22)* and gains of chromosome 7 or 7q (or portions thereof) *(23,24)*, where both HGF and Met reside (7q21.1 and 7q31.2, respectively), have been occasionally detected in human liver tumors. HGF expression in human HCC is not consistently upregulated *(21,25)*; however, in vivo experimental models of HGF production in mouse hepatocytes demonstrate that HGF has HCC promoting activity in an autocrine manner in transgenic mice *(26)*.

2.2. EGF and TGF-α

Both EGF and the closely related molecule TGF-α bind to and activate the EGF receptor (EGFR), a tyrosine kinase-bearing transmembrane protein *(27)*. Like HGF, EGF also stimulates hepatocyte motlility *(11)*, and EGF and TGF-α induce morphogenic changes in hepatocytes *(12)*. This growth factor pair is postulated to provide growth signals to hepatocytes as well as to other hepatic constituents during the regenerative process *(9)*.

Studies have demonstrated enhanced EGF mRNA and/or protein expression in regenerative hepatic nodules *(28)* and in HCCs *(29)*, but analysis of six human HCC cell lines revealed only very low expression of EGF by tumor cells *(30)*. Much data, however, implicate TGF-α in HCC. Mice overexpressing TGF-α in the liver develop HCC after 12 months of age *(31,32)*. Collectively, more than 55% (54 of 94) of human HCCs stained strongly for TGF-α protein as compared to nontumorous adjacent tissue *(33–35)*. TGF-α mRNA abundance was also elevated in HCC tissues and was correlated with HBV infection *(36)*. Hsia et al. *(33)* observed a similar correlation with TGF-α protein and HBV infection. Contradictory data regarding EGFR levels in human HCCs exist, however; levels were reportedly increased in some studies *(37,38)* but unchanged in others *(39,40)*.

2.3. Insulin-Like Growth Factors

The growth and pro-survival substances known as IGF-I and IGF-II have been implicated in hepatic tumor development; as mentioned, they can effect hepatocyte DNA synthesis in cultured cells *(10)*. The IGFs are secreted peptide factors whose relative extracellular concentrations and activities are determined by their interaction with insulin growth factor-binding proteins (IGFBPs) *(41)*. The IGFs signal primarily through the tyrosine kinase containing IGF-I receptor (IGFIR) *(42)*. Tyrosine kinase activity stimulated by IGFs is in part propagated by insulin receptor substrates (IRS-1 through IRS-4) *(43)*.

The human IGF-II gene is genomically imprinted with expression proceeding from only one allele (the paternal allele) in adult tissues *(44)*, except for the liver where biallelic expression is seen *(45)*. The reappearance of monoallelic IGF-II gene expression *(46,47)* with IGF-II fetal-type promoter usage and production of fetal-type transcripts *(48,49)* in human HCCs suggests that IGF-II gene regulation is aberrant in hepatic tumors. Enhanced IGF-II protein and mRNA expression was also detected in human HCCs *(48,49)* and appeared to positively correlate with HBV status *(50)*.

Another mechanism to regulate the function of IGFs in human HCCs may involve altering the relative abundance of IGF-binding proteins; for example, reduced mRNA levels for IGFBPs (IGFBP-1, -3, and -4) *(51–53)* have been detected in human HCCs. Because of the dual effects some IGFBPs like IGFBP3 may have on IGFs *(41)*, it is unclear whether reduced

IGFBP expression in HCCs potentiates or inhibits IGF activity. However, IGFBP3 is a particularly attractive target to be downregulated in tumors given its ability to inhibit IGF-mediated survival as well as inhibit cell growth in an IGF-independent manner. To this end, reduced plasma levels of IGFBP3 are generally associated with an increased risk of some cancers *(42)*.

IRSs are intracellular proteins that become tyrosine phosphorylated after associating with stimulated receptors such as IGFIR; they then couple with effector molecules to activate the mitogen-activated protein kinase (MAPK) and phosphatidylinositol-3-kinases (PI3K) pathways to promote cell survival mechanisms *(43)*. In the liver, IRS-1 is phosphorylated during liver regeneration in the rat *(54)*, and 3-month-old mice overexpressing human IRS-1 in the liver under the direction of the albumin promoter showed enhanced hepatocyte DNA synthesis but no tumor formation *(55)*. Regarding human liver tumors, the human homologue of IRS-1 was originally cloned from human hepatocellular carcinoma cells and showed upregulated mRNA expression in HCC tumor tissues as compared to adjacent liver *(56)*.

3. THE PI3K–AKT/PKB PATHWAY IN HCC

PI3Ks comprise a large family of lipid kinases that phosphorylate the inositol moiety in phosphoinositides (PI). Class Ia PI3K signaling stimulated by interaction with tyrosine kinases launches pro-survival, -proliferation, -growth, -motility and -metabolic programs in cells. PI3Ks in this subclass consist of heterodimers containing one of three p110 enzymatic subunits (α, β, or δ) which is regulated by a p85 subunit (α or β); PI3K can also associate with ras *(57)*. Activation of PI3K in cells causes phosphorylation of the D3 position in the inositol ring of $PI(4,5)P_2$ leading to a rise in $PI(3,4,5)P_3$ levels, which in turn recruits and stimulates Akt/protein kinase B (Akt/PKB), a serine/threonine kinase that is responsible for amplifying and specifying signals from PI3K *(58)*. For full enzymatic activation of Akt/PKB, phosphorylation by protein-dependent kinase (PDK) is required *(59)*. Phosphatidylinositide phosphatases (PIPases) such as phosphatase and tensin homolog (PTEN) and SH2-containing inositol 5'-phosphatases (SHIPs) control the level of $PI(3,4,5)P_3$ generated by PI3K *(60)*. PTEN is a lipid and protein phosphatase that reduces the amount of $PI(3,4,5)P_3$ by dephosphorylating this phospholipid at the 3' position *(61)*. SHIPs are also lipid phosphatases, but they convert $PI(3,4,5)P_3$ to $PI(3,4)P_2$ *(60)*.

Studies demonstrate that the PI3K-Akt/PKB pathway becomes activated in normal cultured hepatocytes and liver under various conditions such as in response to growth factor stimulation *(62)* and during liver regeneration following partial hepatectomy *(63)*, respectively. Interestingly, mice that have been engineered to produce no p85 α-species die perinatally of liver necrosis and other findings *(64)*. In human HCC, a role for the PI3K–Akt/PKB pathway in tumor growth and survival is supported *(65)*. For example, mutation of the PTEN gene, the major PIPase that downregulates the levels of PI3K-generated phospholipids, has been found in some human HCCs *(66)*, whereas analysis of 60 human HCCs and paired nontumorous liver tissues demonstrated diminished PTEN mRNA levels in the malignant component of most cases as determined by Northern blot *(67)*. In other studies, more than 40% (43 of 105) of human HCCs were found to have reduced or absent levels of PTEN protein by immunohistochemistry as compared to adjacent liver tissue. Reduced PTEN staining correlated with higher tumor grade, poorer survival, and increased recurrence *(68)*. Similarly, mice with targeted disruption of one PTEN allele developed tumors in the liver and other organs *(69)*.

4. WNT/β-CATENIN SIGNALING IN HCC

The Wnt/β-catenin signaling pathway is critical to proper embryonic axis development and organogenesis *(70)*. In the adult rat liver, partial hepatectomy stimulates β-catenin nuclear translocation *(71)* suggesting that it regulates physiologic hepatocyte growth. β-Catenin is a multifunctional protein that complexes with a seemingly diverse array of proteins including the cell adhesion molecule, E-cadherin; several proteins involved in β-catenin degradation consisting of axin, glycogen synthase kinase-3 β, protein phosphatase 2A, and adenomatous polyposis coli (APC) protein; transcription factors including lymphoid-enhancing factor (LEF)/T-cell factor (Tcf) *(72)*; the Met tyrosine kinase receptor *(73)*, and others.

The amount of unbound free β-catenin in the cytosol is tightly regulated by its degradation by GSK-3 β through serine/threonine phosphorylation of β-catenin's N-terminal domain *(72)*. Wnt protein, when present, binds to its cell surface receptor frizzled and, via dishevelled, GSK3β-mediated phosphorylation of β-catenin is inhibited. Thus, β-catenin protein dissociates from the axin-containing complex, accumulates in the cytoplasm, and then translocates to the nucleus *(70)*. There, it associates with LEF/Tcf to stimulate transcription of target genes such as *c-myc* (74) and cyclin D1 *(75)*.

Several mechanisms that lead to the reactivation of the Wnt/β-catenin-signaling pathway in human HCC have been proposed. The first is through mutation of the β-catenin gene in exons encoding for the GSK-

3β phosphorylation sites, especially exon 3. This is seen in up to 44% of human HCCs examined by single-strand conformational polymorphism (SSCP) *(76,77)*; however, other estimates of the β-catenin mutation rate place it at about 22% on average in human HCCs *(8)*. Interestingly, a study of 25 dysplastic hepatocellular nodules showed no detectable mutations in the β-catenin gene nor enhanced β-catenin cytoplasmic or nuclear staining *(78)*. β-Catenin gene mutation is particularly common in HCCs from HCV-infected patients *(76)* and, in a separate study, from non-HBV-positive patients *(77)*; it is also associated with a favorable prognosis *(77)*. However, examination of 23 HCC tumors from Malaysian patients showed no β-catenin mutations suggesting that the β-catenin gene may be differentially targeted for mutation depending on the underlying HCC risk factor(s) and/or genetic composition of the population *(79)*.

Nuclear accumulation of β-catenin protein has also been identified in the absence of β-catenin gene mutation. Although the APC gene is frequently lost or mutated in solid tumors such as colon carcinoma and has been linked to abnormal accumulation of β-catenin, APC is not considered to be a major target in HCCs *(80)*; however, Piao et al. *(81)* noted that 20% of human HCC cases had LOH of the APC gene. Interestingly, a case report has documented a patient harboring a germline mutation for APC as the only risk factor for development of HCC. The tumor showed somatic mutation of the remaining APC allele suggesting that patients who inherit an APC mutation may be at risk of developing HCC *(82)*. Because APC may not be a common target for mutation in human HCC, axin has been evaluated. Studies of human HCC have shown that the chromosome arm that harbors the axin1 gene (16p) often displays LOH, although mutation (consisting of point mutations, small deletions, or small insertions) of the axin1 allele has been identified in less than 10% of cases *(83,84)*.

Augmentation of the Wnt/β-catenin-signaling pathway may occur through modifying β-catenin's transactivating properties. To this end, a scaffolding protein known as EBP50 was recently shown to associate with β-catenin and enhance β-catenin's transcriptional activity in in vitro assays. Immunohistochemical staining revealed that EBP50 was overexpressed in 21 of 38 (55%) human HCC tumors as compared to adjacent nontumorous tissues and that increased EBP50 protein accumulation correlated positively with nuclear β-catenin immunostaining (85) suggesting that EBP50 and β-catenin could cooperate in promoting liver tumorigenesis.

Another mechanism for abnormal intracellular accumulation of β-catenin protein has been proposed by Cui et al. (76) who described an enhanced *in situ* hybridization signal for β-catenin mRNA in the cytoplasm of some human HCCs lacking β-catenin gene mutations in exon 3. They suggest that translational activity of abnormally high levels of β-catenin mRNA in HCCs results in an overabundance of β-catenin protein, which ultimately overwhelms the GSK-3β ubiquitination pathway and promotes β-catenin accumulation.

Reactivation of the Wnt/β-catenin-signaling pathway may also occur through downregulation of E-cadherin. Human HCCs commonly show allelic imbalance on chromosome 16q, particularly in the vicinity of the E-cadherin gene (16q22.1) *(86,87)*, and downregulation of E-cadherin protein expression has been seen in HCCs as well *(87,88)*. Although no mutations of the E-cadherin gene have been reported, CpG methylation of the E-cadherin promoter in HCC *(89)*, increased expression of a putative transcriptional repressor (i.e., Snail) of the E-cadherin gene in HCC cell lines *(90)* and polymorphic differences in E-cadherin-promoter nucleotides *(91)* as possible means of downregulating its gene expression have been postulated.

Currently available transgenic mouse models of β-catenin expression in the liver unfortunately do not clarify the role of β-catenin in hepatic tumorigenesis. Studies have demonstrated that stabilized forms of β-catenin either lacking the N-terminus including the GSK-3β phosphorylation and the α-catenin-binding sites *(92)* or engineered to undergo deletion of the third exon containing the GSK-3β phoshorylation sites through cre-mediated recombination *(93)* are associated with hepatomegaly related to increased hepatocyte proliferation in one model *(92)* and mitochondrial dysfunction in the other *(93)* as compared to control animals. Because of enhanced morbidity and limited survival of either set of transgenic animals (3 to 4 weeks for those with N-terminal deletion of β-catenin and more than 6 months for the animals undergoing adenovirus-mediated cre recombination), the mice could not be fully evaluated for the development of hepatic tumors *(92,93)*; however, Harada et al. *(93)* speculate, based on their findings in mice expressing a dominant form of β-catenin lacking the GSK-3β phosphorylation sites via deletion of exon 3, that stabilized β-catenin expression alone is insufficient to induce liver tumors. These results will require further in vivo evaluation.

5. THE RAS SUPERFAMILY IN HCC

The superfamily of small GTP-binding proteins including ras and rho family members is involved in regulation of normal cell proliferation by controlling the expression and activities of regulatory molecules such as cyclin D1, p21Waf1/Cip1, and p27Kip1 following exposure to mitogens or other stimuli *(94)*. Regarding normal liver, ras is involved in hepatocyte replication under in vitro culturing conditions *(95)* as well as during regeneration following partial hepatectomy in rodents *(96,97)*.

Three closely related members, H-, K- and N-*ras*, make up the immediate family of ras molecules and are all commonly targeted in human cancer. Of the three members, the gene for K-*ras* is more often found to be mutated than the others *(98)*. Humans occupationally exposed to vinyl chloride may develop HCC as a consequence *(99)*, and K-*ras* mutation may be an integral step in the process. HCC tumors from individuals exposed to vinyl chloride were examined for K-*ras* mutation, and 33% (6 of 18) of cases were found to be positive. In two of six cases of suspected vinyl chloride-induced HCC that harbored K-*ras* mutation, adjacent liver tissue showed K-*ras* mutation as well. HCCs from patients with other known etiologies (viral infection or ethanol) showed a K-*ras* mutation rate of 15% in this study *(100)*. However, other researchers have rarely detected K-*ras* mutations in human HCC *(101,102)*.

Mutation of the H-ras gene, like the K-*ras* gene, is uncommonly detected in human HCCs *(102,103)*; surprisingly, however, LOH in the vicinity of the H-ras locus on the short arm of chromosome 11 (11p15.5) was found to be prevalent in one study of human HCC, seen in about 42% of cases by Southern blot analysis *(103)*. Others have shown that the intensity of immunostaining for ras in human HCCs appears to be diminished in more poorly differentiated lesions as compared to cirrhotic liver or well-differentiated tumors *(104,105)*, suggesting that ras plays a role in the early stages of carcinogenesis.

Deletions of human chromosome 8p, particularly at 8p21.3-22 *(106)*, are frequently identified in HCC and are associated with the presence of metastatic hepatocellular carcinoma *(107)*, suggesting that a tumor-suppressor gene involved in aggressive HCC behavior resides in the region. To this end, cloning of a possible target gene in the region 8p21.3-22 named deleted in liver cancer-1 (DLC-1) was carried out *(108)*. DLC-1 is related to the rat p122 RhoGAP gene, the product of which negatively regulates the activity of rho. Approximately 50% of human HCCs examined showed loss of heterozygosity of the DLC-1 gene *(108)*, whereas in other studies, 20 to 67% of cases lacked mRNA expression of DLC-1 in tumors *(109,110)*. Enhanced methylation at a CpG island 5' to the DLC-1 gene, which may account for reduced DLC-1 gene transcription, was found in 24% (6 of 25) of HCC cases as compared to adjacent liver tissues *(110)*. A homolog to DLC-1, deleted in liver cancer-2 (DLC-2), has been identified. It likewise has signatures of RhoGAP. The gene for DLC-2 is localized to 13q12.3 in humans, a site commonly found to undergo LOH in HCC *(111)*. More than 35% of informative human HCC cases showed

LOH for two markers flanking DLC-2, whereas reverse transcriptase polymerase chain reaction carried out on those samples showing LOH demonstrated a reduction in DLC-2 mRNA levels in about 18% of tumors compared to adjacent liver tissues *(112)*. Recently, gene expression profiling of human HCCs revealed that the expression of a gene for a small GTPase known as ARHC (RhoC) and a gene for a putative small GTPase-regulating protein known as ARHGAP8 (RhoGAP8) were preferentially up- and downregulated, respectively, in a survey of invasive HCCs as compared to noninvasive tumors *(52)* suggesting that vascular invasion of HCC cells may involve the uncontrolled activity of Rho proteins.

6. C-MYC IN HCC

The myc family of nuclear proteins, to which c-myc belongs, has a wide repertoire of biological functions including growth control, apoptosis, and differentiation, and when deregulated, tumorigenesis. How the members carry out their routine functions is complex and may involve regulation of histone acetylation/deacetylation in the promoter regions of target genes as well as sequestration and inhibition of transcriptional activators *(113)*. Through these interactions, it is proposed that myc, under normal circumstances, protects cells from unregulated growth by simultaneously promoting proliferation while sensitizing cells to apoptosis without directly activating the apoptotic cascade *(114)*.

In the liver, *c-myc* gene expression has been extensively studied in in vitro and in vivo models. Rat HCCs induced by various carcinogenic regimens often show amplification of the *c-myc* gene *(115,116)* and, when *c-myc* was overexpressed in the livers of transgenic mice under an inducible promoter, HCCs resulted *(117)*. In the woodchuck model of HCC, which is induced by infection with woodchuck hepatitis virus (WHV), integration of WHV DNA into the woodchuck genome is often seen in the vicinity of the *N-myc (118)* and *c-myc (119)* genes resulting in their gene activation.

In humans, a fairly robust percentage of HCCs demonstrate gain of genetic material on chromosome 8q by comparative genomic hybridization (CGH) *(8)*. An increase in gene copy number for *c-myc*, which resides at 8q24 was seen cumulatively in about 39% (24 of 62) of human HCCs, and was associated with a poor prognosis and with moderately and poorly differentiated tumors *(120, 121)*. Analysis of *c-myc* mRNA and protein levels demonstrated a progressive increase from normal liver, nontumorous liver, cirrhotic liver, well-differentiated HCC to poorly differentiated HCC *(122)*, but another study did not observe this pattern *(123)*.

7. CELL CYCLE REGULATORS IN HCC

Progression through the cell cycle is a highly orchestrated event employing numerous regulatory proteins. Some of the most well known of these proteins, such as p53 and Rb, are also clearly involved in tumorigenesis of various organs. Cyclin-dependent kinases (cdks), cyclins and cdk inhibitors such as p27 Kip1, p21Waf1/Cip1, and p16INK4A drive the cell cycle through phosphorylation and/or degradation of key substrates *(124)*. As the identities and functions of other cell cycle regulators are revealed, it is becoming obvious that they too can participate in tumor development.

7.1. p53

In human HCC, the short arm of chromosome 17 is perhaps the most frequent chromosome targeted for deletion *(6)*, particularly at 17p13, which harbors the gene for the tumor suppressor molecule p53. Under normal circumstances, cell cycle arrest or apoptosis can result from p53 activation following cellular stress, and this is owing in part to p53-mediated transcriptional regulation of target genes such as p21Waf1/Cip1, 14-3-3σ and Bax *(125)*. Loss of heterozygosity at the p53 locus was seen in 57% (8 of 14) of human HCCs in one study, and more than half (63%) of the cases displaying p53 LOH in tumors showed allelic loss of p53 in adjacent liver tissues as well *(126)*. Mutation of the p53 gene occurs with some regularity in HCCs and is associated with higher grade lesions *(127)*, vascular invasion *(128)*, and lower survival rate *(129)*, although the latter is under question *(130)*. In human HCCs worldwide, p53 gene mutation has been reported to occur in about 28% of cases on average *(8)*, but this incidence increases in certain geographic areas. In patients from regions of China and Africa, HCCs harbor p53 mutations in an estimated 55% of cases with specific mutation at codon 249 (G to T transversion) of p53, accounting for up to 82% of all p53 mutations in these populations *(6)*. It is suspected that aflatoxin, a carcinogenic compound produced by certain members of the *Aspergillus* genus of fungi, contaminates food grains from these regions and induces DNA adducts in hepatocyte DNA following consumption. Codon 249 of the p53 gene is believed to be particularly susceptible to aflatoxin-induced mutagenesis *(6,131)*. HBV infection, which is highly prevalent in these geographic areas, may synergize with aflatoxin to promote hepatocarcinogenesis *(132)*. To this end, Hbx, an HBV-encoded protein, has been shown to bind to and inhibit the activity of p53 *(133,134)* and DNA repair proteins *(135)*, which may allow the DNA of infected hepatocytes to accumulate mutations *(6)*, but this remains speculative.

Although mutation in the coding region of the p53 gene is not uncommon, other rare mechanisms for inactivating p53 such as promoter methylation *(136)* and mutation of the p53 gene at the intron-exon boundary *(137)* have been reported. Altered activity or expression of p53-modulating proteins is another mechanism to affect wild-type p53 function. As mentioned, the viral protein Hbx can reduce p53 action through physical association; murine double minute clone 2 (mdm-2) protein is another candidate. It binds to p53 masking its transactivation domain and targets it for degradation; mdm-2 also associates with other proteins such as Rb and E2F1 and may modulate gene expression *(125)*. The abundances of mdm-2 mRNA *(138)* and protein *(139)* are noted to be increased in about a 25 to 50% of human HCC cases, and increased mdm-2 expression appears to correlate with reduced survival. Interestingly, the abundance of mdm-2 mRNA in tumor tissues as compared to adjacent nontumorous tissues was found to be particularly elevated in tumors lacking p53 gene mutation at codon 249 as compared to those with p53 gene mutation at this location, supporting the hypothesis that mdm-2 is upregulated to inhibit wild-type p53 in tumors lacking mutant p53 *(138)*.

7.2. Rb

Allelic imbalance is observed on chromosome 13q in about 30% of human HCCs *(8)*. Because the Rb tumor suppressor gene (13q14) resides on this chromosomal arm, much attention has been focused on whether Rb participates in HCC development. Rb regulates cell cycle progression into *S*-phase following growth stimulation, is linked to apoptosis induction through a p53-dependent pathway, and is a common target in cancer development *(140)*. Two studies show that 42 to 73% of human HCCs harbor specific loss of one Rb allele *(141,142)*. This was notably accompanied by LOH of Rb in surrounding cirrhotic tissues in about 70% (8 of 11) of HCC cases *(142)*. Identification of genetic alterations in cirrhotic tissues is supported by others: Roncalli et al. *(143)* identified losses of chromosome 13q, as well as 1p, 4q, and 18q, in the cirrhotic livers of patients who later went on to develop HCC, demonstrating that hepatocytes in cirrhotic nodules already take on clonal characteristics and suggesting that the involved chromosomal regions harbor genes important to the early stages of neoplastic transformation.

Given the prevalence of LOH at the Rb locus, mechanisms to inactivate the other allele have been identified. Mutation (in the form of small deletions) of the second Rb allele has rarely been detected in human HCCs displaying LOH for Rb *(141)*. Mutation of the Rb gene promoter may be an unlikely contributor to loss of Rb expression in HCCs *(144)*, but a recent study suggests that 24 of 100 (24%) human HCCs of differing etiology (HCV, HBV, or alcohol-induced) harbored aberrant Rb gene-promoter methylation *(145)*. Other mechanisms, such as increased degradation of Rb protein, have been proposed as means of reducing Rb levels in tumor cells, and one protein, gankyrin, an oncogenic molecule that induces Rb phosphorylation and speeds its destruction through the ubiquitin–proteasome pathway, may play such a role. This is particularly true in HCC, where gankyrin is reportedly overexpressed in all cases studied *(146)*. Recently, this finding was confirmed; 97% (62 of 64) of human HCC samples showed moderately to markedly increased gankyrin mRNA abundance as compared to adjacent nontumorous liver tissues using Northern blot analysis *(147)*.

Although Rb protein loss is observed in about one-fourth of human HCCs (collectively 27 of 102 cases *[141,148]*), an increase in its abundance in liver tumor tissues has been noted with nearly equal frequency (ranging from 18 to 58% of tumors *[148,149]*). Hui et al. *(148)* found that alterations in Rb levels in human HCCs, regardless of whether increased or lost, were associated with later tumor stages or with the presence of HCC metastases.

Rb controls *S*-phase entry by associating with the E2F family of transcription factors such as E2F1. This interaction is mediated in a phosphorylation-dependent manner by a complex containing a cdk and a cyclin, particularly the cdk-4/Cyclin D1 complex. Phosphorylated Rb no longer binds to and sequesters E2F1, which is then free to alter transcription of cell cycle-related genes *(140)*. p16INK4A is an inhibitor of cdks such as cdk-4 and as such indirectly reduces Rb phosphorylation. The p16INK4A gene resides on human chromosome 9p21, an area that is lost in some human HCC cell lines *(150)*. Germ-line mutation of the p16INK4A gene in humans is associated with familial melanoma *(151)*, and in rodent models, gene knockout studies in mice show that biallelic loss of the p16INK4A homologue results in B-cell lymphomas and soft-tissue sarcomas *(152)*. p14ARF/p19ARF, a regulator of mdm-2, shares exons of the p16INK4A gene, and its expression is induced by E2F1, thus linking the Rb and p53 pathways *(153)*. Homozygous deletion of the p16INK4A locus could therefore interfere with both Rb- (via cdk-4-mediated inactivation) and p53- (via mdm-2-mediated inhibition of p53) dependent mechanisms.

Evaluation of p16INK4A in human HCCs has revealed an absence of functional p16INK4A in up to 70% of cases *(154,155)*. Homozygous deletion of the p16INK4A locus was detected in 60% of human HCCs in one study *(156)*. About 50% of HCCs examined for p16INK4A mRNA and protein levels showed reductions *(155,157)*, with abundances gradually decreasing with increasing tumor stage *(157,158)*. Additional mechanisms to downregulate p16INK4A, such as gene promoter hypermethylation, somatic p16INK4 gene mutation, reduced p16INK4A gene transcription through enhanced Id-1 transcriptional repressor expression, and posttranscriptional mechanisms have been proposed *(145,157,159,160)*. Interestingly, four patients with HCC were found to harbor germ-line mutation of one p16INK4A allele, and in two of the patients, loss of the remaining p16INK4A allele in the tumor was detected, suggesting that those with inherited mutations at the p16INK4A locus are at risk for developing HCC *(159)*.

At least two other cdk inhibitors (CDKIs) p21Waf1/Cip1 and p27Kip1 have been linked to human HCC. p21Waf1/Cip1 is a multifunctional protein that modulates diverse cellular functions including cell cycle progression through direct interactions with cyclins, cdks, and E2F; DNA synthesis by binding to proliferating cell nuclear antigen (PCNA); apoptosis by binding to and inhibiting pro-caspase 3; and cell differentiation *(161)*. Levels of p21Waf1/Cip1 mRNA and protein have been examined in human HCCs. Amounts of p21Waf1/Cip1 mRNA tended to be reduced in tumor tissues as compared to adjacent nontumorous tissues *(162–165)*. p21Waf1/Cip1 protein overabundance, on the other hand, was detected in 33 to 64% of HCCs *(149,165)*.

Expression of the CDKI p27Kip1 *(166)*, a protein that is structurally related to p21Waf1/Cip1 and similarly targets the cdk-2/Cyclin E complex in particular for negative regulation *(167)*, has also been investigated in HCCs. Unlike p21Waf1/Cip1 mRNA levels that seem to be markedly downregulated in HCCs, p27Kip1 mRNA abundance appears to remain roughly unchanged or slightly increased in tumor tissues as compared to adjacent nontumorous tissues *(168)*. However, multiple laboratories *(168–170)* demonstrated reduced p27Kip1 protein levels in some HCCs, particularly those having aggressive features such as higher tumor stage *(168)*, portal invasion, poor differentiation, and large size *(169)*. Moreover, these groups *(168–170)* also independently demonstrated a correlation between reduced tumor staining for p27Kip1 protein and poor patient outcome. That decreased p27Kip1 protein staining in HCCs repeatedly correlated with poor patient outcome is a consistent finding for tumors originating in other tissues such as carcinoma of the breast *(171)*.

Amplification of the long arm of chromosome 11 has been identified in human HCC *(172)*. On this chromosomal arm resides the gene for cyclin D1 (11q13), and up to 18% of HCC cases harbor an increased gene copy number for cyclin D1 *(145,173,174)*. Evaluation of cyclin D1 mRNA or protein expression showed enhanced protein levels in HCC tumors that displayed gene amplification as compared to tumors lacking amplification or normal liver, which both demonstrated weak or negative staining.

The presence of cyclin D1 gene amplification was identified in advanced stage tumors with rapid growth suggesting a role for this cell cycle regulator in promoting aggressive neoplastic behavior in some HCCs *(174)*. It should be noted, however, that reduced cyclin D1 gene expression was observed by two groups analyzing global gene expression in human HCCs by cDNA microarray *(52)* and serial analysis of gene expression *(175)* techniques. Nonetheless, the oncogenic potential of cyclin D1 in the liver has been verified in a transgenic mouse model in which the cyclin D1 gene was placed under the control of the rat liver fatty acid-binding protein promoter directing transgene expression to the liver and intestines. Liver abnormalities characterized by hyperplastic changes at 3 months of age, hepatomegaly and dysplasia by 6 months, and adenomas by 9 months were observed in the transgenic animals culminating in HCC development in 31% of mice by 17 months *(176)*.

8. GROWTH INHIBITORS AND APOPTOSIS MEDIATORS IN HCC

Apoptosis is important to tissue homestasis and morphogenesis, and when deregulated, can contribute to carcinogenesis *(177)*. At least two cellular pathways mediate apoptotic signals: the mitochondrial or intrinsic pathway and the death receptor or extrinsic pathway. Numerous pro- and anti-apoptotic molecules such as bad, bax, and survivin appear to modulate the final outcome *(178)*. Under experimental conditions in vitro and/or in vivo, normal hepatocytes are sensitive to growth inhibition and/or apoptosis induced through activation of the Fas death receptor *(179,180)*, by exposure to TGF-β *(181)*, or via other mechanisms.

8.1 TGF-β

TGF-β is cleaved intracellularly and secreted as a latent molecule. Activation of TGF-β may involve interaction with plasmin, metalloproteinases, or the M6P/IGFII receptor, among other molecules. The signaling receptor system for active TGF-β is a heterodimer consisting of the serine/threonine kinase containing TGF-β receptors I and II (TGF-βRI and II). Intracellular signaling is mediated mostly by Smad proteins (such as Smad2, 3, and 4) which target the nucleus to alter gene transcription of cell cycle regulating and other genes in the capacity of co-activators *(182)*.

Experiments with cultured rodent liver epithelial cells demonstrated that they undergo neoplastic transformation in the presence of TGF-β presumably through selection of TGF-β resistant clones *(183)*, and more than half (59%) of transgenic mice overexpressing TGF-β in the liver spontaneously develop hepatic tumors by about 16 months of age *(184)*. In humans, HCCs have been shown to overexpress TGF-β *(185)*, and plasma levels of TGF-β in patients with HCC are elevated *(186)*. Expression of TGF-βRI and II mRNA and protein are reduced by 49 and 60%, respectively, in human HCCs as compared to the adjacent tissue *(187)* and mutation of the TGF-βRII *(188,189)* and Smad (Smads2 and 4) genes *(190)* occasionally occurs.

Analysis of the long arm of chromosome 6 (6q) in human HCCs has shown that LOH is a common occurrence and may be associated with a poor prognosis *(84)*. Most work has centered on the region of 6q25-27, which harbors the M6P/IGFIIR, a cell surface protein that promotes activation of latent TGF-β *(191)* and facilitates lysomal degradation of IGF-II *(192)*. Several studies have shown that up to 64% of HCCs demonstrate LOH in this region *(193–195)*, although another study noted no LOH at the M6P/IGFIIR locus in the examined cases *(196)*. Concomitant missense mutations or major amino acid substitutions were identified in the remaining M6P/IGFIIR allele in approx 25% of cases showing 6q25-27 LOH in one study *(197)*. M6P/IGFIIR protein levels were also reduced in about 65% of human HCCs examined *(187)*.

8.2. Fas

The death receptor Fas (CD95) and its ligand, FasL, are well-characterized mediators of apoptosis in a variety of cell types and may also be involved in liver disease *(198)*. Cultured human HCC cells are resistant to Fas-mediated apoptosis *(199)*; however, in human HCCs, Fas, and FasL expression levels are reportedly variable *(200–203)*. Interestingly, Lee et al. *(202)* saw LOH at the Fas locus on human chromosome 10q24.1 in 15% (5 of 34) of informative HCC cases, but no Fas gene mutations were identified.

8.3. Other Apoptosis and Survival Regulators

The expression levels of a variety of other apoptosis regulating molecules have also been examined in human HCCs. Anti-apoptotic molecules such as soluble Fas *(202)*, Fas-associated phosphatase-1 *(202)*, Bcl-xL *(204)*, and survivin *(205)* were found to be expressed at normal or elevated levels in human HCCs, whereas the expression of pro-apoptic molecules such as bcl-2 *(202)*, bid *(206)*, and caspase 3 *(207)* were found to be moderately reduced or absent (as in the case of bcl-2).

Because conventional therapeutic agents often rely on an intact apoptotic mechanism to kill tumor cells *(208)*, deregulated apoptosis in

HCCs may provide one explanation as to why these agents are less than successful in curtailing tumor growth.

9. EXTRACELLULAR PROTEASES IN HCC

The hepatocyte is normally surrounded by and secured to a scant meshwork of extracellular matrix (ECM) proteins consisting mostly of tenascin, fibronectin, and collagen types I, III, and IV *(209,210)*. Integrins anchor hepatocytes and other cells to the ECM *(211)* and regulate cellular functions such as migration, survival, and anoikis by transmitting signals to the nucleus from extracellular cues *(212,213)*. These pathways may be targeted in malignant transformation of cells to promote survival and invasion *(213)*. In the cirrhotic liver and in HCC, the composition of the ECM is altered primarily through the enhanced deposition of collagen type I *(214)* in the former, with addition of collagen type IV *(215)* and laminin *(216)* in the latter; upregulation of the laminin receptor (integrin-α6) on the hepatocyte surface is also seen in dysplasia and carcinoma *(215,216)*.

ECM remodeling appears to be a feature of the liver as it undergoes repair and regeneration following loss of liver mass such as after partial hepatectomy *(210)*. In hepatocarcinogenesis, as in other tumors, degradation/remodeling of the ECM is considered to be an integral step in the development of intrahepatic and distant metastases *(217,218)*. Occasionally, even small HCCs have been shown to metastasize following resection *(219)*, suggesting that some hepatocytes aggressively acquire the necessary repertoire of gene expression to effect growth, invasion, and motility early in neoplastic development *(220)*.

Numerous proteases such as the plasminogen activators (PAs) and matrix metalloproteinsases (MMPs) have been implicated in ECM remodeling in the liver during the regenerative response *(221,222)*. Some of these same proteases may also play a role in growth and invasion of hepatic tumors *(218)*. Urokinase-type plasminogen activator (uPA) and the MMPs, particularly MMP-2 and -9, appear to be involved in both processes. uPA is a serine protease that generates plasmin from plasminogen *(223)* and activates HGF *(224)*. uPA activity is regulated by PA inhibitors (PAI)-1 and PAI-2 *(223)*. Plasmin, meanwhile, can activate MMPs *(225)*, which in turn degrade ECM proteins and activate growth factors, among other functions *(226)*.

The expression of the uPA receptor (uPAR), a protein that promotes uPA activation and may mediate intracellular signals *(223)*, has been shown to be upregulated in human HCCs, and 75% of patients with high uPAR expression in their tumors vs about 15% of those lacking uPAR tumor expression had HCC recurrence in one study *(227)* suggesting that expression of uPAR by HCCs may be involved in development of recurrent disease. Several investigators have found that MMP-9 mRNA levels are also upregulated in human HCCs *(228–230)*. Giannelli et al. *(231)* surveyed patients with and without metastatic HCC for the expression of MMP-2 and tissue inhibitor of metalloproteinase (TIMP)-2 in primary and/or metastatic HCC tissues as well as patients' sera. They found that, while MMP-2 levels in HCC tissues or serum were not statistically different between those with or without metastases, the levels of TIMP-2 were significantly elevated in tissues and sera of those lacking metastases and correlated positively with survival outcome

10. PRO- AND ANTI-ANGIOGENIC FACTORS IN HCC

Blood vessel formation is essential to the expansion of solid tumors *(232)*. Numerous pro- and anti-angiogenic factors are known, and the interplay between them may be a key component of HCC tumor angiogenesis *(233)*. As HCCs are highly vascular lesions, new blood vessel formation is often exuberant. Early in HCC development the blood supply is often derived from the portal circulation and vascularity is less prominent, but as tumors enlarge and lose their differentiation, the feeding vessels become more pronounced and receive blood from the hepatic artery *(233)*. Two endothelial-specific pro-angiogenic classes of growth factors have been identified: the vascular endothelial growth factor family consisting of six members currently (VEGF-A through E, and placenta growth factor) and the angiopoietins (Ang1 through 4) *(233,234)*. Three endothelial-expressed tyrosine kinase cell surface receptors exist for VEGF including flt-1, KDR/flk-1, and flt-4. The activities of VEGF-A appear to be mediated primarily through KDR/flk-1 *(235)*.

In human HCCs, most studies suggest that VEGF expression is upregulated *(236–239)*, whereas data on the expression of its receptors are less clear. For example, KDR/flk-1 mRNA abundance was upregulated in tumor tissues in one study *(240)*, but Ng et al. *(236)* saw preferential upregulation of Flt-1 mRNA rather than KDR/flk-1 mRNA in their cases of human HCC.

Angiopoietins (Ang) were recently discovered as ligands of the Tie2/Tek vascular endothelium-specific receptor. Although Ang-1 can activate the Tie2/Tek receptor, Ang-2 appears to be an antagonist of Ang-1 and is incapable of inducing Tie2/Tek receptor phosphorylation *(241)*. Enhanced mRNA levels of Ang-2 were noted in HCC tumor tissues and positively correlated with the degree of tumor vascularity as determined presurgically by angiographic studies. Ang-1 mRNA levels were roughly equal between tumorous and nontumorous tissue *(242)*. Others have shown that Ang-2 protein expression as determined by immunohistochemistry was upregulated in human HCCs as compared to normal liver tissue from patients undergoing liver resection or autopsy for nonliver-related disease and was most highly expressed in poorly differentiated highly vascularized HCCs *(239)*. These findings are consistent with the proposed roles of Angs in angiogenesis in some organs: Ang-2 expression correlates with formation of nascent vessels, whereas that of Ang-1 is associated with blood vessel stabilization *(241)*. Evalulation of Tie2/Tek expression by immunohistochemistry in human HCCs showed that the vascular endothelium present in moderately and poorly differentiated tumors stained more intensely than that of well-differentiated tumors. Tie2/Tek-positive tumors also tended to be larger than Tie2/Tek-negative tumors *(243)*.

Endogenous anti-angiogenic factors have been discovered that inhibit tumor vasculogensis. Interestingly, one protein with anti-angiogenic properties is angiostatin, which is derived from plasminogen by enzymatic cleavage *(244)*. MMP-12/human macrophage metalloelastase (HME) *(245)* is one of several enzymes that cleave plasminogen to produce angiostatin. MMP-12/HME mRNA and angiostatin protein were found to be expressed in more than half of HCC tumor samples. In patients whose tumors were negative for both MMP-12/HME and angiostatin, poorer survival was seen *(246)*.

11. MOLECULAR TARGETS OF HCC THERAPY

If untreated, hepatocellular carcinoma has a dismal prognosis with death usually occurring within 6 months of diagnosis *(3)*. Presently, perhaps the best hope for extended survival in patients with small HCC and cirrhosis is liver transplantation because it may effectively eliminate the tumor(s), the risk of developing metachronous lesions in a cirrhotic liver, and end-stage liver disease all at once *(247)*; however, resection remains a viable option, as well, for select patients *(3)*. For those with advanced disease, current treatment protocols have not been very successful in improving patient outcome *(248)*. Thus, other methods of prevention and therapy are desperately needed.

Because viruses (HBV and/or HCV) commonly underlie the development of human HCC *(3)*, preventing viral infection or curtailing viral replication and progression to cirrhosis are logical long-term solutions, and it has been suggested that serious effort be directed at the former *(249)*. These ideas have been placed into practice with promising results. In Taiwan where HBV is prevalent and perinatal maternal–infant and horizontal childhood transmission are common routes of infection, implementation of a universal childhood vaccination program for HBV begun in 1984 resulted in a drop in the average annual incidence of and mortality from HCC in children by roughly 50% in 13 years *(250)*.

Unfortunately, vaccines for HCV have not yet been developed. One treatment protocol for those with HCV infection is therapy with interferon (IFN)-α, which is believed to inhibit viral replication and modulate the immune response *(251)*. Initially, IFN-α was used as a monotherapy; however, combination therapy with ribavirin may be superior in achieving biochemical and virological responses *(252)*. Evidence suggests that treatment with IFN-α causes a reduction in progression of liver fibrosis as well as HCC development; however, the effect on HCC has not been noted by all investigators *(251)*. Thus, long-term randomized clinical trials are needed to evaluate the role of IFN in human HCC development.

Administration of acyclic retinoids to patients in the hopes of preventing recurrent and metachronous HCCs following hepatic resection or percutaneous ethanol therapy has been carried out in Japan. Improved survival and a reduction in second primary lesions were seen in patients receiving acyclic retinoids *(253,254)*. Possible mechanisms explaining the inhibitory effect of acyclic retinoids on development of second primary HCCs include induction of apoptosis and differentiation which has been observed in human HCC cells cultured in the presence of these compounds. The effects of acyclic retinoids on tumor cells may be mediated by retinoid X receptor(RXR)-α, a nuclear hormone receptor involved in gene transcriptional regulation, which appears to become aberrantly phosphorylated and inactivated in HCC cells and tissues. Phosphorylation coupled with reduction of endogenous retinoids in HCCs may inhibit RXR-α-mediated transcription resulting in cell proliferation and dedifferentiation, which is overcome by treatment with acyclic retinoids *(255)*.

With the burgeoning of molecular information about human HCCs from numerous research domains, there is hope that current therapies will be improved and new treatments will be discovered. Albeit rare at this point in time, this has clearly been the case with tumors of other organ systems. For example, the fact that many different tumors show activation of the c-kit tyrosine kinase receptor, particularly through mutation, led to the discovery and clinical use of an inhibitor of kit tyrosine kinase, STI571. Therapeutic responses have been seen in some patients with kit-positive tumors such as gastrointestinal stromal tumors (GISTs) after STI571 administration *(256)* and suggests that these types of pharmacogenetic approaches may be avenues for HCC researchers to pursue. To this end, some of the pathways that appear to be involved in HCC development are already the focus of studies by researchers assessing pharmacological and genetic interventions for other tumors.

Although gene therapy protocols for the treatment of human tumors like HCC initially generated great excitement, enthusiasm has been tempered somewhat by waning expression of transgenes, poor transfection efficiency and specificity, and safety concerns *(257)*. Hepatic tumors are also innately difficult to transduce owing to formation of a blood–tumor barrier that blocks vector diffusion to neoplastic cells *(258)*. Because of the various limitations of gene therapy that need to be overcome, targeting key components of pathways important to neoplastic transformation with small molecular inhibitors like STI571 in GISTs *(256)* or human-mouse chimeric antibodies such as herceptin, an anti-Her-2/neu antibody, in metastatic breast cancer *(259)* is currently the trend. The modifiers discussed here are examples of agents that may prove to be useful in human HCC therapy, but this remains to be seen.

More than half of human HCCs overexpress TGF-α while simultaneously expressing normal or elevated levels of the EGFR, suggesting that an autocrine loop between TGF-α and its receptor may operate in HCC tumor development in the majority of cases. Thus, inhibition of EGFR signaling may be one mechanism to regulate tumor growth. To this end, a humanized chimeric antibody has been developed which appears to bind to the EGFR, inhibit kinase activation, promote receptor internalization, and increase p27KIP1 protein levels resulting in G1 cell cycle arrest. Its administration to patients with various cancers yielded promising results, and further studies are underway. A small molecule inhibitor of EGFR kinase activity has likewise been demonstrated to have some clinical utility and is being investigated *(260)*.

Normal apoptotic and cell cycle control mechanisms seem to be routinely circumvented in human HCCs, notably through mutation and loss of the p53 and Rb genes as well as through alteration of the TGF-β- and Fas-mediated pathways. One promising strategy that may be pertinent to HCC therapy is the use of pharmacological molecules that promote normalized function of mutant p53 proteins through their stabilization resulting in growth arrest *(208)*. Another strategy may be to inhibit the cdks-1 and -2 by 7-hydroxystaurosporine or flavopiridol, both of which are currently under evaluation in humans with various cancers. They may work particularly well in combination with conventional chemotherapeutic drugs *(124)*.

The mechanisms causing hypervascularity and invasion of HCCs may likewise provide good targets for small molecule therapy. Multiple endogenous and synthetic anti-angiogenic molecules exist, and one of the synthetic molecules has received considerable attention and is currently being evaluated in humans with hematological as well as other malignancies *(261)*. This molecule was also shown to significantly inhibit tumor growth in rat models of HCC *(262)*, particularly during early phases of HCC development. ECM remodeling and tumor growth and invasion appear to be modulated by MMPs in human HCC *(263)*. Despite promise in animal models including those of HCC *(264)*, metalloproteinase inhibitors have not been shown to be effective anti-tumor agents in humans and, in fact, resulted in reduced patient survival in some instances *(265)*.

12. CONCLUSIONS

Due to the rising incidence of HCC combined with the large number of patients who present with advanced disease and the poor response rate of these patients to current treatments, a search for alternative therapies to HCC is underway. Molecular characterization of human HCCs has pointed to numerous aberrant signaling and regulatory pathways, and dissecting these pathways should provide a logical framework for new drug development. To this end, a plethora of molecular agents that target some of them are being clinically evaluated in patients with various tumors. For HCC as well as other tumor types, it may be that a combinatorial approach using new and established agents or multiple new agents, rather than the administration of any single anti-cancer agent, will prove to be most effective because tumor resistance to some small molecule monotherapies has been noted. Melding the knowledge from molecular studies of HCC with the output of promising novel therapies into targeted therapeutic strategies for those with HCC should ultimately have a positive effect on patient care and outcome.

13. REFERENCES

1. El-Serag HB, Mason AC. Rising incidence of hepatocellular carcinoma in the United States. *N Engl J Med* 1999;340:745–750.
2. Taylor-Robinson SD, Foster GR, Arora S, Hargreaves S, Thomas HC. Increase in primary liver cancer in the UK, 1979-94. *Lancet* 1997;350:1142–1143.
3. Hussain SA, Ferry DR, El-Gazzaz G, et al. Hepatocellular carcinoma. Ann Oncol 2001;12:161–172.
4. Di Bisceglie AM, Carithers RL, Jr., Gores GJ. Hepatocellular carcinoma. *Hepatology* 1998;28:1161–1165.
5. Thorgeirsson SS. Mechanism(s) of hepatocarcinogensis: insight from transgenic mouse models. In: *TheLiver Biology and Pathobiology* (Arias IM, ed.), Lippincott Williams & Wilkins, Philadelphia,2001, 1013–1028.
6. Puisieux A, Ozturk M. TP53 and hepatocellular carcinoma. *Pathologie et Biologie* 1997;45:864–870.
7. Salvucci M, Lemoine A, Saffroy R, et al. Microsatellite instability in European hepatocellular carcinoma. *Oncogene* 1999;18:181–187.
8. Buendia MA. Genetics of hepatocellular carcinoma. *Semin Cancer Biol* 2000;10:185–200.
9. Michalopoulos GK, DeFrances MC. Liver regeneration. *Science* 1997;276:60–66.
10. Kimura M, Ogihara M. Effects of insulin-like growth factor I and II on DNA synthesis and proliferation in primary cultures of adult rat hepatocytes. *Eur J Pharmacol* 1998;354:271–281.
11. Stolz DB, Michalopoulos GK. Comparative effects of hepatocyte growth factor and epidermal growth factor on motility, morphology, mitogenesis, and signal transduction of primary rat hepatocytes. *J Cell Biochem* 1994;55:445–464.

12. Michalopoulos GK, Bowen WC, Zajac VF, et al. Morphogenetic events in mixed cultures of rat hepatocytes and nonparenchymal cells maintained in biological matrices in the presence of hepatocyte growth factor and epidermal growth factor. *Hepatology* 1999;29:90–100.
13. Webster CR, Anwer MS. Phosphoinositide 3-kinase, but not mitogen-activated protein kinase, pathway is involved in hepatocyte growth factor-mediated protection against bile acid-induced apoptosis in cultured rat hepatocytes. *Hepatology* 2001;33:608–615.
14. Wang X, DeFrances MC, Dai Y, et al. A mechanism of cell survival: sequestration of Fas by the HGF receptor Met. *Molecular Cell* 2002;9:411–421.
15. Naldini L, Vigna E, Narsimhan RP, et al. Hepatocyte growth factor (HGF) stimulates the tyrosine kinase activity of the receptor encoded by the proto-oncogene c-MET. *Oncogene* 1991;6:501–504.
16. Uehara Y, Minowa O, Mori C, et al. Placental defect and embryonic lethality in mice lacking hepatocyte growth factor/scatter factor. *Nature* 1995;373:702–705.
17. Schmidt C, Bladt F, Goedecke S, et al. Scatter factor/hepatocyte growth factor is essential for liver development. *Nature* 1995;373:699–702.
18. Bladt F, Riethmacher D, Isenmann S, Aguzzi A, Birchmeier C. Essential role for the c-met receptor in the migration of myogenic precursor cells into the limb bud. *Nature* 1995;376:768–771.
19. Suzuki K, Hayashi N, Yamada Y, et al. Expression of the c-met protooncogene in human hepatocellular carcinoma. *Hepatology* 1994;20:1231–1236.
20. Ueki T, Fujimoto J, Suzuki T, Yamamoto H, Okamoto E. Expression of hepatocyte growth factor and its receptor c-met proto-oncogene in hepatocellular carcinoma. *Hepatology* 1997;25:862–866.
21. Tavian D, De Petro G, Benetti A, Portolani N, Giulini SM, Barlati S. u-PA and c-MET mRNA expression is co-ordinately enhanced while hepatocyte growth factor mRNA is down-regulated in human hepatocellular carcinoma. *Int J Cancer* 2000;87:644–649.
22. Park WS, Dong SM, Kim SY, et al. Somatic mutations in the kinase domain of the Met/hepatocyte growth factor receptor gene in childhood hepatocellular carcinomas. *Cancer Res* 1999;59:307–310.
23. Collonge-Rame MA, Bresson-Hadni S, Koch S, et al. Pattern of chromosomal imbalances in non-B virus related hepatocellular carcinoma detected by comparative genomic hybridization. *Cancer Genet Cytogenet* 2001;127:49–52.
24. Rao UN, Gollin SM, Beaves S, Cieply K, Nalesnik M, Michalopoulos GK. Comparative genomic hybridization of hepatocellular carcinoma: correlation with fluorescence *in situ* hybridization in paraffin-embedded tissue. *Molecular Diag* 2001;6:27–37.
25. Kiss A, Wang NJ, Xie JP, Thorgeirsson SS. Analysis of transforming growth factor (TGF)-alpha/epidermal growth factor receptor, hepatocyte growth Factor/c-met,TGF-beta receptor type II, and p53 expression in human hepatocellular carcinomas. *Clin Cancer Res* 1997;3:1059–1066.
26. Bell A, Chen Q, DeFrances MC, Michalopoulos GK, Zarnegar R. The five amino acid-deleted isoform of hepatocyte growth factor promotes carcinogenesis in transgenic mice. *Oncogene* 1999;18:887–895.
27. Brown KD. The epidermal growth factor/transforming growth factor-alpha family and their receptors. *Eur J Gastroenterol Hepatol* 1995;7:914–922.
28. Komuves LG, Feren A, Jones AL, Fodor E. Expression of epidermal growth factor and its receptor in cirrhotic liver disease. *J Histochem Cytochem* 2000;48:821–830.
29. Motoo Y, Sawabu N, Nakanuma Y. Expression of epidermal growth factor and fibroblast growth factor in human hepatocellular carcinoma: an immunohistochemical study. *Liver* 1991;11:272–277.

30. Hisaka T, Yano H, Haramaki M, Utsunomiya I, Kojiro M. Expressions of epidermal growth factor family and its receptor in hepatocellular carcinoma cell lines: relationship to cell proliferation. *Int J Oncol* 1999;14:453–460.
31. Lee GH, Merlino G, Fausto N. Development of liver tumors in transforming growth factor alpha transgenic mice. *Cancer Res* 1992;52:5162–5170.
32. Webber EM, Wu JC, Wang L, Merlino G, Fausto N. Overexpression of transforming growth factor-alpha causes liver enlargement and increased hepatocyte proliferation in transgenic mice. *Am J Pathol* 1994;145:398–408.
33. Hsia CC, Axiotis CA, Di Bisceglie AM, Tabor E. Transforming growth factor-alpha in human hepatocellular carcinoma and coexpression with hepatitis B surface antigen in adjacent liver. *Cancer* 1992;70:1049–1056.
34. Collier JD, Guo K, Gullick WJ, Bassendine MF, Burt AD. Expression of transforming growth factor alpha in human hepatocellular carcinoma. *Liver* 1993;13:151–155.
35. Schaff Z, Hsia CC, Sarosi I, Tabor E. Overexpression of transforming growth factor-alpha in hepatocellular carcinoma and focal nodular hyperplasia from European patients. *Hum Pathol* 1994;25:644–651.
36. Chung YH, Kim JA, Song BC, et al. Expression of transforming growth factor-alpha mRNA in livers of patients with chronic viral hepatitis and hepatocellular carcinoma. *Cancer* 2000;89:977–982.
37. Harada K, Shiota G, Kawasaki H. Transforming growth factor-alpha and epidermal growth factor receptor in chronic liver disease and hepatocellular carcinoma. *Liver* 1999;19:318–325.
38. Ito Y, Takeda T, Sakon M, et al. Expression and clinical significance of erb-B receptor family in hepatocellular carcinoma. *Br J Cancer* 2001;84:1377–1383.
39. Morimitsu Y, Hsia CC, Kojiro M, Tabor E. Nodules of less-differentiated tumor within or adjacent to hepatocellular carcinoma: relative expression of transforming growth factor-alpha and its receptor in the different areas of tumor. *Hum Pathol* 1995;26:1126–1132.
40. Hamazaki K, Yunoki Y, Tagashira H, Mimura T, Mori M, Orita K. Epidermal growth factor receptor in human hepatocellular carcinoma. *Cancer Detect Prev* 1997;21:355–360.
41. Baxter RC. Insulin-like growth factor (IGF)-binding proteins: interactions with IGFs and intrinsic bioactivities. *Am J Physiol Endocrinol Metab* 2000;278:E967–E976.
42. Yu H, Rohan T. Role of the insulin-like growth factor family in cancer development and progression. *J Nat Cancer Inst* 2000;92:1472–1489.
43. Giovannone B, Scaldaferri ML, Federici M, et al. Insulin receptor substrate (IRS) transduction system: distinct and overlapping signaling potential. *Diabetes Metab Res Rev* 2000;16:434–441.
44. Jirtle RL. Genomic imprinting and cancer. *Exp Cell Res* 1999;248:18–24.
45. Kalscheuer VM, Mariman EC, Schepens MT, Rehder H, Ropers HH. The insulin-like growth factor type-2 receptor gene is imprinted in the mouse but not in humans. *Nat Genet* 1993;5:74–78.
46. Takeda S, Kondo M, Kumada T, et al. Allelic-expression imbalance of the insulin-like growth factor 2 gene in hepatocellular carcinoma and underlying disease. *Oncogene* 1996;12:1589–1592.
47. Aihara T, Noguchi S, Miyoshi Y, et al. Allelic imbalance of insulin-like growth factor II gene expression in cancerous and precancerous lesions of the liver. *Hepatology* 1998;28:86–89.
48. Sohda T, Yun K, Iwata K, Soejima H, Okumura M. Increased expression of insulin-like growth factor 2 in hepatocellular carcinoma is primarily regulated at the transcriptional level. *Lab Invest* 1996;75:307–311.
49. Ng IO, Lee JM, Srivastava G, Ng M. Expression of insulin-like growth factor II mRNA in hepatocellular carcinoma. *J Gastroenterol Hepatol* 1998;13:152–157.

50. D'Errico A, Grigioni WF, Fiorentino M, et al. Expression of insulin-like growth factor II (IGF-II) in human hepatocellular carcinomas: an immunohistochemical study. Pathol *Int* 1994;44:131–137.
51. Gong Y, Cui L, Minuk GY. The expression of insulin-like growth factor binding proteins in human hepatocellular carcinoma. *Mol Cell Biochem* 2000;207:101–104.
52. Okabe H, Satoh S, Kato T, et al. Genome-wide analysis of gene expression in human hepatocellular carcinomas using cDNA microarray: identification of genes involved in viral carcinogenesis and tumor progression. *Cancer Res* 2001;61:2129–2137.
53. Hanafusa T, Yumoto Y, Nouso K, et al. Reduced expression of insulin-like growth factor binding protein-3 and its promoter hypermethylation in human hepatocellular carcinoma. *Cancer Lett* 2002;176:149–158.
54. Sasaki Y, Zhang XF, Nishiyama M, Avruch J, Wands JR. Expression and phosphorylation of insulin receptor substrate 1 during rat liver regeneration. *J Biol Chem* 1993;268:3805–3808.
55. Tanaka S, Mohr L, Schmidt EV, Sugimachi K, Wands JR. Biological effects of human insulin receptor substrate-1 overexpression in hepatocytes. *Hepatology* 1997;26:598–604.
56. Nishiyama M, Wands JR. Cloning and increased expression of an insulin receptor substrate-1-like gene in human hepatocellular carcinoma. *Biochem Biophys Res Comm* 1992;183:280–285.
57. Fry MJ. Structure, regulation and function of phosphoinositide 3-kinases. *Biochim Biophys Acta* 1994;1226:237–268.
58. Vivanco I, Sawyers CL. The phosphatidylinositol 3-kinase AKT pathway in human cancer. *Nat Rev Cancer* 2002;2:489–501.
59. Toker A, Newton AC. Cellular signaling: pivoting around PDK-1. *Cell* 2000;103:185–188.
60. West KA, Castillo SS, Dennis PA. Activation of the PI3K/Akt pathway and chemotherapeutic resistance. *Drug Res Updates* 2002;5:234–248.
61. Sun H, Lesche R, Li DM, et al. PTEN modulates cell cycle progression and cell survival by regulating phosphatidylinositol 3,4,5,-trisphosphate and Akt/protein kinase B signaling pathway. *Proc Nat Acad Sci USA* 1999;96:6199–6204.
62. Skouteris GG, Georgakopoulos E. Hepatocyte growth factor-induced proliferation of primary hepatocytes is mediated by activation of phosphatidylinositol 3-kinase. *Biochem Biophys Res Comm* 1996;218:229–233.
63. Hong F, Nguyen VA, Shen X, Kunos G, Gao B. Rapid activation of protein kinase B/Akt has a key role in antiapoptotic signaling during liver regeneration. *Biochem Biophys Res Comm* 2000;279:974–979.
64. Fruman DA, Mauvais-Jarvis F, Pollard DA, et al. Hypoglycaemia, liver necrosis and perinatal death in mice lacking all isoforms of phosphoinositide 3-kinase p85 alpha. *Nat Genet* 2000;26:379–382.
65. Thorgeirsson SS, Teramoto T, Factor VM. Dysregulation of apoptosis in hepatocellular carcinoma. *Semin Liver Dis* 1998;18:115–122.
66. Yao YJ, Ping XL, Zhang H, et al. PTEN/MMAC1 mutations in hepatocellular carcinomas. *Oncogene* 1999;18:3181–3185.
67. Wan XW, Jiang M, Cao HF, et al. The alteration of PTEN tumor suppressor expression and its association with the histopathological features of human primary hepatocellular carcinoma. *J Cancer Res Clin Oncol* 2003;129:100–106.
68. Hu TH, Huang CC, Lin PR, et al. Expression and prognostic role of tumor suppressor gene PTEN/MMAC1/TEP1 in hepatocellular carcinoma. *Cancer* 2003;97:1929–1940.
69. Podsypanina K, Ellenson LH, Nemes A, et al. Mutation of Pten/Mmac1 in mice causes neoplasia in multiple organ systems. *Proc Nat Acad Sci USA* 1999;96:1563–1568.
70. Smalley MJ, Dale TC. Wnt signalling in mammalian development and cancer. *Cancer Metastasis Rev* 1999;18:215–230.

71. Monga SP, Pediaditakis P, Mule K, Stolz DB, Michalopoulos GK. Changes in WNT/beta-catenin pathway during regulated growth in rat liver regeneration. *Hepatology* 2001;33:1098–1109.
72. Behrens J. Control of beta-catenin signaling in tumor development. *Ann NY Acad Sci* 2000;910:21–33; discussion 33–35.
73. Monga SP, Mars WM, Pediaditakis P, et al. Hepatocyte growth factor induces Wnt-independent nuclear translocation of beta-catenin after Met-beta-catenin dissociation in hepatocytes. *Cancer Res* 2002;62:2064–2071.
74. He TC, Sparks AB, Rago C, et al. Identification of c-MYC as a target of the APC pathway. *Science* 1998;281:1509–1512.
75. Tetsu O, McCormick F. Beta-catenin regulates expression of cyclin D1 in colon carcinoma cells. *Nature* 1999;398:422–426.
76. Cui J, Zhou X, Liu Y, Tang Z. Mutation and overexpression of the beta-catenin gene may play an important role in primary hepatocellular carcinoma among Chinese people. *J Cancer Res Clin Oncol* 2001;127:577–581.
77. Hsu HC, Jeng YM, Mao TL, Chu JS, Lai PL, Peng SY. Beta-catenin mutations are associated with a subset of low-stage hepatocellular carcinoma negative for hepatitis B virus and with favorable prognosis. *Am J Pathol* 2000;157:763–770.
78. Prange W, Breuhahn K, Fischer F, et al. Beta-catenin accumulation in the progression of human hepatocarcinogenesis correlates with loss of E-cadherin and accumulation of p53, but not with expression of conventional WNT-1 target genes. *J Pathol* 2003;201:250–259.
79. Ban KC, Singh H, Krishnan R, Seow HF. GSK-3beta phosphorylation and alteration of beta-catenin in hepatocellular carcinoma. *Cancer Lett* 2003;199:201–208.
80. Chen TC, Hsieh LL, Ng KF, Jeng LB, Chen MF. Absence of APC gene mutation in the mutation cluster region in hepatocellular carcinoma. *Cancer Lett* 1998;134:23–28.
81. Piao Z, Kim H, Jeon BK, Lee WJ, Park C. Relationship between loss of heterozygosity of tumor suppressor genes and histologic differentiation in hepatocellular carcinoma. *Cancer* 1997;80:865–872.
82. Su LK, Abdalla EK, Law CH, Kohlmann W, Rashid A, Vauthey JN. Biallelic inactivation of the APC gene is associated with hepatocellular carcinoma in familial adenomatous polyposis coli. *Cancer* 2001;92:332–339.
83. Satoh S, Daigo Y, Furukawa Y, et al. AXIN1 mutations in hepatocellular carcinomas, and growth suppression in cancer cells by virus-mediated transfer of AXIN1. *Nat Genet* 2000;24:245–250.
84. Laurent-Puig P, Legoix P, Bluteau O, et al. Genetic alterations associated with hepatocellular carcinomas define distinct pathways of hepatocarcinogenesis. *Gastroenterology* 2001;120:1763–1773.
85. Shibata T, Chuma M, Kokubu A, Sakamoto M, Hirohashi S. EBP50, a beta-catenin-associating protein, enhances Wnt signaling and is over-expressed in hepatocellular carcinoma. *Hepatology* 2003;38:178–186.
86. Slagle BL, Zhou YZ, Birchmeier W, Scorsone KA. Deletion of the E-cadherin gene in hepatitis B virus-positive Chinese hepatocellular carcinomas. *Hepatology* 1993;18:757–762.
87. Matsumura T, Makino R, Mitamura K. Frequent down-regulation of E-cadherin by genetic and epigenetic changes in the malignant progression of hepatocellular carcinomas. *Clin Cancer Res* 2001;7:594–599.
88. Endo K, Ueda T, Ueyama J, Ohta T, Terada T. Immunoreactive E-cadherin, alpha-catenin, beta-catenin, and gamma-catenin proteins in hepatocellular carcinoma: relationships with tumor grade, clinicopathologic parameters, and patients' survival. *Hum Pathol* 2000;31:558–565.
89. Kanai Y, Ushijima S, Hui AM, et al. The E-cadherin gene is silenced by CpG methylation in human hepatocellular carcinomas. *Int J Cancer* 1997;71:355–359.

90. Jiao W, Miyazaki K, Kitajima Y. Inverse correlation between E-cadherin and Snail expression in hepatocellular carcinoma cell lines in vitro and in vivo. *Br J Cancer* 2002;86:98–101.
91. Li LC, Chui RM, Sasaki M, et al. A single nucleotide polymorphism in the E-cadherin gene promoter alters transcriptional activities. *Cancer Res* 2000;60:873–876.92. Cadoret A, Ovejero C, Saadi-Kheddouci S, et al. Hepatomegaly in transgenic mice expressing an oncogenic form of beta-catenin. *Cancer Res* 2001;61:3245–3249.
93. Harada N, Miyoshi H, Murai N, et al. Lack of tumorigenesis in the mouse liver after adenovirus-mediated expression of a dominant stable mutant of beta-catenin. *Cancer Res* 2002;62:1971–1977.
94. Pruitt K, Der CJ. Ras and Rho regulation of the cell cycle and oncogenesis. *Cancer Lett* 2001;171:1–10.
95. Auer KL, Contessa J, Brenz-Verca S, et al. The Ras/Rac1/Cdc42/SEK/JNK/c-Jun cascade is a key pathway by which agonists stimulate DNA synthesis in primary cultures of rat hepatocytes. *Mol Biol Cell* 1998;9:561–573.
96. Cruise JL, Muga SJ, Lee YS, Michalopoulos GK. Regulation of hepatocyte growth: alpha-1 adrenergic receptor and ras p21 changes in liver regeneration. *J Cell Physiol* 1989;140:195–201.
97. Ng YK, Taborn G, Ahmad I, Radosevich J, Bauer K, Iannaccone P. Spatiotemporal changes in Ha-ras p21 expression through the hepatocyte cell cycle during liver regeneration. *Dev Biol* 1992;150:352–362.
98. Ellis CA, Clark G. The importance of being K-Ras. *Cell Signal* 2000;12:425–434.
99. Evans DM, Williams WJ, Kung IT. Angiosarcoma and hepatocellular carcinoma in vinyl chloride workers. *Histopathology* 1983;7:377–388.
100. Weihrauch M, Benicke M, Lehnert G, Wittekind C, Wrbitzky R, Tannapfel A. Frequent k- ras -2 mutations and p16(INK4A)methylation in hepatocellular carcinomas in workers exposed to vinyl chloride. *Br J Cancer* 2001;84:982–989.
101. Tada M, Omata M, Ohto M. Analysis of ras gene mutations in human hepatic malignant tumors by polymerase chain reaction and direct sequencing. *Cancer Res* 1990;50:1121–1124.
102. Leon M, Kew MC. Analysis of ras gene mutations in hepatocellular carcinoma in southern African blacks. *Anticancer Res* 1995;15:859–861.
103. Ogata N, Kamimura T, Asakura H. Point mutation, allelic loss and increased methylation of c-Ha-ras gene in human hepatocellular carcinoma. *Hepatology* 1991;13:31–37.
104. Nonomura A, Ohta G, Hayashi M, et al. Immunohistochemical detection of ras oncogene p21 product in liver cirrhosis and hepatocellular carcinoma. *Am J Gastroenterol* 1987;82:512–518.
105. Jagirdar J, Nonomura A, Patil J, Thor A, Paronetto F. ras oncogene p21 expression in hepatocellular carcinoma. *J Exper Pathol* 1989;4:37–46.
106. Emi M, Fujiwara Y, Ohata H, et al. Allelic loss at chromosome band 8p21.3-p22 is associated with progression of hepatocellular carcinoma. *Genes Chromosomes Cancer* 1993;7:152–157.
107. Qin LX, Tang ZY, Sham JS, et al. The association of chromosome 8p deletion and tumor metastasis in human hepatocellular carcinoma. *Cancer Res* 1999;59:5662–5665.
108. Yuan BZ, Miller MJ, Keck CL, Zimonjic DB, Thorgeirsson SS, Popescu NC. Cloning, characterization, and chromosomal localization of a gene frequently deleted in human liver cancer (DLC-1) homologous to rat RhoGAP. *Cancer Res* 1998;58:2196–2199.
109. Ng IO, Liang ZD, Cao L, Lee TK. DLC-1 is deleted in primary hepatocellular carcinoma and exerts inhibitory effects on the proliferation of hepatoma cell lines with deleted DLC-1. *Cancer Res* 2000;60:6581–6584.
110. Wong CM, Lee JM, Ching YP, Jin DY, Ng IO. Genetic and epigenetic alterations of DLC-1 gene in hepatocellular carcinoma. *Cancer Res* 2003;63:7646–7651.

111. Lin YW, Sheu JC, Liu LY, et al. Loss of heterozygosity at chromosome 13q in hepatocellular carcinoma: identification of three independent regions. *Eur J Cancer* 1999;35:1730–1734.
112. Ching YP, Wong CM, Chan SF, et al. Deleted in liver cancer (DLC) 2 encodes a RhoGAP protein with growth suppressor function and is underexpressed in hepatocellular carcinoma. *J Biol Chem* 2003;278:10,824—10,830.
113. Eisenman RN. Deconstructing myc. *Genes Develop* 2001;15:2023–2030.
114. Pelengaris S, Rudolph B, Littlewood T. Action of Myc in vivo - proliferation and apoptosis. Current Opinion in *Genet Develop* 2000;10:100–105.
115. Chandar N, Lombardi B, Locker J. c-myc gene amplification during hepatocarcinogenesis by a choline-devoid diet. *Proc Nat Acad Sci USA* 1989;86:2703–2707.
116. Pascale RM, De Miglio MR, Muroni MR, et al. c-myc amplification in pre-malignant and malignant lesions induced in rat liver by the resistant hepatocyte model. *Int J Cancer* 1996;68:136–142.
117. Cartier N, Miquerol L, Tulliez M, et al. Diet-dependent carcinogenesis of pancreatic islets and liver in transgenic mice expressing oncogenes under the control of the L-type pyruvate kinase gene promoter. *Oncogene* 1992;7:1413–1422.
118. Fourel G, Trepo C, Bougueleret L, et al. Frequent activation of N-myc genes by hepadnavirus insertion in woodchuck liver tumours. *Nature* 1990;347:294–298.
119. Hsu T, Moroy T, Etiemble J, et al. Activation of c-myc by woodchuck hepatitis virus insertion in hepatocellular carcinoma. *Cell* 1988;55:627–635.
120. Abou-Elella A, Gramlich T, Fritsch C, Gansler T. c-myc amplification in hepatocellular carcinoma predicts unfavorable prognosis. *Mod Pathol* 1996;9:95–98.
121. Kawate S, Fukusato T, Ohwada S, Watanuki A, Morishita Y. Amplification of c-myc in hepatocellular carcinoma: correlation with clinicopathologic features, proliferative activity and p53 overexpression. *Oncology* 1999;57:157–163.
122. Gan FY, Gesell MS, Alousi M, Luk GD. Analysis of ODC and c-myc gene expression in hepatocellular carcinoma by in situ hybridization and immunohistochemistry. *J Histochem Cytochem* 1993;41:1185–1196.
123. Yuen MF, Wu PC, Lai VC, Lau JY, Lai CL. Expression of c-Myc, c-Fos, and c-jun in hepatocellular carcinoma. *Cancer* 2001;91:106–112.
124. Sampath D, Plunkett W. Design of new anticancer therapies targeting cell cycle checkpoint pathways. *Curr Opin Oncol* 2001;13:484–490.
125. Daujat S, Neel H, Piette J. MDM2: life without p53. *Trends Genet* 2001;17:459–464.
126. Kishimoto Y, Shiota G, Kamisaki Y, et al. Loss of the tumor suppressor p53 gene at the liver cirrhosis stage in Japanese patients with hepatocellular carcinoma. *Oncology* 1997;54:304–310.
127. Tanaka S, Toh Y, Adachi E, Matsumata T, Mori R, Sugimachi K. Tumor progression in hepatocellular carcinoma may be mediated by p53 mutation. *Cancer Res* 1993;53:2884–2887.
128. Park NH, Chung YH, Youn KH, et al. Close correlation of p53 mutation to microvascular invasion in hepatocellular carcinoma. *J Clin Gastroenterol* 2001;33:397–401.
129. Yano M, Asahara T, Dohi K, Mizuno T, Iwamoto KS, Seyama T. Close correlation between a p53 or hMSH2 gene mutation in the tumor and survival of hepatocellular carcinoma patients. *Int J Oncol* 1999;14:447–451.
130. Ng IO, Fan ST. Is the p53 gene mutation of prognostic value in hepatocellular carcinoma? [letter; comment.]. *Arch Surg* 2000;135:1476.
131. Bressac B, Kew M, Wands J, Ozturk M. Selective G to T mutations of p53 gene in hepatocellular carcinoma from southern Africa. *Nature* 1991;350:429–431.
132. Ozturk M. p53 mutation in hepatocellular carcinoma after aflatoxin exposure. *Lancet* 1991;338:1356–1359.

133. Feitelson MA, Zhu M, Duan LX, London WT. Hepatitis B x antigen and p53 are associated in vitro and in liver tissues from patients with primary hepatocellular carcinoma. *Oncogene* 1993;8:1109–1117.
134. Wang XW, Forrester K, Yeh H, Feitelson MA, Gu JR, Harris CC. Hepatitis B virus X protein inhibits p53 sequence-specific DNA binding, transcriptional activity, and association with transcription factor ERCC3. *Proc Nat Acad Sci USA* 1994;91:2230–2234.
135. Becker SA, Lee TH, Butel JS, Slagle BL. Hepatitis B virus X protein interferes with cellular DNA repair. *J Virol* 1998;72:266–272.
136. Pogribny IP, James SJ. Reduction of p53 gene expression in human primary hepatocellular carcinoma is associated with promoter region methylation without coding region mutation. *Cancer Lett* 2002;176:169–174.
137. Bourdon JC, D'Errico A, Paterlini P, Grigioni W, May E, Debuire B. p53 protein accumulation in European hepatocellular carcinoma is not always dependent on p53 gene mutation. *Gastroenterology* 1995;108:1176–1182.
138. Qiu SJ, Ye SL, Wu ZQ, Tang ZY, Liu YK. The expression of the mdm2 gene may be related to the aberration of the p53 gene in human hepatocellular carcinoma. *J Cancer Res Clin Oncol* 1998;124:253–258.
139. Endo K, Ueda T, Ohta T, Terada T. Protein expression of MDM2 and its clinicopathological relationships in human hepatocellular carcinoma. *Liver* 2000;20:209–215.
140. Nevins JR. The Rb/E2F pathway and cancer. *Hum Mol Genet* 2001;10:699–703.
141. Zhang X, Xu HJ, Murakami Y, et al. Deletions of chromosome 13q, mutations in Retinoblastoma 1, and retinoblastoma protein state in human hepatocellular carcinoma. *Cancer Res* 1994;54:4177–4182.
142. Ashida K, Kishimoto Y, Nakamoto K, et al. Loss of heterozygosity of the retinoblastoma gene in liver cirrhosis accompanying hepatocellular carcinoma. *J Cancer Res Clin Oncol* 1997;123:489–495.
143. Roncalli M, Borzio M, Bianchi P, Laghi L. Comprehensive allelotype study of hepatocellular carcinoma. *Hepatology* 2000;32:876.
144. Hada H, Koide N, Morita T, et al. Promoter-independent loss of mRNA and protein of the Rb gene in a human hepatocellular carcinoma. *Hepatogastroenterology* 1996;43:1185–1189.
145. Edamoto Y, Hara A, Biernat W, et al. Alterations of RB1, p53 and Wnt pathways in hepatocellular carcinomas associated with hepatitis C, hepatitis B and alcoholic liver cirrhosis. *Int J Cancer* 2003;106:334–341.
146. Higashitsuji H, Itoh K, Nagao T, et al. Reduced stability of retinoblastoma protein by gankyrin, an oncogenic ankyrin-repeat protein overexpressed in hepatomas. *Nat Med* 2000;6:96–99.
147. Fu XY, Wang HY, Tan L, Liu SQ, Cao HF, Wu MC. Overexpression of p28/gankyrin in human hepatocellular carcinoma and its clinical significance. *W J Gastroenterol* 2002;8:638–643.
148. Hui AM, Li X, Makuuchi M, Takayama T, Kubota K. Over-expression and lack of retinoblastoma protein are associated with tumor progression and metastasis in hepatocellular carcinoma. *Int J Cancer* 1999;84:604–608.
149. Naka T, Toyota N, Kaneko T, Kaibara N. Protein expression of p53, p21WAF1, and Rb as prognostic indicators in patients with surgically treated hepatocellular carcinoma. *Anticancer Res* 1998;18:555–564.
150. Zimonjic DB, Keck CL, Thorgeirsson SS, Popescu NC. Novel recurrent genetic imbalances in human hepatocellular carcinoma cell lines identified by comparative genomic hybridization. *Hepatology* 1999;29:1208–1214.
151. Hussussian CJ, Struewing JP, Goldstein AM, et al. Germline p16 mutations in familial melanoma. *Nat Genet* 1994;8:15–21.

152. Serrano M, Lee H, Chin L, Cordon-Cardo C, Beach D, DePinho RA. Role of the INK4a locus in tumor suppression and cell mortality. *Cell* 1996;85:27–37.
153. Bates S, Phillips AC, Clark PA, et al. p14ARF links the tumour suppressors RB and p53. *Nature* 1998;395:124–125.
154. Liew CT, Li HM, Lo KW, et al. High frequency of p16INK4A gene alterations in hepatocellular carcinoma. *Oncogene* 1999;18:789–795.
155. Jin M, Piao Z, Kim NG, et al. p16 is a major inactivation target in hepatocellular carcinoma. *Cancer* 2000;89:60–68.
156. Piao Z, Park C, Lee JS, Yang CH, Choi KY, Kim H. Homozygous deletions of the CDKN2 gene and loss of heterozygosity of 9p in primary hepatocellular carcinoma. *Cancer Lett* 1998;122:201–207.
157. Hui AM, Sakamoto M, Kanai Y, et al. Inactivation of p16INK4 in hepatocellular carcinoma. *Hepatology* 1996;24:575–579.
158. Hui AM, Shi YZ, Li X, Takayama T, Makuuchi M. Loss of p16(INK4) protein, alone and together with loss of retinoblastoma protein, correlate with hepatocellular carcinoma progression. *Cancer Lett* 2000;154:93–99.
159. Chaubert P, Gayer R, Zimmermann A, et al. Germ-line mutations of the p16INK4(MTS1) gene occur in a subset of patients with hepatocellular carcinoma. *Hepatology* 1997;25:1376–1381.
160. Lee TK, Man K, Ling MT, et al. Over-expression of Id-1 induces cell proliferation in hepatocellular carcinoma through inactivation of p16INK4a/RB pathway. *Carcinogenesis* 2003;24:1729–1736.
161. Dotto GP. p21(WAF1/Cip1): more than a break to the cell cycle? *Biochim et Biophys Acta* 2000;1471:M43–M56.
162. Hui AM, Kanai Y, Sakamoto M, Tsuda H, Hirohashi S. Reduced p21(WAF1/CIP1) expression and p53 mutation in hepatocellular carcinomas. *Hepatology* 1997;25:575–579.
163. Furutani M, Arii S, Tanaka H, et al. Decreased expression and rare somatic mutation of the CIP1/WAF1 gene in human hepatocellular carcinoma. *Cancer Lett* 1997;111:191–197.
164. Kobayashi S, Matsushita K, Saigo K, et al. P21WAF1/CIP1 messenger RNA expression in hepatitis B, C virus-infected human hepatocellular carcinoma tissues. *Cancer* 2001;91:2096–2103.
165. Qin LF, Ng IO. Expression of p27(KIP1) and p21(WAF1/CIP1) in primary hepatocellular carcinoma: clinicopathologic correlation and survival analysis. *Hum Pathol* 2001;32:778–784.
166. Sherr CJ, Roberts JM. CDK inhibitors: positive and negative regulators of G1-phase progression. *Genes Develop* 1999;13:1501–1512.
167. Philipp-Staheli J, Payne SR, Kemp CJ. p27(Kip1): regulation and function of a haploinsufficient tumor suppressor and its misregulation in cancer. *Exper Cell Res* 2001;264:148–168.
168. Tannapfel A, Grund D, Katalinic A, et al. Decreased expression of p27 protein is associated with advanced tumor stage in hepatocellular carcinoma. *Int J Cancer* 2000;89:350–355.
169. Ito Y, Matsuura N, Sakon M, et al. Expression and prognostic roles of the G1-S modulators in hepatocellular carcinoma: p27 independently predicts the recurrence. *Hepatology* 1999;30:90–99.
170. Fiorentino M, Altimari A, D'Errico A, et al. Acquired expression of p27 is a favorable prognostic indicator in patients with hepatocellular carcinoma. *Clin Cancer Res* 2000;6:3966–3972.
171. Catzavelos C, Bhattacharya N, Ung YC, et al. Decreased levels of the cell-cycle inhibitor p27Kip1 protein: prognostic implications in primary breast cancer. *Nat Med* 1997;3:227–230.

172. Kusano N, Shiraishi K, Kubo K, Oga A, Okita K, Sasaki K. Genetic aberrations detected by comparative genomic hybridization in hepatocellular carcinomas: their relationship to clinicopathological features. *Hepatology* 1999;29:1858–1862.
173. Zhang YJ, Jiang W, Chen CJ, et al. Amplification and overexpression of cyclin D1 in human hepatocellular carcinoma. *Biochem Biophys Res Commun* 1993;196:1010–1016.
174. Nishida N, Fukuda Y, Komeda T, et al. Amplification and overexpression of the cyclin D1 gene in aggressive human hepatocellular carcinoma. *Cancer Res* 1994;54:3107–3110.
175. Yamashita T, Kaneko S, Hashimoto S, et al. Serial analysis of gene expression in chronic hepatitis C and hepatocellular carcinoma. *Biochem Biophys Res Commun* 2001;282:647–654.
176. Deane NG, Parker MA, Aramandla R, et al. Hepatocellular carcinoma results from chronic cyclin D1 overexpression in transgenic mice. *Cancer Res* 2001;61:5389–5395.
177. Evan GI, Vousden KH. Proliferation, cell cycle and apoptosis in cancer. *Nature* 2001;411:342–348.
178. Gupta S. Molecular steps of death receptor and mitochondrial pathways of apoptosis. *Life Sci* 2001;69:2957–2964.
179. Ni R, Tomita Y, Matsuda K, et al. Fas-mediated apoptosis in primary cultured mouse hepatocytes. *Exper Cell Res* 1994;215:332–337.
180. Ogasawara J, Watanabe-Fukunaga R, Adachi M, et al. Lethal effect of the anti-Fas antibody in mice. *Nature* 1993;364:806–809.
181. Oberhammer FA, Pavelka M, Sharma S, et al. Induction of apoptosis in cultured hepatocytes and in regressing liver by transforming growth factor beta 1. *Proc Natl Acad Sci USA* 1992;89:5408–5412.
182. Bissell DM, Roulot D, George J. Transforming growth factor beta and the liver. *Hepatology* 2001;34:859–867.
183. Zhang X, Wang T, Batist G, Tsao MS. Transforming growth factor beta 1 promotes spontaneous transformation of cultured rat liver epithelial cells. *Cancer Res* 1994;54:6122–6128.
184. Factor VM, Kao CY, Santoni-Rugiu E, Woitach JT, Jensen MR, Thorgeirsson SS. Constitutive expression of mature transforming growth factor beta 1 in the liver accelerates hepatocarcinogenesis in transgenic mice. *Cancer Res* 1997;57:2089–2095.
185. Ito N, Kawata S, Tamura S, et al. Elevated levels of transforming growth factor beta messenger RNA and its polypeptide in human hepatocellular carcinoma. *Cancer Res* 1991;51:4080–4083.
186. Shirai Y, Kawata S, Tamura S, et al. Plasma transforming growth factor-beta 1 in patients with hepatocellular carcinoma. Comparison with chronic liver diseases. *Cancer* 1994;73:2275–2279.
187. Sue SR, Chari RS, Kong FM, et al. Transforming growth factor-beta receptors and mannose 6-phosphate/insulin-like growth factor-II receptor expression in human hepatocellular carcinoma. *Ann Surg* 1995;222:171–178.
188. Furuta K, Misao S, Takahashi K, et al. Gene mutation of transforming growth factor beta1 type II receptor in hepatocellular carcinoma. *Int J Cancer* 1999;81:851–853.
189. Kawate S, Takenoshita S, Ohwada S, et al. Mutation analysis of transforming growth factor beta type II receptor, Smad2, and Smad4 in hepatocellular carcinoma. *Int J Oncology* 1999;14:127–131.
190. Yakicier MC, Irmak MB, Romano A, Kew M, Ozturk M. Smad2 and Smad4 gene mutations in hepatocellular carcinoma. *Oncogene* 1999;18:4879–4883.
191. Dennis PA, Rifkin DB. Cellular activation of latent transforming growth factor beta requires binding to the cation-independent mannose 6-phosphate/insulin-like growth factor type II receptor. *Proc Natl Acad Sci USA* 1991;88:580–584.

192. Dahms NM, Lobel P, Kornfeld S. Mannose 6-phosphate receptors and lysosomal enzyme targeting. *J Biol Chem* 1989;264:12,115—12,118.
193. De Souza AT, Hankins GR, Washington MK, Fine RL, Orton TC, Jirtle RL. Frequent loss of heterozygosity on 6q at the mannose 6-phosphate/insulin-like growth factor II receptor locus in human hepatocellular tumors. *Oncogene* 1995;10:1725–1729.
194. Piao Z, Choi Y, Park C, Lee WJ, Park JH, Kim H. Deletion of the M6P/IGF2r gene in primary hepatocellular carcinoma. *Cancer Lett* 1997;120:39–43.
195. Yamada T, De Souza AT, Finkelstein S, Jirtle RL. Loss of the gene encoding mannose 6-phosphate/insulin-like growth factor II receptor is an early event in liver carcinogenesis. *Proc Natl Acad Sci USA* 1997;94:10,351—10,355.
196. Wada I, Kanada H, Nomura K, Kato Y, Machinami R, Kitagawa T. Failure to detect genetic alteration of the mannose-6-phosphate/insulin-like growth factor 2 receptor (M6P/IGF2R) gene in hepatocellular carcinomas in Japan. *Hepatology* 1999;29:1718–1721.
197. De Souza AT, Hankins GR, Washington MK, Orton TC, Jirtle RL. M6P/IGF2R gene is mutated in human hepatocellular carcinomas with loss of heterozygosity. *Nat Genet* 1995;11:447–449.
198. Kaplowitz N. Cell death at the millennium. Implications for liver diseases. *Clin Liver Dis* 2000;4:1–23, v.
199. Natoli G, Ianni A, Costanzo A, et al. Resistance to Fas-mediated apoptosis in human hepatoma cells. *Oncogene* 1995;11:1157–1164.
200. Ito Y, Monden M, Takeda T, et al. The status of Fas and Fas ligand expression can predict recurrence of hepatocellular carcinoma. *Br J Cancer* 2000;82:1211–1217.
201. Kubo K, Matsuzaki Y, Okazaki M, Kato A, Kobayashi N, Okita K. The Fas system is not significantly involved in apoptosis in human hepatocellular carcinoma. *Liver* 1998;18:117–123.
202. Lee SH, Shin MS, Lee HS, et al. Expression of Fas and Fas-related molecules in human hepatocellular carcinoma. *Hum Pathol* 2001;32:250–256.
203. Roskams T, Libbrecht L, Van Damme B, Desmet V. Fas and Fas ligand: strong co-expression in human hepatocytes surrounding hepatocellular carcinoma; can cancer induce suicide in peritumoural cells? *J Pathol* 2000;191:150–153.
204. Takehara T, Hayashi N. Fas and fas ligand in human hepatocellular carcinoma. *J Gastroenterol* 2001;36:727–728.
205. Ito T, Shiraki K, Sugimoto K, et al. Survivin promotes cell proliferation in human hepatocellular carcinoma. *Hepatology* 2000;31:1080–1085.
206. Chen GG, Lai PB, Chan PK, et al. Decreased expression of Bid in human hepatocellular carcinoma is related to hepatitis B virus X protein. *Eur J Cancer* 2001;37:1695–1702.
207. Fujikawa K, Shiraki K, Sugimoto K, et al. Reduced expression of ICE/caspase1 and CPP32/caspase3 in human hepatocellular carcinoma. *Anticancer Res* 2000;20:1927–1932.
208. Johnstone RW, Ruefli AA, Lowe SW. Apoptosis: a link between cancer genetics and chemotherapy. *Cell* 2002;108:153–164.
209. Rojkind MaG, Patricia. The extracellular matrix of the liver. In: Arias IM, ed. *The Liver Biology and Pathobiology*. New York: Raven Press, 1994:843–868.
210. Martinez-Hernandez A, Delgado FM, Amenta PS. The extracellular matrix in hepatic regeneration. Localization of collagen types I, III, IV, laminin, and fibronectin. *Lab Invest* 1991;64:157–166.
211. Ruoslahti E. Integrins. *J Clin Invest* 1991;87:1–5.
212. Roskelley CD, Srebrow A, Bissell MJ. A hierarchy of ECM-mediated signalling regulates tissue-specific gene expression. *Curr Opin Cell Biol* 1995;7:736–747.
213. Frisch SM, Screaton RA. Anoikis mechanisms. *Curr Opin Cell Biol* 2001;13:555–562.

214. Rojkind MaG, Patricia. Pathophysiology fo liver fibrosis. In: Arias IM, ed. *The Liver Biology and Pathobiology*. Philadelphia: Lippincott Williams & Wilkins, 2001:721–738.
215. Le Bail B, Faouzi S, Boussarie L, Balabaud C, Bioulac-Sage P, Rosenbaum J. Extracellular matrix composition and integrin expression in early hepatocarcinogenesis in human cirrhotic liver. *J Pathol* 1997;181:330–337.
216. Torimura T, Ueno T, Kin M, et al. Coordinated expression of integrin alpha6beta1 and laminin in hepatocellular carcinoma. *Hum Pathol* 1997;28:1131–1138.
217. Murphy G, Gavrilovic J. Proteolysis and cell migration: creating a path? *Curr Opin Cell Biol* 1999;11:614–621.
218. Giannelli G, Bergamini C, Fransvea E, Marinosci F, Quaranta V, Antonaci S. Human hepatocellular carcinoma (HCC) cells require both alpha3beta1 integrin and matrix metalloproteinases activity for migration and invasion. *Lab Invest* 2001;81:613–627.
219. Nakashima O, Kojiro M. Recurrence of hepatocellular carcinoma: multicentric occurrence or intrahepatic metastasis? A viewpoint in terms of pathology. *J Hepatobiliary Pancreat Surg* 2001;8:404–409.
220. Kirimlioglu H, Dvorchick I, Ruppert K, et al. Hepatocellular carcinomas in native livers from patients treated with orthotopic liver transplantation: biologic and therapeutic implications. *Hepatology* 2001;34:502–510.
221. Rudolph KL, Trautwein C, Kubicka S, et al. Differential regulation of extracellular matrix synthesis during liver regeneration after partial hepatectomy in rats. *Hepatology* 1999;30:1159–1166.
222. Kim TH, Mars WM, Stolz DB, Michalopoulos GK. Expression and activation of pro-MMP-2 and pro-MMP-9 during rat liver regeneration. *Hepatology* 2000;31:75–82.
223. Andreasen PA, Kjoller L, Christensen L, Duffy MJ. The urokinase-type plasminogen activator system in cancer metastasis: a review. *Int J Cancer* 1997;72:1–22.
224. Mars WM, Zarnegar R, Michalopoulos GK. Activation of hepatocyte growth factor by the plasminogen activators uPA and tPA. *Am J Pathol* 1993;143:949–958.
225. Nagase H. Activation mechanisms of matrix metalloproteinases. *Biol Chem* 1997;378:151–160.
226. McCawley LJ, Matrisian LM. Matrix metalloproteinases: they're not just for matrix anymore! *Curr Opin Cell Biol* 2001;13:534–540.
227. Morita Y, Hayashi Y, Wang Y, et al. Expression of urokinase-type plasminogen activator receptor in hepatocellular carcinoma. *Hepatology* 1997;25:856–861.
228. Ashida K, Nakatsukasa H, Higashi T, et al. Cellular distribution of 92-kd type IV collagenase/gelatinase B in human hepatocellular carcinoma. *Am J Pathol* 1996;149:1803–1811.
229. Arii S, Mise M, Harada T, et al. Overexpression of matrix metalloproteinase 9 gene in hepatocellular carcinoma with invasive potential. *Hepatology* 1996;24:316–322.
230. Sakamoto Y, Mafune K, Mori M, et al. Overexpression of MMP-9 correlates with growth of small hepatocellular carcinoma. *Int J Oncol* 2000;17:237–743.
231. Giannelli G, Bergamini C, Marinosci F, et al. Clinical role of MMP-2/TIMP-2 imbalance in hepatocellular carcinoma. *Int J Cancer* 2002;97:425–431.
232. Carmeliet P, Jain RK. Angiogenesis in cancer and other diseases. *Nature* 2000;407:249–257.
233. Sugimachi K, Tanaka S, Terashi T, Taguchi K, Rikimaru T. The mechanisms of angiogenesis in hepatocellular carcinoma: angiogenic switch during tumor progression. *Surgery* 2002;131:S135—S141.
234. Yancopoulos GD, Davis S, Gale NW, Rudge JS, Wiegand SJ, Holash J. Vascular-specific growth factors and blood vessel formation. *Nature* 2000;407:242–248.
235. Ferrara N, Davis-Smyth T. The biology of vascular endothelial growth factor. *Endocrine Rev* 1997;18:4–25.

236. Ng IO, Poon RT, Lee JM, Fan ST, Ng M, Tso WK. Microvessel density, vascular endothelial growth factor and its receptors Flt-1 and Flk-1/KDR in hepatocellular carcinoma. *Am J Clin Pathol* 2001;116:838–845.
237. Miura H, Miyazaki T, Kuroda M, et al. Increased expression of vascular endothelial growth factor in human hepatocellular carcinoma. *J Hepatol* 1997;27:854–861.
238. Chow NH, Hsu PI, Lin XZ, et al. Expression of vascular endothelial growth factor in normal liver and hepatocellular carcinoma: an immunohistochemical study. *Hum Pathol* 1997;28:698–703.
239. Moon WS, Rhyu KH, Kang MJ, et al. Overexpression of VEGF and angiopoietin 2: a key to high vascularity of hepatocellular carcinoma? *Mod Pathol* 2003;16:552–557.
240. Shimamura T, Saito S, Morita K, et al. Detection of vascular endothelial growth factor and its receptor expression in human hepatocellular carcinoma biopsy specimens. *J Gastroenterol Hepatol* 2000;15:640–646.
241. Loughna S, Sato TN. Angiopoietin and Tie signaling pathways in vascular development. *Matrix Biol* 2001;20:319–325.
242. Tanaka S, Mori M, Sakamoto Y, Makuuchi M, Sugimachi K, Wands JR. Biologic significance of angiopoietin-2 expression in human hepatocellular carcinoma. *J Clin Invest* 1999;103:341–345.
243. Tanaka S, Sugimachi K, Yamashita Yi Y, et al. Tie2 vascular endothelial receptor expression and function in hepatocellular carcinoma. *Hepatology* 2002;35:861–867.
244. Soff GA. Angiostatin and angiostatin-related proteins. *Cancer Metastasis Rev* 2000;19:97–107.
245. Dong Z, Kumar R, Yang X, Fidler IJ. Macrophage-derived metalloelastase is responsible for the generation of angiostatin in Lewis lung carcinoma. *Cell* 1997;88:801–810.
246. Gorrin Rivas MJ, Arii S, Furutani M, et al. Expression of human macrophage metalloelastase gene in hepatocellular carcinoma: correlation with angiostatin generation and its clinical significance. *Hepatology* 1998;28:986–993.
247. Suehiro T, Terashi T, Shiotani S, Soejima Y, Sugimachi K. Liver transplantation for hepatocellular carcinoma. *Surgery* 2002;131:S190—S194.
248. Bergsland EK, Venook AP. Hepatocellular carcinoma. *Curr Opin Oncol* 2000;12:357–361.
249. Okuda K. Hepatocellular carcinoma. *J Hepatol* 2000;32:225–237.
250. Chang MH, Chen CJ, Lai MS, et al. Universal hepatitis B vaccination in Taiwan and the incidence of hepatocellular carcinoma in children. Taiwan Childhood Hepatoma Study Group. *N Engl J Med* 1997;336:1855–1859.
251. Omata M, Shiratori Y. Long-term effects of interferon therapy on histology and development of hepatocellular carcinoma in hepatitis C. *J Gastroenterol Hepatol* 2000;15:E134–E140.
252. Scott LJ, Perry CM. Interferon-alpha-2b plus ribavirin: a review of its use in the management of chronic hepatitis C. *Drugs* 2002;62:507–556.
253. Muto Y, Moriwaki H, Ninomiya M, et al. Prevention of second primary tumors by an acyclic retinoid, polyprenoic acid, in patients with hepatocellular carcinoma. Hepatoma Prevention Study Group. *N Engl J Med* 1996;334:1561–1567.
254. Muto Y, Moriwaki H, Saito A. Prevention of second primary tumors by an acyclic retinoid in patients with hepatocellular carcinoma. *N Engl J Med* 1999;340:1046–1047.
255. Okuno M, Sano T, Matsushima-Nishiwaki R, et al. Apoptosis induction by acyclic retinoid: a molecular basis of 'clonal deletion' therapy for hepatocellular carcinoma. *Japan J Clin Oncol* 2001;31:359–362.
256. Heinrich MC, Blanke CD, Druker BJ, Corless CL. Inhibition of KIT tyrosine kinase activity: a novel molecular approach to the treatment of KIT-positive malignancies. *J Clin Oncol* 2002;20:1692–1703.

257. Scollay R. Gene therapy: a brief overview of the past, present, and future. *Ann NY Acad Sci* 2001;953:26–30.
258. Qian C, Drozdzik M, Caselmann WH, Prieto J. The potential of gene therapy in the treatment of hepatocellular carcinoma. *J Hepatol* 2000;32:344–351.
259. Baselga J, Albanell J. Mechanism of action of anti-HER2 monoclonal antibodies. *Ann Oncol* 2001;12:S35–S41.
260. Ciardiello F, Tortora G. A novel approach in the treatment of cancer: targeting the epidermal growth factor receptor. *Clin Cancer Res* 2001;7:2958–2970.
261. Liekens S, De Clercq E, Neyts J. Angiogenesis: regulators and clinical applications. *Biochem Pharmacol* 2001;61:253–270.
262. Kin M, Torimura T, Ueno T, et al. Angiogenesis inhibitor TNP-470 suppresses the progression of experimentally-induced hepatocellular carcinoma in rats. *Int J Oncol* 2000;16:375–382.
263. Ikebe T, Yamamoto T, Kubo S, et al. Suppressive effect of the angiogenesis inhibitor TNP-470 on the development of carcinogen-induced hepatic nodules in rats. *Japan J Cancer Res* 1998;89:143–149.
264. Bu W, Tang ZY, Sun FX, et al. Effects of matrix metalloproteinase inhibitor BB-94 on liver cancer growth and metastasis in a patient-like orthotopic model LCI-D20. *Hepatogastroenterology* 1998;45:1056–1061.
265. Coussens LM, Fingleton B, Matrisian LM. Matrix metalloproteinase inhibitors and cancer: trials and tribulations. *Science* 2002;295:2387–2392.

3 Clinical Features and Diagnostic Evaluation of Hepatocellular Carcinoma

David A. Sass, MD and Kapil B. Chopra, MD

CONTENTS

1. INTRODUCTION

The diagnosis of hepatocellular carcinoma (HCC) can be difficult and often requires the use of serum markers, one or more imaging methods, and histological confirmation. HCC frequently is diagnosed late in its course because of the absence of pathognomonic symptoms and the liver's large functional reserve *(1)*. As a result, many patients have untreatable disease when first diagnosed. The clinical presentation generally varies in different parts of the world. Many patients with HCC related to chronic hepatitis B virus (HBV) or hepatitis C virus (HCV) infection in high-incidence locations, for example, in sub-Saharan Africa and in Asia, have severe hepatic decompensation at presentation. However, the common presentation in low-incidence areas such as the United States and other Western countries may follow routine laboratory screening for HCC before symptoms are prominent *(2)*, because approx 40% of patients are asymptomatic at the time of diagnosis *(3)*.

From: *Current Clinical Oncology: Hepatocellular Cancer: Diagnosis and Treatment*
Edited by: B. I. Carr © Humana Press Inc., Totowa, NJ

2. CLINICAL FEATURES

2.1. Asymptomatic Presentation

Increasingly, because of screening programs for cirrhotic patients or during the liver transplantation evaluation process, tumors are being detected at an asymptomatic stage. These tumors tend to be smaller (with current imaging methods, tumors as small as 0.5 cm can be detected) and, therefore, are more amenable to potentially curative therapies such as resection, transplantation, and tumor ablation. The frequency of asymptomatic diagnosis is entirely dependent on the intensity of the screening program; for example, in a series of 461 Italian patients with HCC, 23% were asymptomatic *(4)*.

2.2. Hepatic Decompensation

Another common scenario for the presentation of HCC is sudden hepatic decompensation in a patient known to have cirrhosis. New-onset ascites, recurrent variceal hemorrhage, or progressive encephalopathy should always raise suspicion for HCC in the differential diagnosis. The ascites may be difficult to control with standard diuretic therapy and often is bloodstained.

2.3. Gastrointestinal Hemorrhage

Approximately 10% of patients have gastrointestinal bleeding at presentation. In 40% of these patients, the bleeding is the result of esophageal varices resulting from portal vein invasion and elevated portal pressure. Peptic ulcer disease and other benign causes account for the remaining 60% of cases involving bleeding. Rarely, the tumor directly may invade the gastrointestinal tract, causing bleeding *(5)*.

2.4. The "Classic Triad"

Historically, this method of presentation, although uncommon in clinical practice, has been described to be the triad of right upper quadrant abdominal pain, weight loss, and hepatomegaly (*see* Table 1). Patients with these symptoms at presentation usually have a tumor larger than 6 cm. The pain frequently is described as a dull continuous ache that intensifies late in the course of the illness, when Glisson's capsule is affected. The pain may be referred to the shoulder. Firm, often massive, hepatomegaly is an invariable feature of symptomatic malignant liver tumors. An arterial vascular bruit (resulting from increased vascularity) may be a useful diagnostic pointer. It is present in 25% of cases, occurs in systole, is rough in character, and is not affected by changing the position of the patient. Although not pathognomonic, it rarely occurs with hepatic metastases *(6)*. Less often, a friction rub is heard over the tumor, although this sign is more typical of hepatic metastases or abscesses *(7)*.

Table 1
Frequency of Clinical Features of HCC

Symptoms	*(%)*	*Physical signs*	*(%)*
Abdominal pain	59–95	Hepatomegaly	54–98
Weight loss	34–71	Hepatic bruit	6–25
Weakness	22–53	Ascites	35–61
Abdominal swelling	28–43	Splenomegaly	27–42
Nonspecific symptoms	25–28	Jaundice	4–35
Jaundice	5–26	Wasting	25–41
		Fever	11–54

(Reprinted from: Kew MC. Hepatic tumors and cysts. In: *Gastrointestinal and Liver Disease* [Feldman M, Friedman LS, Sleisenger MH, eds.], WB Saunders, Philadelphia, 2002, p. 1578.)

2.5. Tumor Rupture: "Hemoperitoneum"

Spontaneous rupture is a rare and catastrophic complication of HCC that may occur if a large vascular tumor on the periphery of the liver outstrips its blood supply. This type of rupture may occur spontaneously or with minor blunt abdominal trauma. The clinical presentation is that of severe abdominal pain, vascular collapse, and signs of peritoneal irritation. Although hemoperitoneum is a frequent event late in the course of the disease, it is a presenting feature in less than 5% of cases. The diagnosis is established by paracentesis, which reveals bloodstained fluid. Angiography and embolization of the bleeding vessel can be an effective method for managing this life-threatening complication *(8)*.

2.6. Extrahepatic Endocrine and Paraneoplastic Syndromes

These systemic sequelae result, directly or indirectly, from synthesis and secretion of biologically active substances by the tumor. Although rare, an awareness of these presentations may prevent the diagnosis from being delayed or even missed (*see* Table 2).

Advances have been made in understanding the mechanisms underlying some of these paraneoplastic phenomena. Hypoglycemia (<5% of patients) results from defective processing by malignant hepatocytes of the precursor of insulin-like growth factor II (pro-IGF-II). The resulting big IGF-II circulates in 60-kd complexes that are appreciably smaller than the normal complexes *(9)*. With easier transfer across capillary membranes, the effect is to increase glucose uptake by tissues with resultant hypoglycemia. Polycythemia (<10% of patients) is caused by synthesis of erythropoietin by the tumor *(10)*. Patients with HCC,

Table 2
Paraneoplastic Syndromes Associated With HCC

Hypoglycemia
Polycythemia (erythrocytosis)
Hypercalcemia
Sexual changes: isosexual precocity, gynecomastia, feminization
Systemic arterial hypertension
Watery diarrhea syndrome
Carcinoid syndrome
Osteoporosis
Hypertrophic osteoarthropathy
Thyrotoxicosis
Hypercholesterolemia
Thrombophlebitis migrans
Polymyositis
Neuropathy
Cutaneous manifestations: pityriasis rotunda, Leser-Trelat sign, dermatomyositis, pemphigus foliaceus, porphyria cutanea tarda

(Adapted from: Kew MC. Hepatic tumors and cysts. In: *Gastrointestinal and Liver Disease* [Feldman M, Friedman LS, Sleisenger MH, eds.], WB Saunders, Philadelphia, 2002, p. 1579.)

especially with the sclerosing variety, may present with hypercalcemia in the absence of osteolytic metastases. The probable cause is secretion of parathyroid hormone-related protein by the tumor *(11)*. Arterial hypertension complicating HCC is the consequence of ectopic synthesis of angiotensinogen (with or without ectopic renin production) by malignant hepatocytes *(12)*. Feminization results from the tumor's conversion of circulating dehydroepiandrosterone to estrone and, to a lesser extent, estradiol *(13)*. Hypercholesterolemia is the result of autonomous *de novo* synthesis of cholesterol by the tumor *(14)*. Watery diarrhea, which is occasionally severe and intractable, probably is related to secretion of peptides that promote intestinal secretion, for example, vasoactive intestinal peptide, gastrin, and prostaglandins *(15)*. Several cutaneous manifestations have been described in association with HCC; however, none is specific for the diagnosis. These include dermatomyositis, pemphigus foliaceus, sign of Leser-Trelat, pityriasis rotunda, and porphyria cutanea tarda *(16)*.

2.7. Other Rare Manifestations

HCC has been reported as a cause of fever of unknown origin *(17)*. Massive tense ascites resulting from hepatic vein spread (Budd–Chiari syndrome) *(18)* and obstructive jaundice resulting from bile duct compression are two complications of locally advanced tumor. Other rare presentations may include symptoms referrable to sites of distant metastasis, for example, bone pain (skeletal), sudden paraplegia (with vertebral destruction), and cough or dyspnea (with multiple pulmonary metastases).

3. DIAGNOSTIC METHODS

3.1. Serum Markers

3.1.1. α-Fetoprotein

A large number of candidate markers have been advocated during the last 40 years, but none is more helpful than the first one described, α-fetoprotein (AFP) *(19)*. In 1964, it was first described in the serum of humans with HCC *(20)*, and its use as a serum marker has proved to be a major advance in the diagnosis and management of HCC in clinical practice.

AFP is a glycoprotein that normally is produced during gestation by the fetal liver and yolk sac. Normally, it is present in high concentration in the fetal serum, but in only minute amounts thereafter. Reappearance of high serum levels strongly suggests the diagnosis of HCC *(21)*. AFP is elevated in approx 60–70% of patients with HCC in the United States and Europe *(22)*. The normal range of this serum marker is 0–20 ng/mL, and levels higher than 400 ng/mL are diagnostic of HCC. False-positive results may be caused by acute and chronic benign hepatic diseases with a high degree of necroinflammatory activity, germ cell tumors, or pregnancy. The sensitivity, specificity, and positive predictive value of AFP in three well-performed screening studies for HCC ranged from 39 to 64%, 76 to 91%, and 9 to 32%, respectively *(23)*. The positive predictive value increases significantly when AFP is more than 400 ng/mL, but this comes at the expense of a poor sensitivity.

In countries with a high incidence of HCC, serum AFP concentrations are raised in as many as 90% of patients, and very high levels often are attained *(24)*. AFP production is age-related. Younger patients are more likely to have raised levels and to attain very high concentrations. No difference in AFP production is observed between the sexes; however, there do seem to be racial differences. In a study addressing the clinical usefulness of serum AFP in the diagnosis of HCC in patients with HCV-related cirrhosis from diverse ethnic backgrounds, AFP seemed to be an insensitive test in the African American group *(25)*. There is no obvious correlation between serum AFP concentrations and any clinical or biochemical indices or the survival time after diagnosis *(7)*. Measurement of serum AFP is clinically useful in determining the completeness of surgical resection and in monitoring patients for tumor recurrence.

Because of both false-positive and false-negative results, serum AFP falls short of being an ideal tumor marker. Thus, a number of alternative substances have been suggested, although none have proved to be more useful than AFP.

3.1.2. Fucosylated AFP

AFP is heterogeneous in structure with differences in its asparagine-linked oligosaccharide sidechain. The resultant differential reactivity with lectins is used in diagnosis: reactivity with lens culinaris agglutinin A is helpful in distinguishing HCC from benign hepatic diseases, and, to a lesser extent, reactivity with concanavalin A can help differentiate between HCC and other AFP-producing tumors *(26)*. Measurement of this isoform of AFP has been investigated and has been shown to improve specificity but still has relatively low sensitivity in several retrospective case-control studies *(27)*. The test results are positive in approx 35% of patients with HCC tumors smaller than 2 cm, and this isoform of AFP may be present in serum up to 9 months before the detection of HCC by other methods *(28,29)*. Its cost and availability also has limited its clinical use, especially because the greatest numbers of patients with HCC are found in countries with the least resources.

3.1.3. Des-γ-Carboxy Prothrombin

In 1984, Liebman et al. *(30)* were the first to report an abnormal form of prothrombin in patients with HCC. Malignant hepatocytes seem to lack the ability to carboxylate glutamic acid to form γ-carboxyglutamic acid. The resulting abnormal prothrombin has been referred to as des-γ-carboxyprothrombin (DCP). Because this is the same prothrombin formed by vitamin K absence or antagonism, DCP is also known as PIVKA-II. In the absence of carboxylation, calcium binding fails and prothrombin cannot be activated *(31)*.

Although DCP has demonstrated a greater specificity than AFP (with less than 5% of patients without HCC having levels higher than 100 mAU/mL), it still lacks sensitivity, especially for HCC tumors less than 3 cm in diameter, with sensitivity ranging from 19 to 48% *(32)*. A cross-sectional case-control study recently was conducted comparing DCP and AFP in differentiating HCC from nonmalignant liver disease in 207 patients from the United States. A receiver operating characteristic curve indicated that a DCP value of 125 mAU/mL had the highest accuracy in differentiating HCC from nonmalignant chronic liver disease with a sensitivity of 89%, specificity of 95%, positive predictive value (PPV) of 87%, and negative predictive value (NPV) of 95% *(33)*. Compared with AFP, DCP levels had higher sensitivity and specificity in differentiating HCC from nonmalignant chronic liver disease *(33)*. Certain inadequacies of measuring AFP and DCP levels alone have resulted in an attempt to increase the sensitivity by coupling these tests. One prospective study screening cirrhotic patients for HCC, using cutoff values of 40 ng/mL for AFP and 80 mAU/mL for DCP, showed 65% sensitivity and 85% specificity when both markers were combined *(34)*.

3.1.4. Glypican-3

Glypican-3 is a heparan sulfate proteoglycan that is expressed at a protein level in hepatoma cells but not in normal or dysplastic liver cells. It is detectable in the serum in at least 50% of patients with HCC *(35)*. Although still experimental, it is of interest because it seems to be expressed preferentially in small HCC tumors compared with larger HCC tumors and it may be complementary to other surveillance tools, such as AFP.

3.1.5. Other Markers

Other markers of HCC that have been studied include tumor-associated isoenzymes of γ-glutamyl transpeptidase *(36)*, urinary TGF-β-1 *(37)*, serum levels of circulating intercellular adhesion molecule (ICAM) -1 *(38)*, serum α-L-fucosidase activity *(39)*, and tissue polypeptide-specific antigen *(40)*. None of these diagnostic tests have demonstrated superior accuracy compared with serum AFP. Two tumor markers, abnormal vitamin B_{12}-binding protein and neurotensin, have been linked specifically to the fibrolamellar variant of HCC *(7)*. Although both markers provide useful confirmatory evidence of this variant when present, they have low sensitivity.

3.2. Hepatic Imaging

Imaging studies play a key role in the diagnosis of HCC. The approach to documentation of the presence of a space-occupying lesion within the liver depends on local availability and expertise. There has been a steady evolution in the radiological techniques used to diagnose HCC. Ultrasound, computed tomography (CT), and magnetic resonance imaging (MRI) are the most commonly used methods, although there is also a body of literature describing radionuclide scanning, positron emission tomography (PET), and hepatic arteriography as imaging techniques.

Imaging of the cirrhotic liver poses a formidable challenge to the radiologist. There are several reasons for the inherent difficulty encountered. First, the liver architecture is severely distorted because of fibrosis, necrosis, and numerous regenerating nodules. Second, cirrhosis results in altered portal hemodynamics that ultimately affect any technique that uses intravenous contrast material. These altered hemodynamics result from arterial portal shunting, the physical effect of regenerating nodules, decreased portal venous flow, and portosystemic collaterals. Consequently, detection of HCC in the cirrhotic liver may involve several complementary imaging techniques (*see* Table 3 for a comparison of characteristic features of HCC as seen on ultrasound, CT, and MRI).

Table 3
Imaging Findings Favoring a Diagnosis of HCC

	Ultrasound	*Computed tomography*	*Magnetic resonance imaging*
HCC nodule	Small (<2 cm): hypoechoic Large (>2 cm): heterogeneous	Small (<2 cm): hypoechoic Large (>2 cm): heterogeneous	T1: hypointense T2: hyperintense
Capsule	Peripheral halo	Rim of retained contrast on equilibrium phase	Double layer capsule on T2
Vascular supply	Fine network	Arterial phase enhancement, portal venous washout	Gd-DTPA enhancement
Invasion	Vascular/biliary	Vascular/biliary	Vascular/biliary
Perinodular region	Satellite/daughter lesions	Satellite/daughter lesions	Satellite/daughter lesions

(Reprinted from: Bailey MA, Brunt EM. Hepatocellular carcinoma: predisposing conditions and precursor lesions. *Gastroenterol Clin N Am* 2002;31:641–642.)

3.2.1. Ultrasound

Ultrasonography was introduced in the late 1960s and, by the late 1970s, had superceded radionuclide scanning as first-line hepatic imaging. Its advantages include safety, availability, and cost effectiveness, although it has the drawbacks of being nonstandardized and examiner dependent *(19)*. The sonographic appearance of HCC is highly dependent on the size, composition, and internal characteristics of a given neoplasm. Although ultrasound cannot distinguish HCC tumors from other solid tumors in the liver, it has the benefit of assessing patency of the hepatic blood supply and the presence of vascular invasion by the tumor. Sonographic characteristics of a hepatic lesion that are suggestive of HCC include poorly defined margins and coarse, irregular internal echoes. Small tumors are often hypoechoic, but as the tumor grows, the echo pattern tends to become isoechoic or hyperechoic, and HCC can be difficult to distinguish from the surrounding liver *(41)*. The typical ultrasonographic findings of small HCC tumors are a mosaic pattern, septum formation, peripheral sonolucency (halo), a lateral shadow produced by fibrotic pseudocapsule, and posterior echo enhancement *(42)*.

Recent refinements, such as dynamic contrast-enhanced ultrasonography with intra-arterial infusion of CO_2 microbubbles and intravenous-enhanced color Doppler ultrasonography, have added new dimensions to its diagnostic capabilities *(43)*. Color Doppler ultrasound demonstrates an intralesional tangle of vessels, the basket pattern, in 15% of cases, indicating hypervascularity and tumor shunting *(44)*. Ultrasound has been studied extensively as a screening tool for HCC *(45–47)*. In this setting, ultrasound has been reported to have relatively high sensitivity and specificity. Its use in diagnosis has been largely replaced by CT and MRI, but it remains useful, especially in assessing vascular invasion by HCC.

3.2.2. Computed Tomography

CT relies on differences in X-ray attenuation between tumor tissue and adjacent liver parenchyma. Because this difference often is insufficient for reliable tumor detection, contrast material is used to increase the attenuation of liver tissue but not that of HCC *(48)*. Unenhanced CT scans demonstrate a large, hypodense mass or masses with central areas of lower attenuation that correspond to the tumor necrosis frequently seen in HCC.

There have been several key developments in improving CT imaging of HCC. First, the use of spiral (helical) scanners allows very rapid imaging of the liver after infusion of intravenous contrast agents *(43)*. A second major advancement has been the adoption of better scanning protocols that take into account the increased vascularity of HCC. Because HCC derives most of its blood supply from the hepatic artery, it enhances early during infusion of contrast, whereas the liver parenchyma enhances during the portal venous phase (which takes place 50–90 seconds after infusing contrast). The triphasic CT scan describes the periods of contrast enhancement, including the precontrast, arterial, and portal venous phases. Encapsulated HCC is characterized by a hypodense rim on unenhanced and early enhanced CT scan. It enhances in a delayed fashion after intravenous contrast administration *(49)*. A recent study has shown that in 9% of patients with HCC, tumor is detected only on arterial phase images and is not seen on nonenhanced or portal venous phase images *(50)*. Furthermore, arterial phase imaging has been shown to detect an additional 27% of HCC tumor nodules not seen on nonenhanced and portal venous phase imaging *(51)*. For these reasons, it is paramount that imaging of the cirrhotic liver include an arterial phase enhanced scan; otherwise, small HCCs will be missed.

Despite its improvement in recent years, a substantial number of tumor nodules may still go undetected by CT. In a study by Miller et al. *(52)*, enhanced CT had a sensitivity of 68% and a specificity of 81%; many undetected tumor nodules were found on examination of explanted livers after transplantation. CT scanning in conjunction with hepatic arteriography using iodized poppy seed oil (Lipiodol) also has been used to detect very small tumors. CT hepatic arteriography has been reported to detect up to an additional 66% of HCC tumor nodules not seen by triphasic CT *(51)*. Although there are reports of greater sensitivity *(53)*, this technique is not commonly used given the need for intra-arterial injection.

3.2.3. Magnetic Resonance Imaging

There have been significant recent advances in MRI technology, including scanner hardware, software, and contrast agents. HCC enhances after gadolinium-diethylenetriaminepentaacetic acid (Gd-DTPA) administration. Most tumors appear as high-intensity patterns on T2-weighted images and with a low signal intensity in T1-weighted sequences *(54)*. There is considerable variability in its appearance on T1-weighted images that may be attributed to foci of hemorrhage, accumulation of copper, glycogen, or areas of fatty change. Encapsulated HCC has a rim of low signal intensity on T1-weighted images or a double-layered rim or ring (inner hypointense, outer hyperintense) on T2-weighted images corresponding to the fibrous nature of the capsule *(49)*. A small number of larger tumors contain visible calcifications or a central scar. Vascular invasion by HCC is also readily demonstrated by MRI. MRI is the preferred imaging study at some institutions with similar sensitivity for the diagnosis of HCC as helical CT. Other radiologists still favor CT because of the high cost of MRI and the long duration required to obtain MRI images. MRI may be useful in patients with renal insufficiency or those with an allergy to contrast dye and may be beneficial in cases in which CT results are ambiguous, particularly in an extremely nodular liver, because MRI can differentiate dysplastic nodules from HCC *(55)*.

3.2.4. Radionuclide Scanning and PET

In the present era of MRI and helical CT, scintigraphic scanning has a limited role in hepatic imaging for HCC. This method was based on recording the emission of a radionuclide incorporated into colloidal material and taken up from the bloodstream by Kupffer's cells. The absence of these cells from tumors produced a defect in the liver image *(56)*. Radionuclide scanning lacks good specificity for HCC. PET uses fluorodeoxyglucose (FDG) uptake differences to distinguish between HCC and normal liver tissue. The main use of FDG PET in HCC is in assessing the degree of differentiation and in staging moderately and poorly differentiated tumors rather than in primary lesion detection. Sensitivities of FDG PET for detection of HCC ranged from 50 *(57)* to 70% *(58)*. FDG PET cannot differentiate well-differentiated HCC from a regenerating nodule *(59)*. In addition to tumor differentiation, larger tumor size and higher serum AFP levels are associated with increased tumor visualization on PET.

3.2.5. Hepatic Arteriography

Because the blood supply of HCC is predominantly from the hepatic artery, hepatic arteriography can detect hypervascular tumors as small as 0.5 cm in diameter *(60)*. Tumors are characterized by an enlarged feeding artery, hypervascularity, tumor vascular channels and lakes, arterioportal communications, and capsular radiolucency. With the evolution of less invasive techniques, the diagnostic role of conventional angiography has become more circumscribed.

However, arteriography continues to be used to help delineate the hepatic arterial anatomy when planning surgical intervention, for chemoembolization, and for the infusion of cytotoxic drugs directly into the hepatic artery.

3.2.6. Radiologic Characteristics of Fibrolamellar HCC

Fibrolamellar HCC (FLC) is a variant of HCC that typically occurs in younger patients who often have no underlying liver disease. It is usually a large, well-defined mass, and in approximately one-half of cases, it is notable for a central scar. Focal nodular hyperplasia (FNH) also is seen in younger patients and has similar imaging features, also with a central scar. The central scar of FLC often is calcified, but calcification of the scar of FNH is very rare. With MRI, the central scar of FLC typically is hypointense (dark) on T2-weighted images, whereas the scar of FNH is hyperintense (bright) on T2-weighted images with delayed contrast enhancement *(61)*.

3.3. Histology

Although histological examination of liver tissue is an important element in diagnosing HCC, the routine use of liver biopsy to confirm the diagnosis of HCC is controversial. In some instances, the presence of a hepatic mass with elevated serum AFP may be considered sufficient for diagnosis. Possible risks of percutaneous needle biopsy are bleeding (resulting from the vascular nature of the tumor) and local spread of HCC along the needle track *(62)*. Although the exact frequency of the latter complication is unknown, preliminary evidence suggests occurrence rates of about 1% *(62)*. Because of this concern, some physicians do not advocate performing a needle biopsy before liver resection or transplantation for HCC. When performed, the yield and safety of the procedure can be optimized by using radiologic guidance (either ultrasound or CT). An algorithm for evaluation of patients with suspected HCC is presented in Fig. 1.

4. SCREENING FOR HCC

Programs for detecting subclinical (presymptomatic) HCC are of two kinds: (a) screening entire populations that have a high incidence of tumor and (b) long-term surveillance of persons known to be at high risk for developing HCC. Mass population screening has been attempted in a number of ethnic Chinese and African populations at high risk of developing HCC. The serum AFP was the sole screening method used. Because only 45% of presymptomatic HCCs produce a diagnostic level of this marker *(63)*, an appreciable number of small tumors are missed in programs of this sort.

Patients with cirrhosis have a markedly increased risk of developing HCC. The incidence in well-compensated cirrhosis is approx 3% per year *(64)*. Patients with most forms of chronic hepatitis are not at increased risk until cirrhosis

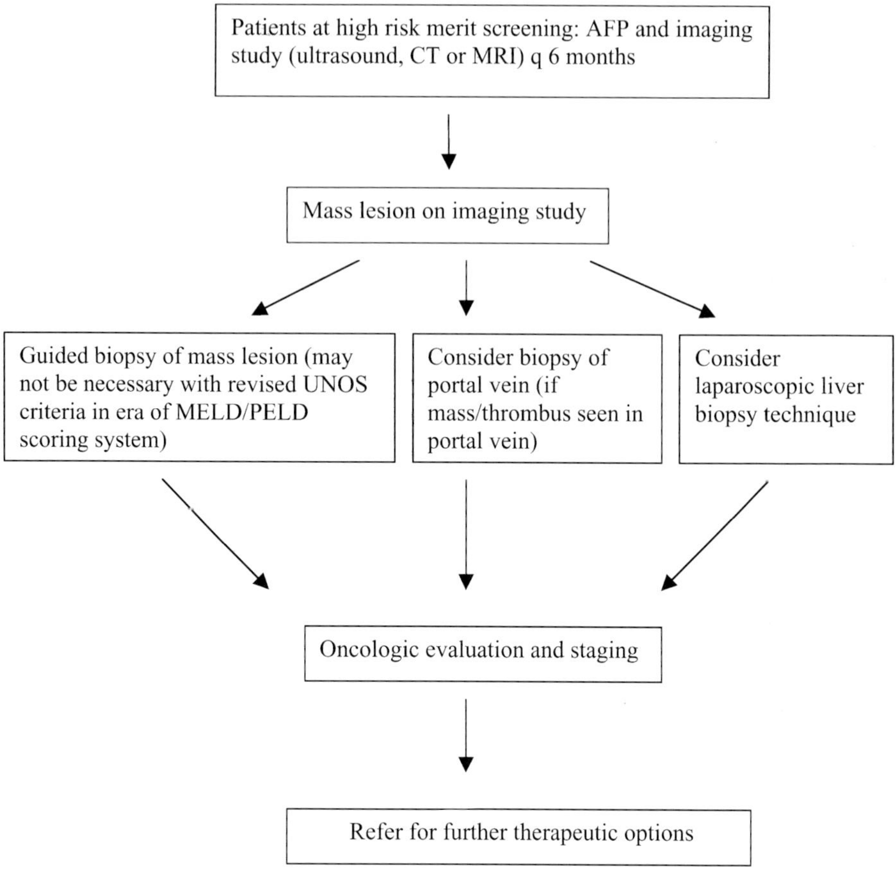

Fig. 1. A proposed algorithm for evaluation of patients with suspected HCC.

develops, an exception to this rule being chronic HBV infection in which HCC can develop in the absence of cirrhosis *(65)*. Certain causes of cirrhosis—namely, HBV, HCV, and genetic hemochromatosis *(66)*—traditionally have been regarded as posing a relatively higher risk for developing HCC compared with, for example, cirrhosis resulting from autoimmune hepatitis *(67)* or Wilson's disease. Primary biliary cirrhosis (PBC) *(68,69)* and nonalcoholic steatohepatitis (NASH) *(70,71)* previously were regarded as carrying low risk for HCC, but there is emerging evidence from recent studies that both late-stage PBC and NASH (or NAFLD) pose higher risks than once appreciated.

The issue of periodic surveillance of patients at risk for HCC remains contentious from the viewpoint of cost effectiveness, because an improvement in survival has not been demonstrated consistently *(23,45)*. Despite the relative lack of clear evidence, surveillance for HCC in patients with cirrhosis has become accepted by most hepatologists *(23)*. Measurement of AFP and performance of an imaging study (usually an ultrasound) frequently are adopted screening strategies in patients with Child–Pugh class A cirrhosis who would be suitable candidates for partial hepatectomy if HCC were discovered and in those patients who are candidates for liver transplantation or percutaneous therapies. The optimal frequency of screening is not known. The median doubling time for HCC is 3–4 months (although this varies widely), which suggests the need for screening every 3–6 months *(72)*.

Few studies have examined specific screening strategies for HCC in patients with advanced HCV. The 2002 National Institutes of Health Consensus Development Statement on the management of hepatitis C addressed this issue *(73)*. It was concluded by the panel that despite the lack of evidence, screening for HCC with AFP testing and hepatic ultrasound at 6-month intervals is a common practice in the United States. However, such routine AFP or imaging screening should not be performed in patients with hepatitis C in the absence of cirrhosis because HCC is so rare in this group *(73)*. Moreover, there is a great need for carefully designed studies on the reliability and benefit of surveillance screening.

Because chronic HBV infection has the propensity to produce HCC in the precirrhotic stage, special practice guidelines have been proposed by the American Association for the Study of Liver Diseases *(74)*. Recommendations for HCC screening in this population group include HBV carriers who are either men older than 45 years, who have established cirrhosis, or who have a family history of HCC; these individuals should undergo periodic screening with both AFP and ultrasound *(74)*. The optimal frequency seems to be every 6 months. Although there are insufficient data to recommend routine screening in low-risk patients with chronic HBV infection, period screening with AFP in carriers from endemic areas should be considered *(74)*.

5. HCC AND LISTING CRITERIA FOR LIVER TRANSPLANTATION IN THE ERA OF THE MELD/PELD SCORING SYSTEM

In November 2001, the United Network for Organ Sharing (UNOS) adopted the MELD/PELD systems into policy for the allocation of livers. In February 2002, UNOS deemed that a prelisting biopsy was not mandatory if the lesion met established imaging criteria *(75)*. In addition, the patient ought to have one of the following: tumor greater than 1 cm with a blush corresponding to the area of suspicion seen on imaging, AFP level greater than 200 ng/mL, an arteriogram confirming a tumor, a biopsy confirming HCC, chemoembolization, radiofrequency, or cryoablation or chemical ablation of the lesion. In addition, the patient should not be a resection candidate. Patients with T1 lesions fulfilling the UNOS policy criteria were given a MELD/PELD score corresponding to a predicted 3-month mortality of 15% (MELD score of 24, PELD score of 31). Those with T2 lesions fulfilling criteria were given a MELD/PELD score corresponding to a 30% 3-month mortality (MELD score of 29, PELD score of 40) *(75)*. Moreover, these patients were entitled to an additional 10% increase in mortality (i.e., MELD score increase by 2 points) every 3 months as long as they remained untransplanted and repeat imaging did not show progression to T3 or T4 lesions *(75)*.

Further MELD/PELD modifications implemented in February 2003 lowered the mortality risks of T1 and T2 lesions to 8 and 15%, respectively, corresponding to MELD/PELD scores of 20/25 and 24/32, respectively, for T1 and T2 lesions. Another important amendment is that patients with chronic liver disease whose AFP is 500 ng/mL or greater on at least one occasion may be listed as having stage 1 HCC although there is no evidence of a tumor based on imaging studies (UNOS, personal communication, February 14, 2003). This again highlights the lack of use of histological confirmation of HCC in the current era of the MELD/PELD scoring system.

REFERENCES

1. Kew MC, Dos Santos HA, Sherlock S. Diagnosis of primary cancer of the liver. *Br Med J* 1971;4:408–411.
2. Craig JR. Tumors of the liver. In: *Hepatology: A Textbook of Liver Disease* (Zakim D, Boyer TD, eds.), WB Saunders, Philadelphia, 2003, pp. 1355–1370.
3. Aguayo A, Patt YZ. Liver cancer [review]. *Clin Liver Dis* 2001;5:479–507.
4. Trevisani F, D'Intino PE, Grazi GL, Caraceni P, Gasbarrini A, Colantoni A, et al. Clinical and pathologic features of hepatocellular carcinoma in young and older Italian patients. *Cancer* 1996;77:2223–2232.
5. Johnson PJ. Malignant tumors of the liver. In: *Comprehensive Clinical Hepatology* (O'Grady JG, Lake JR, Howdle PD, eds.), Harcourt, London, 2000, pp. 25.1–25.18.
6. Kew MC. Clinical manifestations and paraneoplastic syndromes of hepatocellular carcinoma. In: *Neoplasms of the Liver* (Okuda K, Ishak KG, eds.), Springer-Verlag, Tokyo, 1987, p. 199.
7. Kew MC. Hepatic tumors and cysts. In: *Gastrointestinal and Liver Disease* (Feldman M, Friedman LS, Sleisenger MH, eds.) WB Saunders, Philadelphia, 2002, pp. 1577–1602.
8. Chearanai O, Plengvanit U, Asavanich C, Damrongsak D, Sindhvananda K, Boonyapisit S. Spontaneous rupture of primary hepatoma: report of 63 cases with particular reference to the pathogenesis and rationale for treatment by hepatic artery ligation. *Cancer* 1983;51: 1532–1536.
9. Zapf J, Futo E, Peter M, Froesch ER. Can "big" insulin-like growth factor II in serum of tumor patients account for the development of extrapancreatic tumor hypoglycemia? *J Clin Investigation* 1992;90:2574–2584.
10. Kew MC, Fisher JW. Serum erythropoietin concentrations in patients with hepatocellular carcinoma. *Cancer* 1986;58:2485–2488.
11. Yen TC, Hwang SJ, Wang CC, Lee SD, Yeh SH. Hypercalcemia and parathyroid hormone-related protein in hepatocellular carcinoma. *Liver* 1993;13:311–315.
12. Kew MC, Leckie BJ, Greeff MC. Arterial hypertension as a paraneoplastic phenomenon in hepatocellular carcinoma. *Arch Intern Med* 1989;149:2111–2113.

13. Kew MC, Kirschner MA, Abrahams GE, Katz M. Mechanism of feminization in primary liver cancer. *New Engl J Med* 1977;296:1084–1088.
14. Goldberg RB, Bersohn I, Kew MC. Hypercholesterolaemia in primary cancer of the liver. *S Afr Med J* 1975;49:1464–1466.
15. Steiner E, Velt P, Gutierrez O, Schwartz S, Chey W. Hepatocellular carcinoma presenting with intractable diarrhea. A radiologic–pathologic correlation. *Arch Surg* 1986;121:849–851.
16. Gregory B, Ho VC. Cutaneous manifestations of gastrointestinal disorders. Part I [review]. *J Am Acad Dermatol* 1992; 26:153–166.
17. Stein CM, Gelfand M. Hepatocellular carcinoma presenting as a fever of undetermined origin. *Cent Afr J Med* 1985;31:21,22.
18. Okada S. How to manage hepatic vein tumour thrombus in hepatocellular carcinoma [review]. *J Gastroenterol Hepatol* 2000;15:346–348.
19. Kew MC. Hepatocellular cancer. A century of progress [review]. *Clin Liver Dis* 2000; 4:257–268.
20. Tatarinov YS. Presence of embryonal a-globulin in the serum of patients with primary hepatocellular carcinoma. *Vopr Med Khim* 1964;10:90.
21. Alpert E. Human alpha1-fetoprotein (AFP): developmental biology and clinical significance [review]. *Prog Liver Dis* 1976;5:337–349.
22. Carr BI, Flickinger JC, Lotze MT. Hepatobiliary cancers. In: *Cancer: Principles and Practice of Oncology* (DeVita VT, Hellman S, Rosenberg SA, eds.), Lippincott-Raven, Philadelphia, 1997, p. 1087.
23. Collier J, Sherman M. Screening for hepatocellular carcinoma [review]. *Hepatology* 1998;27:273–278.
24. Kew MC. a-fetoprotein in primary liver cancer and other diseases. *Gut* 1974;15:814.
25. Nguyen MH, Garcia RT, Simpson PW, Wright TL, Keeffe EB. Racial differences in effectiveness of alpha-fetoprotein for diagnosis of hepatocellular carcinoma in hepatitis C virus cirrhosis. *Hepatology* 2002;36:410–417.
26. Taketa K, Sekiya C, Namiki M, Akamatsu K, Ohta Y, Endo Y, Kosaka K. Lectin-reactive profiles of alpha-fetoprotein characterizing hepatocellular carcinoma and related conditions. *Gastroenterology* 1990;99:508–518.
27. Sato Y, Nakata K, Kato Y, Shima M, Ishii N, Koji T, et al. Early recognition of hepatocellular carcinoma based on altered profiles of alpha-fetoprotein. *New Engl J Med* 1993;328:1802–1806.
28. Oka H, Saito A, Ito K, Kumada T, Satomura S, Kasugai H, et al. Multicenter prospective analysis of newly diagnosed hepatocellular carcinoma with respect to the percentage of lens culinaris agglutinin-reactive alpha-fetoprotein. *J Gastroenterol Hepatol* 2001;16:1378–1383.
29. Taketa K, Endo Y, Sekiya C, Tanikawa K, Koji T, Taga H, et al. A collaborative study for the evaluation of lectin-reactive alpha-fetoproteins in early detection of hepatocellular carcinoma. *Cancer Res* 1993;53:5419–5423.
30. Liebman HA, Furie BC, Tong MJ, Blanchard RA, Lo KJ, Lee SD, et al. Des-gamma-carboxy (abnormal) prothrombin as a serum marker of primary hepatocellular carcinoma. *New Engl J Med* 1984;310:1427–1431.
31. Weitz IC, Liebman HA. Des-gamma-carboxy (abnormal) prothrombin and hepatocellular carcinoma: a critical review. *Hepatology* 1993;18:990–997.
32. Tanabe Y, Ohnishi K, Nomura F, Iida S. Plasma abnormal prothrombin levels in patients with small hepatocellular carcinoma. *Am J Gastroenterol* 1988;83:1386–1389.
33. Marrero JA, Su GL, Wei W, Emick D, Conjeevaram HS, Fontana RJ, et al. Des-gamma carboxyprothrombin can differentiate hepatocellular carcinoma from non-malignant liver disease in American patients. *Hepatology* 2003;37:1114–1121.
34. Ishii M, Gama H, Chida N, Ueno Y, Shinzawa H, Takagi T, et al. Simultaneous measurements of serum alpha-fetoprotein and protein induced by vitamin K absence for detecting hepatocellular carcinoma. South Tohoku District Study Group. *Am J Gastroenterol* 2000; 95:1036–1040.

35. Capurro M, Wanless IR, Sherman M, Deboer G, Shi W, Miyoshi E, et al. Glypican-3: a novel serum and histochemical marker for hepatocellular carcinoma. *Gastroenterology* 2003;125:89–97.
36. Kew MC, Wolf P, Whittaker D, Rowe P. Tumour-associated isoenzymes of gamma-glutamyl transferase in the serum of patients with hepatocellular carcinoma. *Br J Cancer* 1984; 50:451–455.
37. Tsai JF, Jeng JE, Chuang LY, Yang ML, Ho MS, Chang WY, et al. Clinical evaluation of urinary transforming growth factor-beta1 and serum alpha-fetoprotein as tumour markers of hepatocellular carcinoma. *Br J Cancer* 1997;75:1460–1466.
38. Hamazaki K, Gochi A, Shimamura H, Kaihara A, Maruo Y, Doi Y, et al. Serum levels of circulating intercellular adhesion molecule 1 in hepatocellular carcinoma. *Hepatogastroenterology* 1996;43:229–234.
39. Takahashi H, Saibara T, Iwamura S, Tomita A, Maeda T, Onishi S, et al. Serum alpha-L-fucosidase activity and tumor size in hepatocellular carcinoma. *Hepatology* 1994;19: 1414–1417.
40. Tu DG, Wang ST, Chang TT, Chiu NT, Yao WJ. The value of serum tissue polypeptide specific antigen in the diagnosis of hepatocellular carcinoma. *Cancer* 1999;85:1039–1043.
41. Ishiguchi T, Shimamoto K, Fukatsu H, Yamakawa K, Ishigaki T. Radiologic diagnosis of hepatocellular carcinoma [review]. *Semin Surg Oncol* 1996;12:164–169.
42. Tanaka S, Kitamura T, Imaoka S, Sasaki Y, Taniguchi H, Ishiguro S. Hepatocellular carcinoma: sonographic and histologic correlation. *Am J Roentgenol* 1983;140:701–707.
43. Kudo M. Imaging diagnosis of hepatocellular carcinoma and premalignant/borderline lesions [review]. *Semin Liver Dis* 1999;19:297–309.
44. Tanaka S, Kitamura T, Fujita M, Nakanishi K, Okuda S. Color Doppler flow imaging of liver tumors. *Am J Roentgenol* 1990;154:509–514.
45. Larcos G, Sorokopud H, Berry G, Farrell GC. Sonographic screening for hepatocellular carcinoma in patients with chronic hepatitis or cirrhosis: an evaluation. *Am J Roentgenol* 1998;171:433–435.
46. Dodd GD, Miller WJ, Baron RL, et al. Detection of malignant tumors in end-stage cirrhotic livers: efficacy of sonography as a screening technique. *Am J Roentgenol* 1992;159:727–733.
47. Pateron D, Ganne N, Trinchet JC, Aurousseau MH, Mal F, Meicler C, et al. Prospective study of screening for hepatocellular carcinoma in Caucasian patients with cirrhosis [comment]. *J Hepatol* 1994;20:65–71.
48. Choi BI. CT diagnosis of liver cancer. In: *Liver Cancer* (Okuda K, Tabor E, eds.), Churchill Livingstone, New York, 1997, p. 371.
49. Ros PR, Murphy BJ, Buck JL, Olmedilla G, Goodman Z. Encapsulated hepatocellular carcinoma: radiologic findings and pathologic correlation. *Gastrointest Radiol* 1990;15:233–237.
50 Oliver JH, Baron RL, Federle MP, Rockette HE Jr. Detecting hepatocellular carcinoma: value of unenhanced or arterial phase CT imaging or both used in conjunction with conventional portal venous phase contrast-enhanced CT imaging. *Am J Roentgenol* 1996;167:71–77.
51. Oliver JH, Baron RL, Carr BI. CT imaging of hepatocellular carcinoma: CT-arteriography versus triphasic helical contrast CT. *Radiology* 1997;205:144.
52. Miller WJ, Baron RL, Dodd GD, Federle MP. Malignancies in patients with cirrhosis: CT sensitivity and specificity in 200 consecutive transplant patients. *Radiology* 1994;193:645–650.
53. Ngan H. Lipiodol computerized tomography: how sensitive and specific is the technique in the diagnosis of hepatocellular carcinoma? *Br J Radiol* 1990;63:771–775.
54. Ebara M. MRI diagnosis of hepatocellular carcinoma. In: *Liver Cancer* (Okuda K, Tabor E, eds.), Churchill Livingstone, New York, 1997, p. 361.
55. Lencioni R, Mascalchi M, Caramella D, Bartolozzi C. Small hepatocellular carcinoma: differentiation from adenomatous hyperplasia with color Doppler US and dynamic Gd-DTPA-enhanced MR imaging. *Abdominal Imaging* 1996;21:41–48.

56. Kew MC, Levin J. Scintigraphy in the diagnosis of hepatocellular carcinoma. In: *Neoplasms of the Liver* (Okuda K, Ishak KG, eds.), Springer-Verlag, Tokyo, 1987, p. 239.
57. Trojan J, Schroeder O, Raedle J, Baum RP, Herrmann G, Jacobi V, et al. Fluorine-18 FDG positron emission tomography for imaging of hepatocellular carcinoma. *Am J Gastroenterol* 1999;94:3314–3319.
58. Delbeke D, Martin WH, Sandler MP, Chapman WC, Wright JK Jr, Pinson CW. Evaluation of benign vs malignant hepatic lesions with positron emission tomography. *Arch Surg* 1998;133:510–515.
59. Schroder O, Trojan J, Zeuzem S, Baum RP. Limited value of fluorine-18-fluorodeoxyglucose PET for the differential diagnosis of focal liver lesions in patients with chronic hepatitis C virus infection. *Nuklearmedizin* 1998;37:279–285.
60. Takayasu K. Hepatic angiography. In: *Liver Cancer* (Okuda K, Tabor E, eds.), Churchill Livingstone, New York, 1997, p. 347.
61. Ichikawa T, Federle MP, Grazioli L, Madariaga J, Nalesnik M, Marsh W. Fibrolamellar hepatocellular carcinoma: imaging and pathologic findings in 31 recent cases. Radiology 1999;213:352–361.
62. Durand F, Regimbeau JM, Belghiti J, Sauvanet A, Vilgrain V, Terris B, et al. Assessment of the benefits and risks of percutaneous biopsy before surgical resection of hepatocellular carcinoma. *J Hepatol* 2001;35:254–258.
63. Kew MC. The detection and treatment of small hepatocellular carcinoma. In: *Viral Hepatitis and Liver Disease* (Hollinger FB, Lemon SM, Margolis H, eds.), Williams and Wilkins, Baltimore, 1991, p. 515.
64. Colombo M, de Franchis R, Del Ninno E, Sangiovanni A, De Fazio C, Tommasini M, et al. Hepatocellular carcinoma in Italian patients with cirrhosis. *New Engl J Med* 1991;325: 675–680.
65. Beasley RP, Hwang LY, Lin CC, Chien CS. Hepatocellular carcinoma and hepatitis B virus. A prospective study of 22,707 men in Taiwan. *Lancet* 1981;2:1129–1133.
66. Fargion S, Fracanzani AL, Piperno A, Braga M, D'Alba R, Ronchi G, et al. Prognostic factors for hepatocellular carcinoma in genetic hemochromatosis. *Hepatology* 1994;20:1426–1431.
67. Park SZ, Nagorney DM, Czaja AJ. Hepatocellular carcinoma in autoimmune hepatitis. *Dig Dis Sci* 2000;45:1944–1948.
68. Caballeria L, Pares A, Castells A, Gines A, Bru C, Rodes J. Hepatocellular carcinoma in primary biliary cirrhosis: similar incidence to that in hepatitis C virus-related cirrhosis. *Am J Gastroenterol* 2001;96:1160–1163.
69. Shibuya A, Tanaka K, Miyakawa H, Shibata M, Takatori M, Sekiyama K, et al. Hepatocellular carcinoma and survival in patients with primary biliary cirrhosis. *Hepatology* 2002;35: 1172–1178.
70. Bugianesi E, Leone N, Vanni E, Marchesini G, Brunello F, Carucci P, et al. Expanding the natural history of nonalcoholic steatohepatitis: from cryptogenic cirrhosis to hepatocellular carcinoma. *Gastroenterology* 2002;123:134–140.
71. Marrero JA, Fontana RJ, Su GL, Conjeevaram HS, Emick DM, Lok AS. NAFLD may be a common underlying liver disease in patients with hepatocellular carcinoma in the United States. *Hepatology* 2002;36:1349–1354.
72. Sheu J, Sung J, Chen D, Yang PM, Lai MY, Lee CS, et al. Growth rate of asymptomatic hepatocellular carcinoma and its clinical implications. *Gastroenterology* 1985;89:259–266.
73. Seeff LB, Hoofnagle JH. National Institutes of Health Consensus Development Statement on the management of hepatitis C. *Hepatology* 2002;36:S3–S20.
74. Lok ASF, McMahon BJ. Chronic hepatitis B. *Hepatology* 2001;34:1225–1241.
75. UNOS Policies and Bylaws. Organ distribution: allocation of livers. Policy 3.6.4.4. Liver Transplant Candidates with Hepatocellular Carcinoma. Last revised 2/14/03.

4 Pathological Aspects of Hepatocellular Tumors

Hale Kirimlioglu, MD,
Anthony J. Demetris, MD,
and Michael A. Nalesnik, MD

Contents

1. HEPATOCELLULAR ADENOMA

Hepatocellular adenoma (HA) is an uncommon and benign tumor of the liver, seen most often in young women of childbearing age with a history of oral contraceptive use (Table 1) *(1)*. The longer the duration of intake of oral contraceptives, the higher the risk of developing hepatic adenoma *(2)*. Anabolic steroid use also is associated with HA, and an example of this lesion arising in conjunction with growth hormone therapy for Turner's syndrome has been reported *(3)*. An association of liver cell adenoma and various genetic metabolic disorders (such as glycogen storage diseases types I, III, or IV, galactosemia, tyrosinemia, and, rarely, diabetes mellitus or familial adenomatous polyposis) also has been reported *(4–9)*.

From: *Current Clinical Oncology: Hepatocellular Cancer: Diagnosis and Treatment*
Edited by: B. I. Carr © Humana Press Inc., Totowa, NJ

Table 1
Neoplastic Hepatocellular Lesions: Selected Features

	Clinical features	*Pathological features*
HA	Usually single, rarely multiple; associated with birth control pills; may bleed	Clonal growth of normal appearing hepatocytes with arterial vasculature and otherwise bland trabecular architecture
HCC, usual	Most commonly arises in cirrhotic liver	Single, multiple, or diffuse tumors; cytologically abnormal hepatocytes with arterial vasculature and trabecular to solid architecture
HCC Variants Fibrolamellar HCC	Most often in young adults without cirrhosis; surgical resection may be more efficacious than in case of usual HCC	Large, aberrant hepatocytes with large nucleoli; abundant cytoplasm in variably fibrotic stroma
Clear cell HCC	Similar to HCC	Cytoplasmic clearing of hepatocytes because of lipid or glycogen may cause confusion with similarly appearing tumors arising in other organs
Sclerosing HCC	Reported association with hypercalcemia	Malignant cells in densely fibrous stroma may cause c onfusion with other forms of adenocarcinoma; large cells of fibrolamellar type not seen
Combined HCC/ cholangio-carcinoma	Similar to HCC	Cells resemble a mixture of malignant hepatocytes and bile duct epithelial cells likely representing divergent differentiation from precursor cell
Sarcomatoid HCC	Rare, similar to HCC	Sarcomatous element derives from malignant hepatocellular element

(*Continued*)

Table 1 (*Continued*)
Neoplastic Hepatocellular Lesions: Selected Features

	Clinical features	*Pathological features*
Hepatoblastoma	Most common primary tumor of infancy and childhood; association with several congenital abnormalities	Epithelial, mixed epithelial and mesenchymal patterns

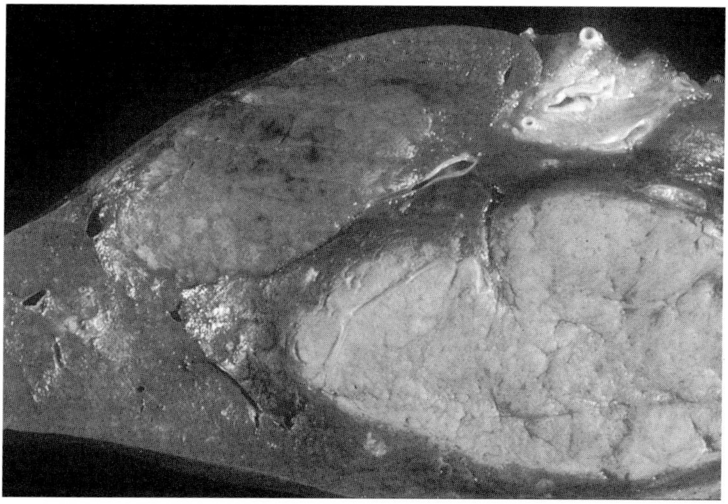

Fig. 1. Two mass lesions arising in a noncirrhotic liver. The large one proved to be a HA, and the smaller one was a focal nodular hyperplasia. The characteristic fibrous scar of the latter is not evident in this photograph (*see* Fig. 3).

The tumor may present as a palpable mass with or without abdominal pain. Bleeding into the tumor may occur, and hemoperitoneum resulting from tumor rupture with free hemorrhage into the peritoneal space is a surgical emergency. Serum α-fetoprotein (AFP) levels are within normal limits.

1.1. Macroscopic Pathology

HA characteristically appears as a well-circumscribed, nonlobulated lesion arising within a noncirrhotic liver (Fig. 1). Adenomas can range from 1 to more than 30 cm, but most are between 5 and 15 cm in diameter. Adenomas typically occur in subcapsular locations and in the right lobe. The tumor may be pedunculated *(10)*. It usually is solitary; however, multiple lesions are seen rarely, particularly in glycogen storage disease type I and in the condition referred to as liver adenomatosis *(4,5,11,12)*. The color varies from yellow to tan and can be variegated because of a combination of intratumoral hemorrhage, infarction, and fatty changes *(4,13)*. Adenomas usually are unencapsulated.

1.2. Microscopic Pathology

HAs contain normal-appearing hepatocytes arranged in a trabecular architecture between one and three cells thick (Fig. 2A,B). There are no portal tracts and, therefore, the normal hepatic microanatomical relationships are lacking. The hepatocyte nuclei are small, round, and uniform. Nucleoli are inconspicuous. Mitoses are absent or few. Cytoplasm is pale or eosinophilic. In some adenomas, clear changes of the cytoplasm may be prominent because of increased storage of glycogen, fat, or both. Cholestasis is not uncommon. The normal reticulin pattern is well-preserved, and Kupffer's cells exist in their usual locations. Small venous and arterial branches are seen throughout the tumor (Fig. 2C). Occasional larger vessels are seen and also may appear as feeding vessels adjacent to the tumor (Fig. 2D). Occasionally, the tumoral hepatocytes may contain periodic acid–Schiff (PAS)-positive, diastase-resistant hyaline globules *(14,15)*, Mallory's hyaline *(16)*, or degenerate-appearing hyperchromatic nuclei *(17)*.

The distinction of HA from well-differentiated hepatocellular carcinoma (HCC) may be difficult or impossible by conventional light microscopy. The clinical context is important in this regard, and the diagnosis of hepatic adenoma outside of the setting of a young woman taking oral contraceptives should be viewed with suspicion. Immunohistochemical markers occasionally may be helpful in distinguishing HA from a well-differentiated HCC.

Investigations should focus on suspicious-looking areas that are characterized by a clonal appearance (referring to a focus of cells that has a distinctly different look from the surrounding adenoma). This may be the result of cytological to architectural differences such as solid growth or formation of pseudoacini. Demonstration of AFP positivity is strong evidence in support of HCC over adenoma. In our experience, foci of carcinoma within an adenoma usually show increased cytological atypia and cell cycle activity, highlighted by the marker Ki-67, in comparison with adjacent adenoma and surrounding liver. Such changes must be interpreted in the context of the overall lesion, that is, the pathologist must make the interpretation as to whether he or she believes that carcinoma, if found, involves the entire lesion or only a portion of the tumor. Other immunostains do not add appreciably to the diagnostic information. Estrogen, progesterone, and androgenic steroid receptors have been detected in 26–73% of adenomas in different series *(18,19)* and also may be seen in HCC. Hepatic progenitor cells are identifiable by immunohistochemical means in a considerable proportion of HAs and support the hypothesis that oval hepatic progenitor cells play a role in

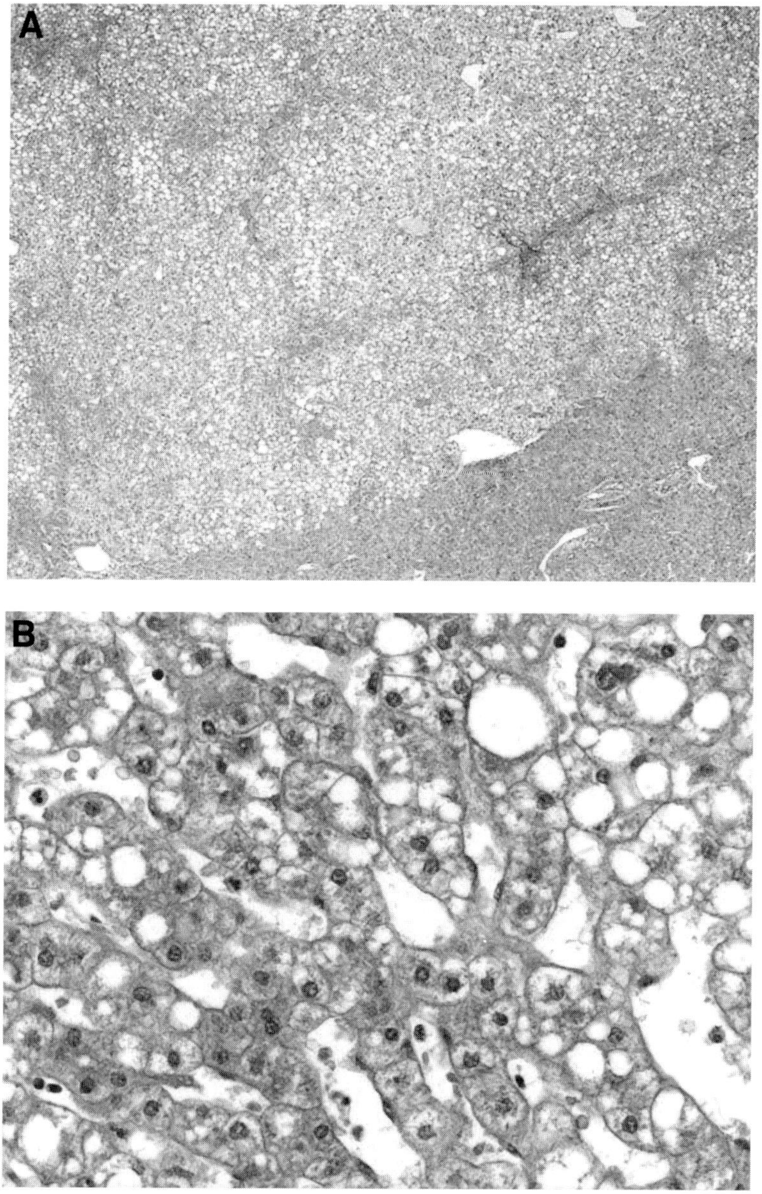

Fig. 2. (A) Interface of HA and normal liver. The adenoma comprises most of the photomicrograph and has numerous white areas at this low magnification because of increased intracellular fat. The normal liver (lower right hand portion) has a more solid appearance. The interface is smooth and no capsule is seen (stain, hematoxylin–eosin; original magnification, ×4). **(B)** High-power view of HA. The bland appearance and trabecular (*continued on pages 76 and 77*)

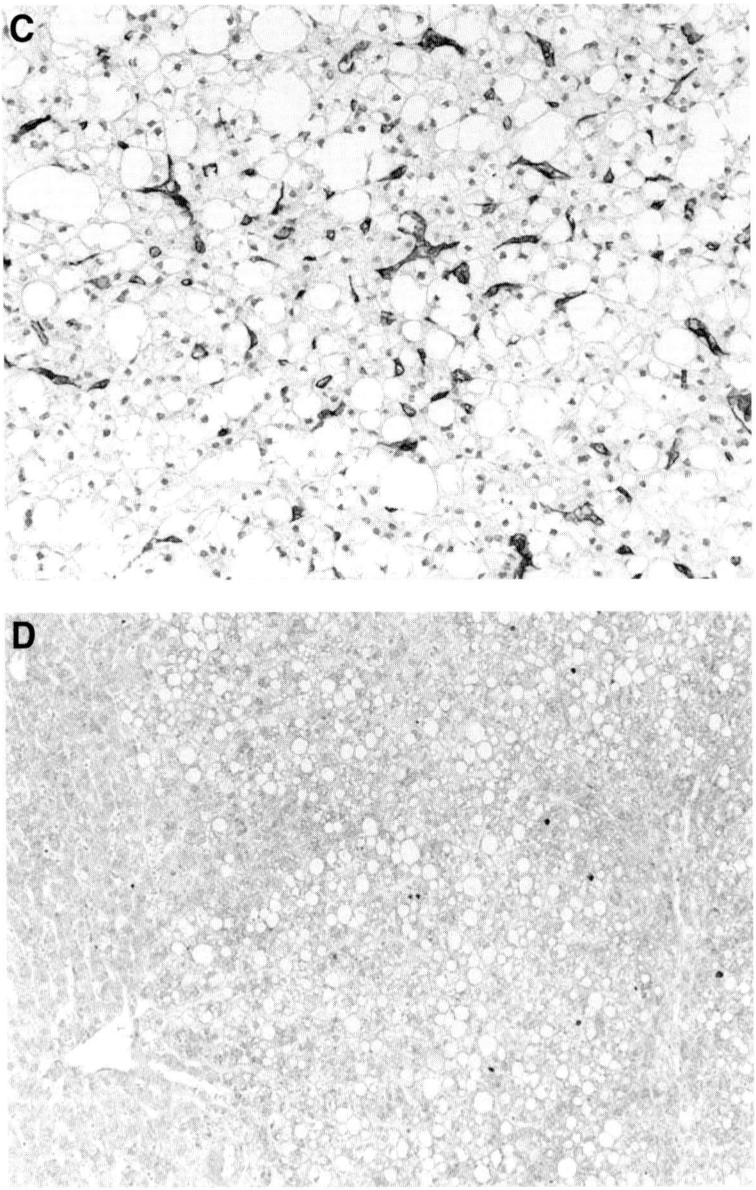

Fig. 2. (*continued from page 75*) arrangement of tumor cells is apparent. Large and small fat vesicles are seen within cell cytoplasm (stain, hematoxylin–eosin; original magnification, ×40). **(C)** Vasculature within HA. Immunostain highlights the dispersed arterial vasculature supplying the adenoma cells (stain, anti-CD31 immunoperoxidase; original magnification, ×20). **(D)** Cell proliferation

the development of hepatic tumors *(20)*. However, their identification does not distinguish benign from malignant tumors.

Comparative genomic hybridization has been suggested as a useful ancillary technique for the distinction of adenoma and carcinoma. Gains and losses of chromosome sites on 1q, 4q, 8p, 8q, 16p, and 17p were found to be the six most frequent alterations in HCC by this approach, and detection of one or more of these has been proposed as evidence in support of the diagnosis of carcinoma *(21)*. These authors have updated this technique by using fluorescent *in situ* hybridization to detect quantitative anomalies of chromosomes 1, 6, 7, and 8, thereby distinguishing HCCs from adenomas and other benign lesions in paraffin-embedded material *(22)*.

The distinction between HA and focal nodular hyperplasia (FNH) has clinical significance, because FNH is a benign condition that does not undergo malignant transformation and rarely ruptures, allowing in some cases for a more conservative approach to management *(23)*. Magnetic resonance imaging, enhanced CT, scintigraphic findings, and angiography show large peripheral vessels with centripetal flow and are diagnostically useful, but the best method for the differentiation of HA and FNH is surgical biopsy *(1,24,25)*.

Histopathologically, both FNH and HA contain benign-appearing hepatocytes. The presence of fibrous bands with artery branches and peripheral ductular hepatocytes in the absence of true bile ducts is characteristic of FNH (Fig. 3). Small vessels are also seen in the lobular portion of FNH, but these derive from the core arteries in the fibrous septa and rapidly diminish in caliber as the distance from the fibrous bands increases. Such a gradient may or may not be apparent in individual adenomas.

One of the major differences between FNH and HA is the presence of cholangioles at the interface zone between the hepatocytes and the connective tissue sheath surrounding the aberrant vascularity. In general, adenomas do not contain cholangioles in this region, whereas mature FNH do. Thus, immunohistochemical stains for cholangiolar cytokeratins, such as CK19 or AE1, highlight the cholangioles in FNH. The only caveat to using this method to distinguish between the two is that very early FNH lesions may lack the interface zone cholangioles, whereas otherwise typical adenomas will show occasional cholangioles. When the distinction becomes impossible, reliance on mutational analysis may be helpful.

Fig. 2. (*continued from page 76*) within HA. Immunolabeling of the nuclear cell cycle marker Ki67 shows scattered individual cells actively traversing the cell cycle. No foci of markedly increased activity are observed (stain, immunoperoxidase; original magnification, ×10).

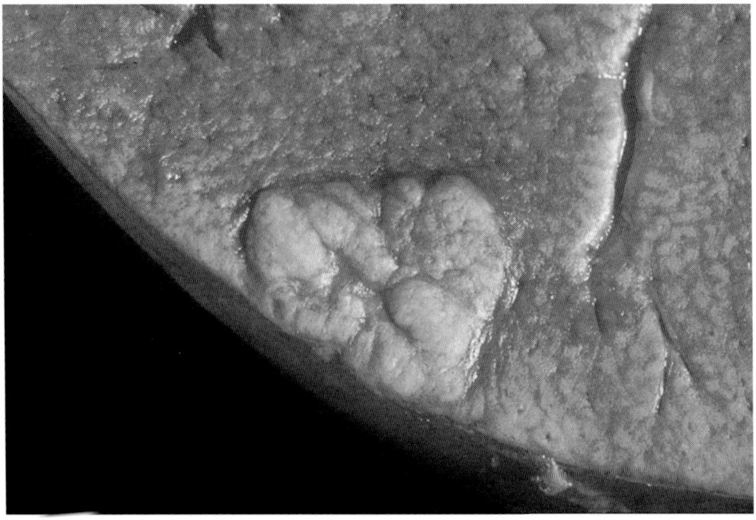

Fig. 3. Focal nodular hyperplasia. This well-circumscribed lesion frequently contains a central stellate depression that corresponds to a central fibrous region with radiating bands of fibrosis containing arterial vessels.

1.3. Clinical Comments

It is our opinion that hepatic adenomas are basically a surgical disease, and resection should be carried out in all HAs larger than 5 cm to reduce the risk of rupture and malignant transformation *(26,27)*.

There have been several reports of tumor regression after withdrawal of oral contraceptives *(28–30)*, and spontaneous regression of HA in a patient with glycogen storage disease type I has been reported *(12)*. However, this behavior is not invariable; HAs may remain the same size, may increase in size, or may undergo hemorrhage, spontaneous rupture, or, rarely, malignant transformation *(31)*.

Multiple lesions are claimed to be more progressive and symptomatic and are more likely to lead to impaired liver function, hemorrhage, and malignant transformation *(25)*. Proven HAs in males were smaller and simpler than those in women, which were more likely to undergo hemorrhage and necrosis, according to one study *(13)*. The users of oral contraceptives in whom HA develops are likely to have larger tumors and higher rates of bleeding and rupture than nonusers with HA *(1)*.

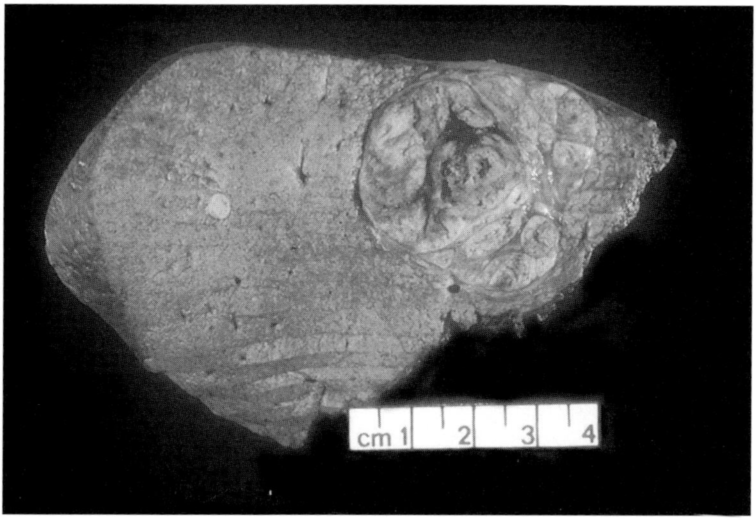

Fig. 4. Hepatocellular carcinoma. A large well-circumscribed nodular tumor appears to be comprised of variably nodular subunits in this macroscopic view. Two smaller satellite nodules are also visible.

2. HEPATOCELLULAR CARCINOMA

2.1. Macroscopic Pathology

In the Western world, most HCCs arise in cirrhotic livers and most frequently involve the right lobe. The tumors are typically soft, vary in color from gray-green-yellow to light brown, are occasionally bile-stained, and often contain foci of hemorrhage or necrosis. The tumors can be single or multiple and range from less than 1 cm to more than 30 cm in diameter with a tendency toward larger sizes when involving noncirrhotic livers *(32)*.

A wide variety of macroscopic patterns of tumor growth exist, but these have few clinical correlates. The traditional classification of Eggel *(33)* distinguishes three patterns of HCCs: multinodular, massive, and diffuse. Multinodular HCC (including solitary nodular HCC; *see* Fig. 4) was the most common type in one series. In this pattern, multiple tumor nodules are scattered throughout the liver *(32,34)*. Multinodular HCC typically is associated with cirrhosis *(32)*. In the massive pattern, a solitary tumor mass occupies much of the liver and may be associated with smaller satellite nodules. This pattern has been associated with noncirrhotic livers *(32)*. The diffuse pattern is the least common and is characterized by numerous widespread small nodules that mimic cirrhotic nodules and virtually replace the entire liver. In cirrhosis, clinically advanced liver disease has been associated with the diffuse or multinodular patterns of HCC *(34,35)*.

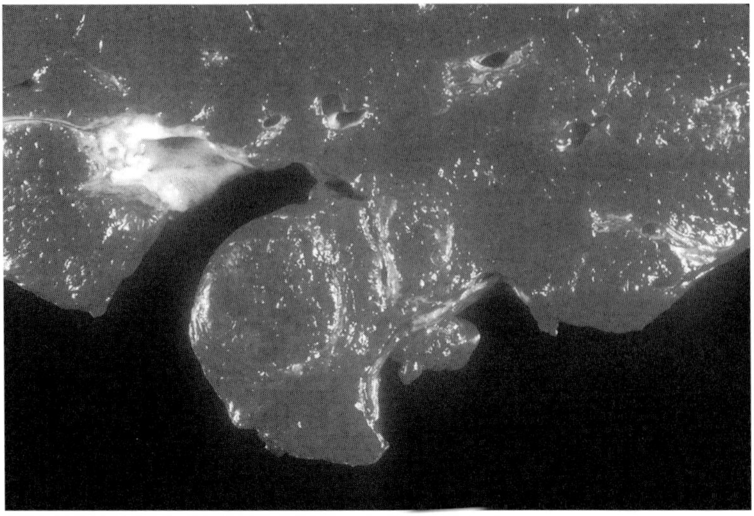

Fig. 5. Hepatocellular carcinoma with portal vein invasion. Despite the small size of this tumor, macroscopic spread into a portal vein branch was apparent. This is seen here as a projection of tissue from the liver surface on the right side of the tumor.

Rarely, HCC may be pedunculated, presumably reflecting an origin within an accessory lobe *(36)*. In one study, it was concluded that pedunculated HCC has an unfavorable prognosis if appropriate surgical procedures are not performed during the early stages of development *(37)*.

In more recent macroscopic classifications, HCCs are subdivided further into two main patterns based on growth characteristics. Expanding or expansive tumors have distinct borders that push aside the adjacent liver, and spreading or infiltrative tumors have poorly defined borders that microscopically invade the adjacent liver *(38,39)*. Kanai et al. *(40)* and Yuki et al. *(41)* subdivided nodular HCC into an additional three subtypes: type 1 is represented by HCC presenting as a single nodule, type 2 is a single nodule with extranodular growth, and type 3 has a contiguous multinodular growth pattern.

Blood groups have been related to macroscopic tumor patterns, and one group suggested that blood group status other than O was an independent risk factor for multinodular pattern HCC in those patients with tumor, and the presence of blood group O was associated with the solitary growth pattern *(32)*.

Portal vein thrombosis occurs in a high proportion of advanced cases *(42)*, and the frequency is lower in small HCC (Fig. 5) *(43)*. However, it has been proposed that curative resection may be possible, even in the presence of portal vein invasion, if the primary tumor is small, that is, early stage *(44)*.

Table 2
Cancer of the Liver Italian Program (CLIP)
Scoring System for HCC

Variable	*Score*
Child–Pugh stage	
A	0
B	1
C	2
Tumor morphologic features	
Uninodular and extension †50%	0
Multinodular and extension †50%	1
Massive or extension	2
AFP	
<400 ng/dL	0
‡400 ng/dL	1
Portal vein thrombosis	
No	0
Yes	1

(From ref. *50*.)

Less frequently, HCC may involve the main hepatic veins, the inferior vena cava, or the right atrium and can even extend into the large bile ducts. The clinical consequences of those involvements include Budd–Chiari syndrome, biliary obstruction, and hemobilia *(45–48)*.

Pathological staging is a primary determinant of prognosis, and the growth pattern does not add additional information. However, the manner of growth, such as diffuse, may make it less likely that the tumor will be detected at an earlier stage, and, by definition, growth patterns such as diffuse or massive are synonymous with advanced disease and associated poor prognosis *(34,35)*.

2.2. Pathological Staging

The International Union against Cancer and the American Joint Committee on Cancer (AJCC/UICC) published the TNM classification of intrahepatic cancers in 1987 (recently modified, *see* below). The major tumor variables in that system were tumor size, vascular invasion, and involvement of left and right hepatic lobes. Several modifications to HCC staging have been introduced since. The Izumi TNM modification *(49)*, The Cancer of the Liver Italian Program (CLIP) scoring system (Table 2) *(50)*, the Barcelona Clinic Liver Cancer (BCLC) staging *(51)*, the Chinese University Prognostic Index (CUPI) *(52)*, and the Prognostic Risk Score (PRS) *(53,54)* all have been proposed as offering more precise prognostic subgrouping and more applicability for patients undergoing hepatic resection or transplantation. The CLIP system (Table 2) uses the Child–Pugh score, tumor morphological features, AFP level, and portal vein thrombosis as independent predictive survival factors *(50)*. The BCLC is based on the presence or absence of symptoms, tumor multinodularity, vascular invasion, and extrahepatic spread *(51)*. The CUPI is constructed by adding liver function variables (total bilirubin, ascites, alkaline phosphatase, AFP, and asymptomatic disease on presentation) into the TNM staging system *(52)*. The PRS is based on vascular invasion (microscopic and macroscopic), lobar distribution, lymph node status, and largest tumor size *(54)*.

Recently, the AJCC updated and simplified its classification of intrahepatic tumors. Most of the revisions were related to categorization of the primary tumor, that is, T stage. A T1 tumor includes solitary tumors of any size without vascular invasion, and a T2 tumor includes solitary tumors of any size with vascular invasion. The older classification further subdivided solitary tumors on the basis of size, but this was not found to be prognostically useful. Nevertheless, tumor size continues to affect classification in the case of multiple tumors. Multiple tumors in the new system are staged as either T2, in which the size of the largest tumor does not exceed 5 cm, or T3, in which the largest tumor does exceed 5 cm in diameter. Factors such as bilateral location of tumors or tumor multifocality vs intrahepatic metastasis of a single tumor are not taken into account when assessing multiple tumors. Any tumor that involves a major branch of the portal vein (including portal vein and right and left branches) or hepatic vein (including right, left, or middle hepatic vein) is staged as T3. Finally, tumors with direct invasion of adjacent organs (excluding gallbladder) or penetration through the visceral peritoneum are staged as T4. A breakdown of TNM staging and stage grouping is provided in Tables 3 and 4.

2.3. Microscopic Pathology

HCCs can show a range of microscopic appearances, most of which recapitulate aspects of normal hepatocyte cytology and architecture. Well-differentiated HCC may be difficult or histologically impossible to distinguish from HA *(55–57)*, and it may likewise be difficult to precisely establish the interface between tumor and normal liver *(56)*. In contrast, poorly differentiated examples of HCC may betray only minor evidence of their hepatocellular origin.

The most common architectural pattern of malignant hepatocytes is an arrangement that caricatures the normal trabecular arrangement of liver lobules (Fig. 6) *(55,58)*. These neoplastic pseudotrabeculae vary from 2 to more than 20 cells in thickness, are irregularly arrayed, have a reduced or absent reticulin framework, and are separated by a vascular network lined by endothelial cells. All of these features distinguish them from normal trabeculae, which are one to two cells thick, evenly arranged, bordered by a well-developed reticulin network, and separated by sinusoids without prominent endothelial cells.

Table 3
American Joint Committee on Cancer Staging for Intrahepatic Tumors: Definitions of TNM

Primary tumor (T)	
TX	Primary tumor cannot be assessed
T0	No evidence of primary tumor
T1	Solitary tumor without vascular invasion
T2	Solitary tumor with vascular invasion or multiple tumors none more than 5 cm
T3	Multiple tumors more than 5 cm or tumor involving a major branch of the portal or hepatic vein(s)
T4	Tumor(s) with direct invasion of adjacent organs other than the gallbladder or with perforation of visceral peritoneum
Regional lymph nodes (N)	
NX	Regional lymph nodes cannot be assessed
N0	No regional lymph node metastasis
N1	Regional lymph node metastasis
Distant metastasis (M)	
MX	Distant metastasis cannot be assessed
M0	No distant metastasis
N1	Distant metastasis

(Used with the permission of the American Joint Committee on Cancer [AJCC], Chicago, Illinois. The original source for this material is the *AJCC Cancer Staging Manual*, Sixth Edition, Springer-Verlag, New York, 2002, www.springer-ny.com.)

Table 4
American Joint Committee on Cancer Staging for Intrahepatic Tumors: Stage Grouping

Stage	*T*	*N*	*M*
I	1	0	0
II	2	0	0
IIIA	3	0	0
IIIB	4	0	0
IIIC	Any	1	0
IV	Any	Any	1

(Used with the permission of the American Joint Committee on Cancer [AJCC], Chicago, Illinois. The original source for this material is the *AJCC Cancer Staging Manual*, Sixth Edition, Springer-Verlag, New York, 2002, www.springer-ny.com.)

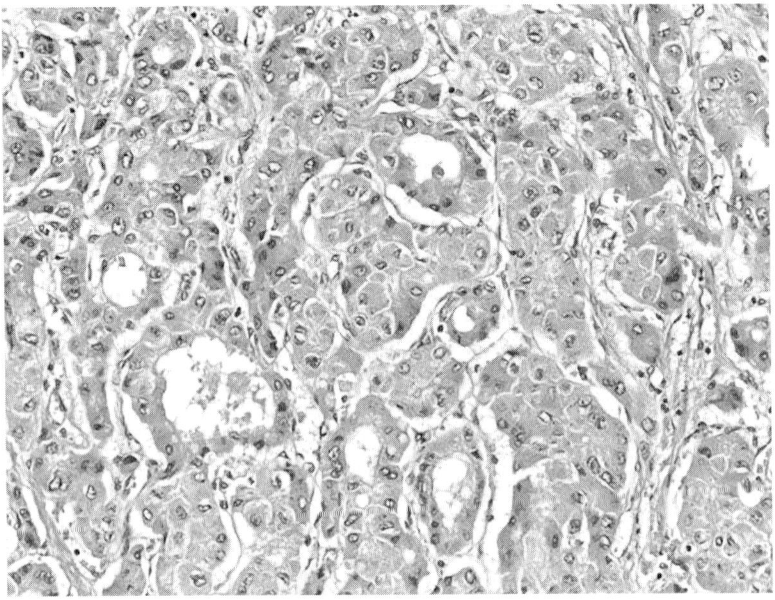

Fig. 6. Hepatocellular carcinoma. The cells arrange as cords or trabeculae of cells that are much broader than those of the normal liver. In addition, the cells may partially separate, leading to open spaces that simulate gland formation (pseudoacini; stain, hematoxylin–eosin; original magnification, ×20).

Other growth patterns of HCC are variations on this basic theme. A pseudoglandular (pseudoacinar) pattern may result either from dilatation of the bile canaliculi between tumor cells or from central lytic degeneration of solid trabeculae (Fig. 6). The gland-like spaces can be empty or can contain PAS-positive cellular debris, lipid-laden macrophages, or bile. Complex pseudoglandular formations can result in pseudopapillary structures and give the appearance of "islands" of tumor cells, usually surrounded by a lining of endothelial cells *(58)*. A compact or solid pattern results when malignant cells appose each other closely, rendering sinusoidal or vascular spaces inapparent. It has been suggested that HCCs with a compact growth pattern have a better prognosis as compared with trabecular and acinar patterns *(59)*.

Tumor cells generally retain a histological resemblance to hepatocytes but have more irregular nuclear membranes, coarser and more irregularly distributed heterochromatin, and slightly higher nuclear-to-cytoplasmic ratios than do their benign counterparts. Mitotic and apoptotic activity are increased in the tumor cell population. As HCC approaches moderately to poorly differentiated phenotypes, there is a corresponding exaggeration of all of these features, with an increase in cell-to-cell heterogeneity and the emergence of giant and bizarre tumor cells in some cases. Different degrees of differentiation can be seen within a single tumor.

A variety of cytological modifications may be seen within a given case of HCC. In general, these have no prognostic relevance, but they can be useful clues for the diagnostic histopathologist. In some cases, clear cells may predominate because of glycogen or lipid accumulation *(60,61)*. Macrovesicular steatosis may be diffuse or focal and seems to be a more frequent finding in small HCC. In one study, it was found that such tumors had fewer vessels than those without fatty change, and it was suggested that these fatty changes may be related to deficient vessel development in early tumors *(62)*.

Bile pigment is noted in approx 20% of HCCs. Bile within the neoplastic cells or bile canaliculi is an important indicator of hepatocellular origin. Bile is usually evident on routine histological analysis, but on occasion it may be necessary to demonstrate bile canaliculi by polyclonal anticarcinoembryonic antigen antibody (which is cross reactive with biliary glycoprotein) or even by electron microscopy.

Various intracellular inclusions can be identified. Dense eosinophilic globular bodies may be intra- or extracellular. These are usually PAS-positive and can contain various proteins, including AFP, α-1-antitrypsin, α-1-antichymotrypsin, albumin, fibrinogen, ferritin, or a combination thereof. Pale bodies are lightly staining, eosinophilic, intracytoplasmic inclusions that correspond to dilated rough endoplasmic reticulum and contain mainly fibrinogen, probably reflecting defective protein transport *(39,63)*. Pale bodies may simulate ground-glass inclusions that are related to hepatitis B virus infection; however, unlike true ground-glass inclusions, they do not contain viral components *(64,65)*. It has been suggested that proteins expressed in intracytoplasmic bodies in some cases may contribute to the malignant phenotype, because in one case p62, a phosphotyrosine-independent ligand of p56 (lck) and putative signal transducer, was identified as the major component of such inclusions *(66)*. Typical Mallory bodies can be seen in approx 20% of HCCs, regardless of underlying disease *(67)*. Megamitochondria, enlarged lysosomes, myelin deposits, abnormal accumulations of glycogen, and degenerative material occasionally are seen and can be identified ultrastructurally. Copper, copper-related protein, and Dubin–Johnson-like pigment all have been described in tumor cells. The latter may impart a black macroscopic appearance to the tumor *(68)*. Rarely, extramedullary hematopoieses and granulomas can be detected.

Kupffer cells often are scanty to absent in HCCs, with the most prominent decreases noted in the most poorly differentiated tumors. However, small, well-differentiated HCC may contain Kupffer cells in nearly normal numbers. For this reason, diagnostic techniques such as enhanced magnetic resonance imaging

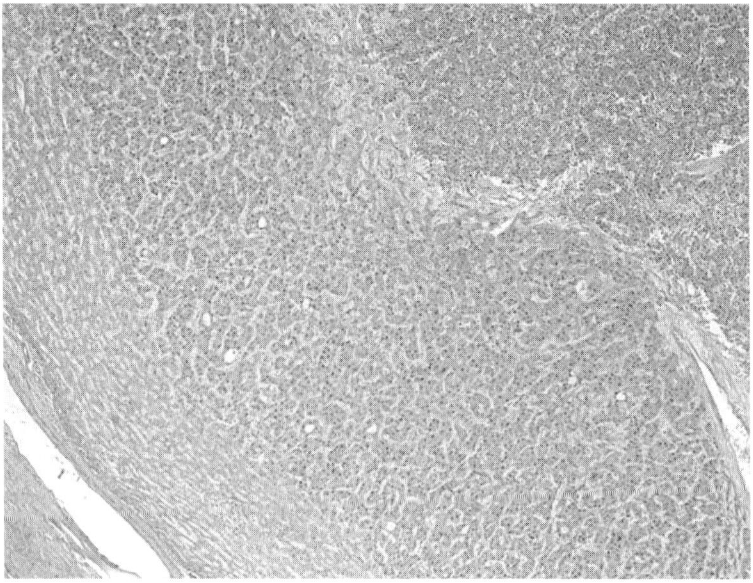

Fig. 7. Hepatocellular carcinoma. The fibrous capsule marking the periphery of this tumor is seen in the lower left-hand corner of the photograph, where it is artifactually split. The outermost third of the tumor consists of a band of attenuated normal hepatocytes, which have a somewhat compressed appearance at low power magnification. The middle third is comprised of hepatocellular carcinoma and shows a distinctly different architectural pattern even at this magnification. The inner third (upper right hand corner) also represents hepatocellular carcinoma. The more compact cell arrangement suggests that a less well differentiated subclone may have arisen within this tumor (stain, hematoxylin–eosin; original magnification, ×4).

(MRI), that are related to phagocytic cell uptake of marker agents, may reach their limits of detection with small HCC *(69–71)*. Reduced Kupffer cell function and cytokine production have been suggested as possible augmenters of HCC progression in an experimental animal model *(70)*.

The stroma of HCC usually is scanty *(55)*. In some cases, there can be a fibrous background, and differentiation from other forms of adenocarcinoma may become problematic.

Tumor nodules are frequently surrounded by grossly and microscopically distinct fibrous capsules, and septum formation can be observed during the development of HCC (Fig. 7). The capsule consists primarily of type III collagen, with type I collagen facing the tumor in more well-developed examples *(72–74)*. Small HCC have a higher proportion of well-encapsulated tumors *(43)*. The

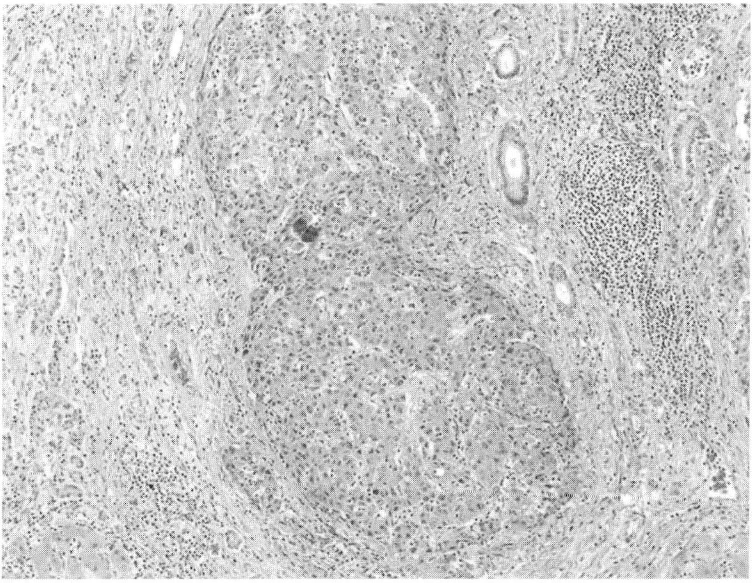

Fig. 8. Hepatocellular carcinoma. The tumor is seen as a vertically oriented aggregate of cells in the center of this photograph. To the right, the bile duct is cut longitudinally in several planes. To the left, a branch of hepatic artery is seen. The tumor itself lies within a portal vein branch within this intrahepatic portal tract (stain, hematoxylin–eosin; original magnification, ×20).

capsule and septa mainly are formed by α-smooth muscle actin-positive mesenchymal cells and can result from interactions between tumor and host liver parenchyma. It is thought by some investigators that the capsule is a manifestation of host defense that can interfere with the growth and invasiveness of HCC *(73,74)*. It has been suggested that tumor infiltration of the peritumoral capsule or of the surrounding parenchyma may correlate with a higher frequency of portal vein invasion (Fig. 8) and intrahepatic metastases *(34)*.

A four-tiered histological grading system originally was devised by Edmondson and Steiner *(75)*, with grades I– IV denoting progressive loss of differentiation. Tumor grades have been shown to correlate with the gross morphological features, DNA content, proliferation markers, metastases, laboratory parameters, and AFP production, but grading is a weak independent prognostic predictor *(34,76–78)*.

The ability to distinguish hepatocellular dysplasia from frank HCC has obvious clinical implications, and this distinction may be challenging for the diagnostic histopathologist. An increased cellular proliferation rate, as reflected by Ki-67 labeling, and the induction of tumor angiogenesis have been found to be helpful in supporting a diagnosis of HCC *(79–81)*. Vasculature can be highlighted by staining with antibodies to smooth muscle actin, with the endothelial markers factor VIII-related antigen, or with CD 34 *(79,82,83)*. HCC-associated angiogenesis patterns can be sinusoid-like or can be comprised of discrete vessels. The frequency of intratumoral arteries was found to be lower in steatotic areas in one study *(62)*. Several studies have attempted to correlate microvascular density to tumor aggressiveness, size, differentiation, or vascular invasion, but the results are not clear at this time *(79,83–85)*.

The differential diagnosis of HCC and HA is addressed in the section on HA (*see* Section 1.2.).

Special staining procedures may be used for the differential diagnosis of HCC and other carcinomas, particularly cholangiocarcinoma, neuroendocrine carcinoma, and metastatic carcinoma. However, none of these stains seem to be completely specific or sensitive. For example, the presence of bile in tumor cells is unambiguous evidence of hepatocellular phenotype but is not sensitive. The specificity of AFP is as high as 97%, but its sensitivity is low. Its expression often is patchy and weak, and it has been suggested that AFP positivity correlates with size and differentiation of the tumor; small, well-differentiated HCCs are less positive than poorly differentiated ones *(86–90)*.

Detection of biliary glycoprotein by the use of crossreactive polyclonal anticarcinoembryonic antigen (CEA) antibody highlights a bile canalicular pattern in 60–90% of HCC and was estimated in one series to be 79% sensitive and 97% specific for these tumors *(86)*. Adenocarcinomas and cholangiocarcinomas can show cytoplasmic staining with these antibodies, a pattern that is less common in HCC. Further, these other tumors also can react with the more specific monoclonal anti-CEA antibodies, a result that is seen only rarely with HCC *(88,89,91)*.

A canalicular pattern of staining in benign and malignant hepatocytes also can be demonstrated with antibody to CD10 (neprilysin) *(92,93)*. In one study, this antibody showed 68% sensitivity and 100% specificity for the differential diagnosis of HCC, although it did not distinguish it from normal liver parenchyma *(92)*.

For the differentiation of HCC from cholangiocarcinoma and metastatic carcinomas, particularly those of colorectal origin, immunostaining for individual cytokeratins may be helpful. Normal adult liver cells contain cytokeratins 8 and 18 as defined in Moll's catalog, and bile duct epithelial cells contain cytokeratins 7, 8, 18, and 19. Because tumors frequently recapitulate the phenotype of their normal counterparts, albeit imperfectly, HCCs often are positive with monoclonal antibodies CAM 5.2 (recognizing cytokeratins 7 and 8) and 35 βH11 (recognizing cytokeratin 8) and negative with the antikeratin antibody clones AE1 and 34 βE12; most cholangiocellular carcinomas are positive with both set of antibodies *(94)*. However, the results must be interpreted with caution, because both of these tumors arise from a common cell type and can coexpress cytokeratin types normally found on the other mature cell type *(95,96)*. Of perhaps more use is the fact that these antibodies can differentiate tumors of hepatocellular origin from colorectal adenocarcinoma. The latter most often are cytokeratin 20^+ 7^-, a pattern rarely seen in either HCC or cholangiocarcinoma *(97)*.

HepPar 1 is a monoclonal antibody that decorates both benign and neoplastic liver cells. It is not absolutely specific for the hepatocyte phenotype, because it rarely may be expressed in other cell types. However in one study, HepPar1 had 82% sensitivity and 90% specificity for the detection of HCCs *(86)*. When it is used as a part of a diagnostic panel, its diagnostic accuracy is enhanced *(86,98)*.

Serum des-carboxy-prothrombin, also known as protein induced by vitamin K absence II (PIVKA-II), is useful as a marker of HCC. Recently, immunohistochemical detection of this protein within the cytoplasm of HCC tumor cells was documented *(99)*. Positive staining did not correlate with tissue levels. Sensitivity and specificity of this stain for the detection of HCC remain to be evaluated, and the authors suggested that it may prove useful in separating small HCC from examples of adenomatous hyperplasia.

Epithelial glycoprotein-2 is a cell surface molecule present on many carcinomas but absent on HCC *(100)*. The glycoprotein is detected by the monoclonal antibody MOC-31, and a positive staining result with this antibody would suggest a tumor other than HCC *(68)*.

Several other proteins have been identified in HCCs, including albumin, α-1-antitrypsin, α-1-chymotrypsin, ferritin, fibrinogen, transferrin receptor, IgG, C-reactive protein, metallothionein, erythropoiesis-associated protein, factor XIII, aromatase, integrins VLA-α1 and VLA-β1, CD15, epidermal growth factor, transforming growth factor-α, and insulin-like growth factor II. They may help to determine liver cell origin in some cases, but their sensitivities and specificities are low. Tumor markers CA19-9 and CA50 are negative in HCC and have been suggested as being helpful in the differential diagnosis of HCC from bile duct carcinoma. Epithelial cell markers such as epithelial membrane antigen (EMA), Leu-M1, tumor-associated glycoprotein 72, and glycoprotein BCA-225 can show positivity in a small proportion of HCCs *(88–91,101–109)*.

Morphometric image analysis has been used to aid in the differential diagnosis of benign vs malignant hepatocellular lesions by determining the mean cell size, nuclear/cytoplasmic ratio, nuclear size and shape, and cell density *(110,111)*. Clinical application of these techniques, although promising, remains limited and awaits the introduction of a more user-friendly and reproducible technical infrastructure.

2.4. Molecular Pathology

Molecular biological techniques have aided our understanding of HCC greatly. Clonal analysis has shown that HCC arises from a single cell *(112)*. With tumor progression, different subclones may evolve, resulting in foci of variant histological growth patterns and degree of cytological differentiation *(77)*.

Multicentric intrahepatic HCC is common, and molecular techniques such as comparative genomic hybridization have shown that in some cases, this can represent independent primary tumor development, whereas in other cases, it reflects intrahepatic metastasis *(113)*. Kubo et al. *(114)* found that hepatitis C virus (HCV) infection was a risk factor for multicentricity in their patients, and this tendency was amplified further if there was evidence of prior hepatitis B virus (HBV) infection. They did not find multicentricity *per se* to be an independent prognostic factor, although molecular analysis of the tumors was not performed. Others also have found that the prognosis after hepatectomy for HCC is not appreciably different among patients regardless of prior HBV or HCV status *(115)*.

DNA ploidy studies have shown intratumoral heterogeneity, suggesting the presence of either cell dedifferentiation or multiple tumor clones. Aneuploidy was observed in one study to correlate inversely with the degree of histological differentiation *(77)*. The *S*-phase fraction of HCC cells was shown to correlate to survival in univariate analysis *(76)*. Interestingly, this latter study also suggested that a high *S*-phase fraction of peritumoral benign hepatocytes was an independent predictor of tumor behavior *(76)*.

Proliferation activity and apoptosis of tumor cells can be assessed by various methods. For determination of the proliferation activity of HCC, counts of silver staining nucleolar organizer regions (AgNORs), proliferating cell nuclear antigen (PCNA/cyclin) expression, and monoclonal antibody Ki-67 (MIB1) have been used *(116,117)*. MIB-1 and PCNA immunostaining and AgNORs have good correlation among themselves and were prognostic indicators in univariate analysis in one study *(116)*. This study found that the mitotic index was an independent prognostic parameter in multivariate analysis, and that apoptosis was unrelated to outcome *(116)*. However, a separate study *(118)* found both Ki67 index and apoptotic index to be independent prognostic factors.

Both apoptotic and proliferative activity are increased as the degree of histological differentiation decreases, and the importance of kinetic imbalance between cell loss and cell proliferation in tumor progression recently has been stressed *(119,120)*. The apoptosis/mitosis ratio reportedly was significantly lower in tumors with clear cell change, giant cells, and tumor necrosis. Both predominant and worst degrees of differentiation correlated with apoptosis, mitosis, and the apoptosis/mitosis ratio. The ratio also decreased with dedifferentiation *(79)*.

Regulation of mitosis and apoptosis through the cell cycle-related proteins p16, p21, p27, and cyclin D1 is an intriguing aspect of liver carcinogenesis *(79,118,121–123)*. Inactivation of p16 by posttranscriptional regulation seems to participate in both tumor formation and progression, whereas reduced p21 expression caused by p53 mutations seems to occur at an early stage. Tumor suppressor genes p53 and Rb have been studied extensively *(124–133)*. Large tumors, poorly differentiated tumors, and dedifferentiated foci more often demonstrate p53 mutations, and Rb dysfunction is associated with malignant progression and metastasis of HCC *(79,119,121,134)*. Protein p73, which is an analog of p53, induces apoptosis and in one study was found to be a correlate of poor prognosis *(78)*.

Reduced expression of p27 protein is associated with advanced tumor stage in HCC and has been suggested as a surrogate marker of late-stage disease *(135)*.

Recent studies have suggested that nuclear β-catenin expression is associated with reduced epithelial expression of E-Cadherin and may contribute to tumor progression by reducing cell adhesion. This may be associated with a poor prognosis according to some investigators *(136,137)*.

Activation of cellular proto-oncogenes *n-ras*, *c-myc*, and *c-fos* has been detected during chemically induced HCC in animal models and in clinical HCC *(138)*. The clinical significance of these changes is not clear; for example, some studies have found amplification of *c-myc* in less well-differentiated tumors, whereas others have noted lower *c-myc* expression in such tumors *(138,139)*.

Telomerase activity has been observed in HCCs. Some studies have noted prominence of this finding in poorly differentiated tumors, whereas one has recorded activity in atypical adenomatous hyperplasia and has suggested an early role for telomerase activation in hepatocarcinogenesis *(140–142)*. Caspase 3 expression segregates with p21(waf-1) expression, and loss of caspase 3 has been suggested as a contributor to hepatocyte neoplasia *(143)*.

Recognition of vascular invasion is a direct indication of tumor aggressiveness and the single most significant predictor of tumor recurrence after transplantation *(79)*. A correlation between the apoptosis/mitosis ratio and the extent of vascular invasion has been reported *(79)*.

Most HCCs seem to begin as small, well-differentiated neoplasms without vascular invasion *(79,144)*. With progression, the tumors enlarge and intratumoral foci lose individual phenotypic features of hepatocytes, that is, "dedifferentiate." The development of variant foci within a tumor is recognized histologically by both a lesser degree of cellular differentiation or architecture, increased histomorphological cell-to-cell heterogeneity, and higher Ki-67 (proliferative) labeling index *(38,79,119,144–146)*. The apoptosis/mitosis ratio also can differ from that in the surrounding tumor *(79,144,147–150)*.

In such cases, less-differentiated foci are surrounded by better differentiated neoplastic hepatocytes *(38,79,144–146)*. Dedifferentiated foci can acquire the ability to invade the vasculature and metastasize, likely attributable to further genetic instability, as histologically reflected by such changes as, for example, tumor giant cells.

Recent studies support the idea of different molecular pathways of hepatocarcinogenesis in those livers with vs those without cirrhosis, each group having different risk factors and clinical characteristics *(151–153)*.

The progenitor cell ultimately giving rise to HCC may be the oval cell, a bipotential liver stem cell able to differentiate into hepatocytes and bile duct epithelial cells. Oval cells have been described in hepatic adenomas *(20)*. In support of a role for oval cells in HCC, it has been shown that p53 deletion leads to immortalization and transformation of oval-like cell lines *(154)*. Others have argued against a primary role for this cell, because experimental HCCs can be induced with regimens associated with minimal oval cell stimulation *(155)*.

The host response to HCC is also being assessed. Recent studies suggest that a T-cell-predominant immune response containing a lesser B-cell component can exist, and several studies have suggested a better outcome in the presence of such immune infiltration *(156,157)*. Enhancement of the immune response is being examined as a means to reduce the risk of HCC recurrence *(158)*.

Our conceptual framework of HCC development, from the standpoint of the surgical pathologist, is sketched in Fig. 9. The cell of origin, whether a resting hepatocyte or oval cell, may develop along several overlapping pathways. Experimental studies have defined so-called foci of altered hepatocytes, which histologically appear as normal hepatocytes with a tendency toward increased cytoplasmic glycogen or basophilia. These cells are considered preneoplastic and rarely are recognized in routine specimens. A more readily recognized preneoplastic cell type that arises from such foci is the dysplastic hepatocyte. It is not known whether hepatocytes may proceed directly to dysplasia without first undergoing a state of physiological alteration. Regardless, the appearance of hepatocellular dysplasia should prompt a systematic search for more advanced foci of neoplasia. In our series *(79)*, most small HCCs arose as well-differentiated lesions, and larger tumors tended to develop dedifferentiated foci of moderately to poorly differentiated HCC. The development of moderately to poorly differentiated areas of HCC correlated well with angiolymphatic invasion and the apoptosis/mitosis ratio in this study. Such correlations are consistent with the concept that hepatocellular carcinogenesis is a multistep process. Importantly, however, approx 15–20% of HCCs seem to develop features of advanced tumor progression rapidly, such as dedifferentiation and angiolymphatic invasion, despite small size. It is not known whether this represents an acceleration of the genetic and epigenetic pathways found in more slowly evolving HCC or if it represents an alternate pathway of carcinogenesis. The practical message to the surgical pathologist is that it is important to assess each tumor for such features as differentiation and microscopic angiolymphatic invasion regardless of tumor size.

HCC also may arise from HAs, as discussed earlier. In our experience, such tumors largely have been well-differentiated HCCs, but there is no reason to think that less well-differentiated HCCs would not arise in this setting.

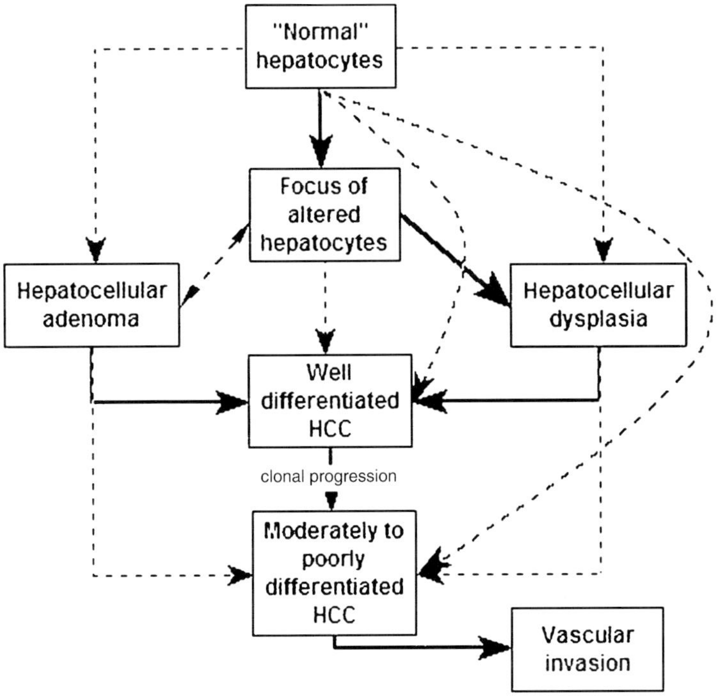

Fig. 9. Hypothetical pathways of hepatocyte neoplastic transformation. Generally accepted paths of cellular alterations are connected by thick lines; more conjectural pathways are connected by dashed lines. Normal hepatocytes undergo physiological alteration and are visible in experimental models as foci of altered hepatocytes. This is thought to be a precursor to hepatocyte dysplasia, which in turn may evolve into well-differentiated hepatocellular carcinoma. Tumor progression occurs as subclones evolve, and this leads to further growth and spread, summarized here as vascular invasion. It is not clear whether foci of altered hepatocytes may proceed directly to a neoplastic state, nor is it known whether hepatocytes may bypass these earlier states and proceed directly to hepatocellular carcinoma. Similarly, although it is known that HA may serve as a substrate for the development of carcinoma, the exact sequence of alteration involved in this process is not yet clear.

3. FIBROLAMELLAR HCC

Fibrolamellar HCC (FL-HCC), also known as oncocytic HCC or polygonal cell type HCC with fibrous stroma, is considered to be an entity separable from ordinary HCC *(159)*. This distinctive variant of HCC is seen predominantly in young patients (90% younger than age 35 years) without cirrhosis *(160)*. This

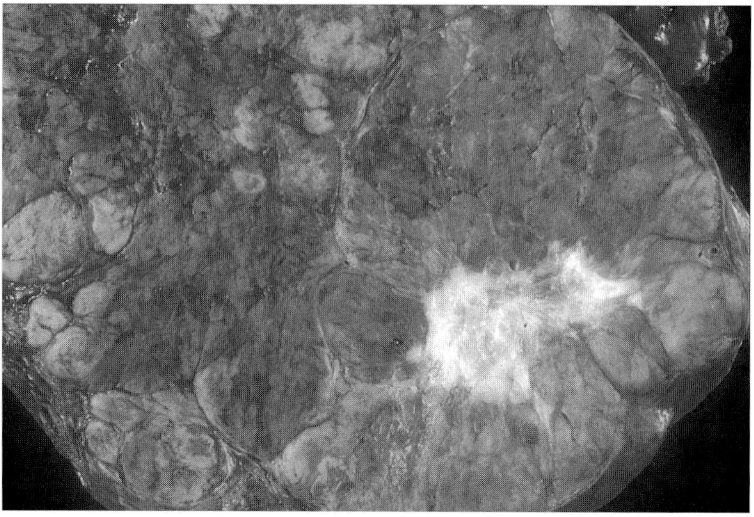

Fig. 10. Hepatocellular carcinoma, fibrolamellar subtype. This large tumor comprises most of the photograph and shows a multilobulated appearance with a large white central scar.

subtype is rare in Asia, and a male predominance has been described in Japan *(161)*. The lesions most often are large and solitary but may be multiple. The fibrous component of FL-HCC often forms a central scar that can be demonstrated by radiological techniques (Fig. 10) *(162)*.

Microscopically, there is usually a compact architectural growth pattern, but trabecular or acinar patterns can also be observed. The neoplastic cells are larger than normal hepatocytes. They are polygonal in shape and possess granular, eosinophilic cytoplasm, a so-called "oncocytic" appearance, resulting from numerous swollen mitochondria *(163)*. Nuclei are vesicular, rounded, and have prominent nucleoli, the latter being a characteristic feature of this tumor. Mitoses are usually sparse, and pleomorphism and multinucleation are infrequent. Tumor cells contain pale bodies that are reactive for fibrinogen. Hyaline globular inclusion bodies also can be seen *(164)*. Within the tumor cells, bile production, fat, glycogen, copper, and copper-associated protein can be detected *(165)*. Clear cell changes have been described in a case of otherwise typical fibrolamellar HCC *(166)*. Tumor cells immunohistochemically demonstrate cytokeratin 8 and 18 expression like conventional HCC and also may contain biliary cytokeratins (cytokeratin 7 and 19) *(95)*. The tumor cells usually are reactive with antibodies to polyclonal CEA, α-1-antitrypsin, ferritin, and C-reactive protein. AFP is present only in occasional cases *(163,167)*, and prominent AFP positivity, particularly when combined with elevated serum levels, suggests that a search for areas of more typical HCC should be undertaken *(168)*.

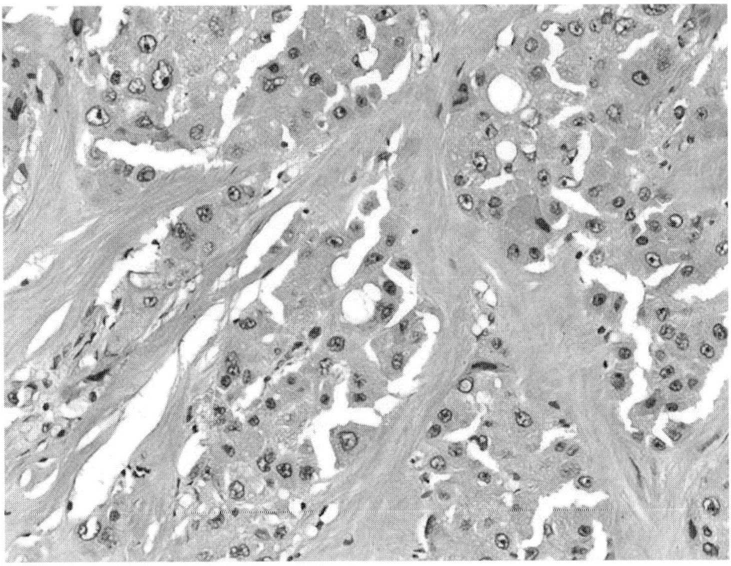

Fig. 11. Hepatocellular carcinoma, fibrolamellar subtype. The large tumor cells are separated by a stringy-appearing or lamellar pattern of fibrosis (stain, hematoxylin–eosin; original magnification, ×40).

A prominent collagenous fibrous stroma that is arranged in thin parallel bands (lamellae) is a characteristic feature of fibrolamellar HCC (Fig. 11), but may be sparse or even absent in some tumors. The collagen is predominantly composed of types I, III, and V *(169)*. It has been suggested that lamellar fibrosis might be the result of the production of collagen by stromal cells, which in turn are stimulated by transforming growth factor (TGF)-β produced by tumor cells *(170)*. Calcification also is a frequent finding in fibrolamellar carcinoma.

As noted earlier, the fibrous tissue may form a central scar, and this can radiate in a stellate fashion, mimicking the pattern of fibrosis seen in the benign condition of focal nodular hyperplasia. It has been suggested previously that fibrolamellar HCC and focal nodular hyperplasia may be pathogenetically related, but most investigators do not subscribe to that concept *(171)*.

Pure fibrolamellar HCC has a better prognosis than ordinary HCC because it often presents as a surgically resectable lesion, and the fibrous component is thought to result in a slower rate of tumor growth. For these reasons, aggressive surgical management has been advocated for this tumor *(172–175)*.

4. CLEAR CELL HCC

Clear cell HCC is comprised of malignant hepatocytes, the large majority of which contain a clear or empty-appearing cytoplasm reflecting the accumulation of intracellular glycogen or lipid *(60,176)*. Such tumors account for approx 9% of HCC in some series, although it is also noted that small numbers of clear cells are a common component of ordinary HCC.

A clinical association of clear cell HCC with nonalcoholic steatohepatitis in a diabetic patient has been seen, and a relationship with hypoglycemia and hypercholesterolemia also has been reported (60, 177). One study uncovered an example of clear cell HCC with a histological appearance similar to that of chromophobe renal cell carcinoma. Because this tumor had significant microsatellite instability in contrast to the remainder of clear cell HCC in that series, the authors concluded that clear cell HCC represents a heterogeneous category of tumors *(178)*. Orsatti et al. *(179)* also pointed to subtypes within this category. They showed that nondiploid clear cell tumors in their series were more pleomorphic and had a higher mitotic rate than diploid clear cell HCC and suggested that differences between these subgroups may account in part for differing opinions regarding the behavior of clear cell HCC.

One source of diagnostic difficulty lies in the possible histologic confusion with other tumors that may present as clear cell neoplasms, in particular renal cell carcinoma and adrenal cortical tumors. Immunohistochemical and ultrastructural studies may be of aid in defining a hepatocellular phenotype of these lesions *(180)*.

There seems to be no clear evidence suggesting that the overall clinical behavior of clear cell HCC differs from usual HCC *(178)*.

5. SCLEROSING HCC

Sclerosing HCC is a rare variant of HCC that usually occurs in older age groups. It is frequently associated with hypercalcemia in cases occurring in the United States, but not in those reported from Japan *(181)*. Parathyroid hormone-related protein was detected by immunohistochemical means in tumor cells of one case, and this was suggested as the cause of tumor-associated hypercalcemia *(182)*. Radiologically, the tumor is well-defined *(183)*. Macroscopically, the mass is usually large, firm, and gray-white. The characteristic histological features of the sclerosing HCC are nonlamellar, extensive fibrosis and a pseudoacinar formation of the tumor cells. Individual tumor cells can demonstrate characteristic cytological features of liver cells, especially at the periphery of the mass *(184)*. A definite sinusoidal vasculature usually is absent, and no tumor capsule is present.

Because of the extreme sclerosis and the apparent glandular configuration of tumor cells, it may be difficult to differentiate this HCC variant from cholangiocarcinoma and metastatic carcinoma *(184)*. Finding the characteristic trabecular growth pattern elsewhere in the tumor, finding immunohistochemical evidence of hepatocellular differentiation, or both are necessary for an unambiguous diagnosis *(55)*. Intracellular mucin is absent in HCC. An immunohistochemical panel incorporating cytokeratins 7, 8, 18, 19, 20, HepPar-1, and AFP also can be helpful in the differential diagnosis *(86,98,108)*.

6. COMBINED HCC AND CHOLANGIOCELLULAR CARCINOMA

Combined HCC and cholangiocellular carcinoma (HCC/CC) is a rare subtype also known as cholangiohepatoma, cholangioma, hepatocholangioma, and mixed cell carcinoma. HCC/CC can present as separate tumors, contiguous tumors, or single lesions incorporating both cell phenotypes. The tumors morphologically consist of mixed populations of hepatocytes, neoplastic cholangiolar cells, and small, undifferentiated oval-like cells on the basis of both light and electron microscopy *(185)*. In one study, these three cell lines were cloned from a single founder cell line and showed the same immunohistochemical and molecular pattern *(186)*.

Characteristically, areas of trabecular HCC are mixed with varying numbers of bile duct-type cells. Generally, the central areas are typical of HCC and the peripheral cells resemble biliary type cells. There may be glomeruli-like cell masses or glandular areas within the tumor. There is a moderate amount of stroma. Rarely, combined HCC/CC can be associated with a pseudosarcomatous component *(185)*.

7. SARCOMATOID HCC

Sarcomatoid HCC is a rare variant of HCC, accounting for less than 4% of cases. Spindle-shaped cells resembling fibrosarcoma or leiomyosarcoma admixed with multinucleated, pleomorphic, cytologically anaplastic giant cells are typical for this subtype. There can be rhabdomyoblastic differentiation, a schwannomatous component, osteoclast-like giant cells, chondro- or osteosarcomatous differentiation. A hepatocellular component also may be apparent *(187–189)*. Sarcomatoid hepatocellular cancers can show positivity for hepatocyte keratin subtypes within the sarcomatoid component in some cases, and immunoreactivity for these markers may be useful to distinguish these neoplasms from primary or metastatic sarcomas *(188,190)*. Hepatocyte markers also were found in a cell line recently derived from sarcomatoid HCC *(191)*.

8. HEPATOBLASTOMA

Hepatoblastoma is the most common primary liver tumor of infancy and childhood. It arises most frequently during the first 3 years of life and, rarely, may be present at birth. A few cases are reported in young adults or even those in old age *(192,193)*. The male/female ratio for hepatoblastoma is approx 2:1, and the tumor can be associated with several congenital abnormalities. Hemihypertrophy, Beckwith–Wiedemann syndrome, Down's syndrome, familial colonic polyposis, cardiac and renal malformations, cleft palate, glycogen storage disease, diaphragmatic hernia, and nephroblastoma have been reported in conjunction with hepatoblastoma *(194–198)*. Cytogenetic abnormalities, especially trisomies 2q and 20, are common *(199,200)*. There is no known relationship with liver cirrhosis.

Clinically, a rapidly enlarging upper quadrant mass, vomiting, fever, or a combination thereof are frequent presenting signs and symptoms. Serum AFP is elevated in 97% of patients. In infants and children with a primary liver tumor, low levels of AFP suggest the presence of either well-differentiated or immature hepatoblastoma, or fibrolamellar HCC *(201)*. In occasional cases, human chorionic gonadotropin (HCG) production may occur and may be sufficient to cause virilization *(202)*.

8.1. Macroscopic Pathology

Macroscopically, the tumor usually presents as a single, well-circumscribed, large mass up to 25 cm. The gross tumor appearance may be heterogeneous because of any combination of necrosis, hemorrhage, calcification, and cystic degeneration.

8.2. Microscopic Pathology

Histologically, there are two main patterns, namely epithelial and mixed epithelial-mesenchymal. The epithelial type is typically more common *(194)* and can be subdivided by the cell appearance into anaplastic (undifferentiated small-cell) *(203)*, anaplastic-mucoid *(204)*, embryonal, fetal, macrotrabecular *(205)*, and teratoid *(206)*. These all likely derive from a single stem-cell precursor *(207)*.

Anaplastic hepatoblastoma contains small round cells that histologically are similar to those seen in neuroblastoma *(199,208,209)*. Enlarged, bizarre cells also may occur. A mucoid stroma can be associated with anaplastic epithelial tumors *(204)*. Embryonal-type cells are small and elongated with hyperchromatic nuclei and scant cytoplasm. Mitoses can be detected easily, and foci of necrosis also can be present. The cells are arranged in ribbons, cords, or rosettes *(210)*. Fetal-type cells are more polygonal and are relatively larger than embryonal type cells. These cells bear a resemblance to normal fetal liver cells with granular cytoplasm, round to oval nuclei, and single small nucleoli. Mitoses are scant. The cytoplasm may contain fat and glycogen. They may assemble in irregular cords that are two cells in thickness and contain bile canaliculi and sinusoids *(198)*. Fetal- and embryonal-type hepatoblastomas in particular commonly show foci of extramedullary hematopoiesis *(211)*. Macrotrabecular hepatoblastoma contains cells that resemble adult HCC. Trabeculae containing fetal and embryonal cells can also be seen *(212)*.

Mixed hepatoblastomas combine the epithelial elements listed above with a mesenchymal component that characteristically has a spindled, undifferentiated appearance. Osteoid also can be present. Other components such as cartilage, bone, striated muscle, neural tissue, respiratory or intestinal epithelial cells, and other mature tissues may occur in some tumors, and this combination of tissues gives rise to the term *teratoid hepatoblastoma (213)*.

Hepatoblastomas express AFP in epithelial cells, especially fetal and embryonal variants. Epithelial components also can express EMA and cytokeratins 8, 18, 7, and 19. HCG positivity can be detected in giant cells *(214)*. Vimentin is positive in anaplastic cells and osteoid. α-1-antytrypsin, S-100 protein, neuron-specific enolase, and chromogranin A can be demonstrated in some cases *(202,207,215)*.

The histological distinction of fetal or macrotrabecular hepatoblastoma from adult HCC may be difficult. Anaplastic and embryonal subtypes need to be distinguished from other small, round cell tumors, and this may require immunohistochemical analysis *(205)*.

The treatments of choice include surgical resection combined with chemotherapy and liver transplantation *(216,217)*. After preoperative chemotherapy, both necrosis and the amount of osteoid increase *(218)*.

The stage of the disease is the most important prognostic parameter *(203)*. A purely fetal subtype was associated with improved prognosis in one series *(219)*. Anaplastic and macrotrabecular subtypes have a poor prognosis *(210)*. In childhood, there is no significant difference in median survival time between hepatoblastoma and HCC. Hepatoblastomas that are mitotically active have a poor prognosis, but necrosis and vascular invasion have not been found to affect outcome *(219)*. DNA content does not significantly affect prognosis *(203)*. Differentiation in hepatoblastoma is a good prognostic parameter *(219)*.

REFERENCES

1. Shortell CK, Schwartz SI. Hepatic adenoma and focal nodular hyperplasia. *Surg Gynecol Obstet* 1991;173:426–431.
2. Rosenberg L. The risk of liver neoplasia in relation to combined oral contraceptive use. *Contraception* 1991;43:643–652.
3. Espat J, Chamberlain RS, Sklar C, Blumgart LH. Hepatic adenoma associated with recombinant human growth hormone therapy in a patient with Turner's syndrome. *Dig Surg* 2000;17:640–643.
4. Grazioli L, Federle MP, Brancatelli G, Ichikawa T, Olivetti L, Blachar A. Hepatic adenomas: imaging and pathologic findings. *Radiographics* 2001;21:877–892; discussion, 892–894.
5. Yoshikawa M, Fukui K, Kuriyama S, et al. Hepatic adenomas treated with percutaneous ethanol injection in a patient with glycogen storage disease type Ia. *J Gastroenterol* 2001;36:52–61.
6. Alshak NS, Cocjin J, Podesta L, et al. Hepatocellular adenoma in glycogen storage disease type IV. *Arch Pathol Lab Med* 1994;118:88–91.

7. Chandra RS, Kapur SP, Kelleher J Jr, Luban N, Patterson K. Benign hepatocellular tumors in the young. A clinicopathologic spectrum. *Arch Pathol Lab Med* 1984;108:168–171.
8. Bala S, Wunsch PH, Ballhausen WG. Childhood hepatocellular adenoma in familial adenomatous polyposis: mutations in adenomatous polyposis coli gene and p53. *Gastroenterology* 1997;112:919–922.
9. Foster JH, Donohue TA, Berman MM. Familial liver-cell adenomas and diabetes mellitus. *N Engl J Med* 1978;299:239–241.
10. Chevallier P, Peten EP, Baldini E, Gugenheim J. Pedunculated hepatic adenoma: sonographic and MR imaging features. *AJR Am J Roentgenol* 1999;172:1146–1147.
11. Balci NC, Sirvanci M, Duran C, Akinci A. Hepatic adenomatosis: MRI demonstration with the use of superparamagnetic iron oxide. *Clin Imaging* 2002;26:35–38.
12. Iijima H, Moriwaki Y, Yamamoto T, Takahashi S, Nishigami T, Hada T. Spontaneous regression of hepatic adenoma in a patient with glycogen storage disease type I after hemodialysis: ultrasonographic and CT findings. *Intern Med* 2001;40:891–895.
13. Hung CH, Changchien CS, Lu SN, et al. Sonographic features of hepatic adenomas with pathologic correlation. *Abdom Imaging* 2001;26:500–506.
14. Palmer PE, Christopherson WM, Wolfe HJ. Alpha-1-antitrypsin, protein marker in oral contraceptive-associated hepatic tumors. *Am J Clin Pathol* 1977;68:736–739.
15. Poe R, Snover DC. Adenomas in glycogen storage disease type 1. Two cases with unusual histologic features. *Am J Surg Pathol* 1988;12:477–483.
16. Heffelfinger S, Irani DR, Finegold MJ. "Alcoholic hepatitis" in a hepatic adenoma. *Hum Pathol* 1987;18:751–754.
17. Tao LC. Oral contraceptive-associated liver cell adenoma and hepatocellular carcinoma. Cytomorphology and mechanism of malignant transformation. Cancer 1991;68(2):341–347.
18. Cohen C, Lawson D, DeRose PB. Sex and androgenic steroid receptor expression in hepatic adenomas. *Hum Pathol* 1998;29:1428–1432.
19. Torbenson M, Lee J, Choti M, et al. Hepatic adenomas: analysis of sex steroid receptor status and the Wnt signaling pathway. *Mod Pathol* 2002;15:189–196.
20. Libbrecht L, De Vos R, Cassiman D, Desmet V, Aerts R, Roskams T. Hepatic progenitor cells in hepatocellular adenomas. *Am J Surg Pathol* 2001;25:1388–1396.
21. Wilkens L, Bredt M, Flemming P, Becker T, Klempnauer J, Kreipe HH. Differentiation of liver cell adenomas from well-differentiated hepatocellular carcinomas by comparative genomic hybridization. *J Pathol* 2001;193:476–482.
22. Wilkens L, Bredt M, Flemming A, et al. Detection of chromosomal aberrations in well-differentiated hepatocellular carcinoma by bright-field in situ hybridization. *Mod Pathol* 2002;15:470–475.
23. Reddy KR, Kligerman S, Levi J, et al. Benign and solid tumors of the liver: relationship to sex, age, size of tumors, and outcome. *Am Surg* 2001;67:173–178.
24. Herman P, Pugliese V, Machado MA, et al. Hepatic adenoma and focal nodular hyperplasia: differential diagnosis and treatment. *World J Surg* 2000;24:372–376.
25. Ichikawa T, Federle MP, Grazioli L, Nalesnik M. Hepatocellular adenoma: multiphasic CT and histopathologic findings in 25 patients. *Radiology* 2000;214:861–868.
26. Terkivatan T, de Wilt JH, de Man RA, et al. Indications and long-term outcome of treatment for benign hepatic tumors: a critical appraisal. *Arch Surg* 2001;136:1033–1038.
27. Closset J, Veys I, Peny MO, et al. Retrospective analysis of 29 patients surgically treated for hepatocellular adenoma or focal nodular hyperplasia. *Hepatogastroenterology* 2000;47:1382–1384.
28. Aseni P, Sansalone CV, Sammartino C, et al. Rapid disappearance of hepatic adenoma after contraceptive withdrawal. *J Clin Gastroenterol* 2001;33:234–236.
29. Steinbrecher UP, Lisbona R, Huang SN, Mishkin S. Complete regression of hepatocellular adenoma after withdrawal of oral contraceptives. *Dig Dis Sci* 1981;26:1045–1050.

30. Buhler H, Pirovino M, Akobiantz A, et al. Regression of liver cell adenoma. A follow-up study of three consecutive patients after discontinuation of oral contraceptive use. *Gastroenterology* 1982;82:775–782.
31. Heeringa B, Sardi A. Bleeding hepatic adenoma: expectant treatment to limit the extent of liver resection. *Am Surg* 2001;67:927–929.
32. Trevisani F, Caraceni P, Bernardi M, et al. Gross pathologic types of hepatocellular carcinoma in Italian patients. Relationship with demographic, environmental, and clinical factors. *Cancer* 1993;72:1557–1563.
33. Eggel H. Uber das primare carcinom der leber. *Beitr Pathol Anat* 1901;30:506–604.
34. Shimada M, Rikimaru T, Hamatsu T, et al. The role of macroscopic classification in nodular-type hepatocellular carcinoma. *Am J Surg* 2001;182:177–182.
35. Stroffolini T, Andreone P, Andriulli A, et al. Gross pathologic types of hepatocellular carcinoma in Italy. *Oncology* 1999;56:189–192.
36. Horie Y, Katoh S, Yoshida H, Imaoka T, Suou T, Hirayama C. Pedunculated hepatocellular carcinoma. Report of three cases and review of literature. *Cancer* 1983;51:746–751.
37. Horie Y, Shigoku A, Tanaka H, et al. Prognosis for pedunculated hepatocellular carcinoma. *Oncology* 1999;57:23–28.
38. Okuda K. Hepatocellular carcinoma. *J Hepatol* 2000;32:225–237.
39. Nakashima O, Sugihara S, Eguchi A, Taguchi J, Watanabe J, Kojiro M. Pathomorphologic study of pale bodies in hepatocellular carcinoma. *Acta Pathol Jpn* 1992;42:414–418.
40. Kanai T, Hirohashi S, Upton MP, et al. Pathology of small hepatocellular carcinoma. A proposal for a new gross classification. *Cancer* 1987;60:810–819.
41. Yuki K, Hirohashi S, Sakamoto M, Kanai T, Shimosato Y. Growth and spread of hepatocellular carcinoma. A review of 240 consecutive autopsy cases. *Cancer* 1990;66:2174–2170.
42. Albacete RA, Matthews MJ, Saini N. Portal vein thromboses in malignant hepatoma. *Ann Intern Med* 1967;67:337–348.
43. Zhou XD, Tang ZY, Yang BH, et al. Experience of 1000 patients who underwent hepatectomy for small hepatocellular carcinoma. *Cancer* 2001;91:1479–1486.
44. Ohkubo T, Yamamoto J, Sugawara Y, et al. Surgical results for hepatocellular carcinoma with macroscopic portal vein tumor thrombosis. *J Am Coll Surg* 2000;191:657–660.
45. Kojiro M, Kawabata K, Kawano Y, Shirai F, Takemoto N, Nakashima T. Hepatocellular carcinoma presenting as intrabile duct tumor growth: a clinicopathologic study of 24 cases. *Cancer* 1982;49:2144–2147.
46. Kojiro M, Nakahara H, Sugihara S, Murakami T, Nakashima T, Kawasaki H. Hepatocellular carcinoma with intra-atrial tumor growth. A clinicopathologic study of 18 autopsy cases. *Arch Pathol Lab Med* 1984;108:989–992.
47. Nakashima T, Okuda K, Kojiro M, et al. Pathology of hepatocellular carcinoma in Japan. Two hundred thirty-two consecutive cases autopsied in ten years. *Cancer* 1983;51:863–877.
48. Tantawi B, Cherqui D, Tran van Nhieu J, Kracht M, Fagniez PL. Surgery for biliary obstruction by tumour thrombus in primary liver cancer. *Br J Surg* 1996;83:1522–1525.
49. Staudacher C, Chiappa A, Biella F, Audisio RA, Bertani E, Zbar AP. Validation of the modified TNM-Izumi classification for hepatocellular carcinoma. *Tumori* 2000;86:8–11.
50. The Cancer of the Liver Italian Program (CLIP) Investigators. Prospective validation of the CLIP score: a new prognostic system for patients with cirrhosis and hepatocellular carcinoma. *Hepatology* 2000;31:840–845.
51. Llovet JM, Bru C, Bruix J. Prognosis of hepatocellular carcinoma: the BCLC staging classification. *Semin Liver Dis* 1999;19:329–338.
52. Leung TW, Tang AM, Zee B, et al. Construction of the Chinese University Prognostic Index for hepatocellular carcinoma and comparison with the TNM staging system, the Okuda staging system, and the Cancer of the Liver Italian Program staging system: a study based on 926 patients. *Cancer* 2002;94:1760–1769.

53. Marsh JW, Dvorchik I, Bonham CA, Iwatsuki S. Is the pathologic TNM staging system for patients with hepatoma predictive of outcome? *Cancer* 2000;88:538–543.
54. Iwatsuki S, Dvorchik I, Marsh JW, et al. Liver transplantation for hepatocellular carcinoma: a proposal of a prognostic scoring system. *J Am Coll Surg* 2000;191:389–394.
55. Kondo Y. Histologic features of hepatocellular carcinoma and allied disorders. *Pathol Ann* 1985;20(Pt 2):405–430.
56. Komatsu T, Kondo Y, Yamamoto Y, Isono K. Hepatocellular carcinoma presenting well differentiated, normotrabecular patterns in peripheral or metastatic loci. Analysis of 103 resected cases. *Acta Pathol Jpn* 1990;40:887–893.
57. Nakashima T, Kojiro M. Pathologic characteristics of hepatocellular carcinoma. *Semin Liver Dis* 1986;6:259–266.
58. Kondo Y, Nakajima T. Pseudoglandular hepatocellular carcinoma. A morphogenetic study. *Cancer* 1987;60:1032–1037.
59. Lauwers GY, Terris B, Balis UJ, et al. Prognostic histologic indicators of curatively resected hepatocellular carcinomas: a multi-institutional analysis of 425 patients with definition of a histologic prognostic index. *Am J Surg Pathol* 2002;26:25–34.
60. Orikasa H, Ohyama R, Tsuka N, Eyden BP, Yamazaki K. Lipid-rich clear-cell hepatocellular carcinoma arising in non-alcoholic steatohepatitis in a patient with diabetes mellitus. *J Submicrosc Cytol Pathol* 2001;33:195–200.
61. Yang SH, Watanabe J, Nakashima O, Kojiro M. Clinicopathologic study on clear cell hepatocellular carcinoma. *Pathol Int* 1996;46:503–509.
62. Kutami R, Nakashima Y, Nakashima O, Shiota K, Kojiro M. Pathomorphologic study on the mechanism of fatty change in small hepatocellular carcinoma of humans. *J Hepatol* 2000;33:282–289.
63. Moon WS, Yu HC, Chung MJ, Kang MJ, Lee DG. Pale bodies in hepatocellular carcinoma. *J Korean Med Sci* 2000;15:516–520.
64. Stromeyer FW, Ishak KG, Gerber MA, Mathew T. Ground-glass cells in hepatocellular carcinoma. *Am J Clin Pathol* 1980;74:254–258.
65. Nakanuma Y, Kono N, Ohta G, et al. Pale eosinophilic inclusions simulating ground-glass appearance of cells of hepatocellular carcinoma. *Acta Pathol Jpn* 1982;32:71–81.
66. Stumptner C, Heid H, Fuchsbichler A, et al. Analysis of intracytoplasmic hyaline bodies in a hepatocellular carcinoma. Demonstration of p62 as major constituent. *Am J Pathol* 1999;154:1701–1710.
67. Jensen K, Gluud C. The Mallory body: morphological, clinical and experimental studies (part 1 of a literature survey). *Hepatology* 1994;20:1061–1077.
68. Dominguez-Malagon H, Gaytan-Graham S. Hepatocellular carcinoma: an update. *Ultrastruct Pathol* 2001;25:497–516.
69. Tanaka M, Nakashima O, Wada Y, Kage M, Kojiro M. Pathomorphological study of Kupffer cells in hepatocellular carcinoma and hyperplastic nodular lesions in the liver. *Hepatology* 1996;24:807–812.
70. Tsujimoto T, Kuriyama S, Yamazaki M, et al. Augmented hepatocellular carcinoma progression and depressed Kupffer cell activity in rat cirrhotic livers. *Int J Oncol* 2001;18:41–47.
71. Imai Y, Murakami T, Yoshida S, et al. Superparamagnetic iron oxide-enhanced magnetic resonance images of hepatocellular carcinoma: correlation with histological grading. *Hepatology* 2000;32:205–212.
72. Okuda K, Musha H, Nakajima Y, et al. Clinicopathologic features of encapsulated hepatocellular carcinoma: a study of 26 cases. *Cancer* 1977;40:1240–1245.
73. Torimura T, Ueno T, Inuzuka S, Tanaka M, Abe H, Tanikawa K. Mechanism of fibrous capsule formation surrounding hepatocellular carcinoma. Immunohistochemical study. *Arch Pathol Lab* Med 1991;115:365–371.
74. Ishizaki M, Ashida K, Higashi T, et al. The formation of capsule and septum in human hepatocellular carcinoma. *Virchows Arch* 2001;438:574–580.

75. Edmondson HA, Steiner PE. Primary carcinoma of the liver. A study of 100 cases among 48,900 necropsies. *Cancer* 1954;7:462–503.
76. Rua S, Comino A, Fruttero A, et al. Flow cytometric DNA analysis of cirrhotic liver cells in patients with hepatocellular carcinoma can provide a new prognostic factor. *Cancer* 1996;78:1195–1202.
77. Oriyama T, Yamanaka N, Fujimoto J, Ichikawa N, Okamoto E. Progression of hepatocellular carcinoma as reflected by nuclear DNA ploidy and cellular differentiation. *J Hepatol* 1998;28:142–149.
78. Tannapfel A, Wasner M, Krause K, et al. Expression of p73 and its relation to histopathology and prognosis in hepatocellular carcinoma. *J Natl Cancer Inst* 1999;91:1154–1158.
79. Kirimlioglu H, Dvorchick I, Ruppert K, et al. Hepatocellular carcinomas in native livers from patients treated with orthotopic liver transplantation: biologic and therapeutic implications. *Hepatology* 2001;34:502–510.
80. Saito Y, Matsuzaki Y, Doi M, et al. Multiple regression analysis for assessing the growth of small hepatocellular carcinoma: the MIB-1 labeling index is the most effective parameter. *J Gastroenterol* 1998;33:229–235.
81. Nolte M, Werner M, Nasarek A, et al. Expression of proliferation associated antigens and detection of numerical chromosome aberrations in primary human liver tumours: relevance to tumour characteristics and prognosis. *J Clin Pathol* 1998;51:47–51.
82. Tanigawa N, Lu C, Mitsui T, Miura S. Quantitation of sinusoid-like vessels in hepatocellular carcinoma: its clinical and prognostic significance. *Hepatology* 1997;26:1216–1223.
83. El-Assal ON, Yamanoi A, Soda Y, et al. Clinical significance of microvessel density and vascular endothelial growth factor expression in hepatocellular carcinoma and surrounding liver: possible involvement of vascular endothelial growth factor in the angiogenesis of cirrhotic liver. *Hepatology* 1998;27:1554–1562.
84. Ker CG, Chen HY, Juan CC, et al. Role of angiogenesis in hepatitis and hepatocellular carcinoma. *Hepatogastroenterology* 1999;46:646–650.
85. Kimura H, Nakajima T, Kagawa K, et al. Angiogenesis in hepatocellular carcinoma as evaluated by CD34 immunohistochemistry. *Liver* 1998;18:14–19.
86. Minervini MI, Demetris AJ, Lee RG, Carr BI, Madariaga J, Nalesnik MA. Utilization of hepatocyte-specific antibody in the immunocytochemical evaluation of liver tumors. *Mod Pathol* 1997;10:686–692.
87. Brumm C, Schulze C, Charels K, Morohoshi T, Kloppel G. The significance of alpha-fetoprotein and other tumour markers in differential immunocytochemistry of primary liver tumours. *Histopathology* 1989;14:503–513.
88. Hurlimann J, Gardiol D. Immunohistochemistry in the differential diagnosis of liver carcinomas. *Am J Surg Pathol* 1991;15:280–288.
89. Ma CK, Zarbo RJ, Frierson HF Jr, Lee MW. Comparative immunohistochemical study of primary and metastatic carcinomas of the liver. *Am J Clin Pathol* 1993;99:551–557.
90. Wu PC, Fang JW, Lau VK, Lai CL, Lo CK, Lau JY. Classification of hepatocellular carcinoma according to hepatocellular and biliary differentiation markers. Clinical and biological implications. *Am J Pathol* 1996;149:1167–1175.
91. Fucich LF, Cheles MK, Thung SN, Gerber MA, Marrogi AJ. Primary vs metastatic hepatic carcinoma. An immunohistochemical study of 34 cases. *Arch Pathol Lab Med* 1994;118:927–930.
92. Borscheri N, Roessner A, Rocken C. Canalicular immunostaining of neprilysin (CD10) as a diagnostic marker for hepatocellular carcinomas. *Am J Surg Pathol* 2001;25:1297–1303.
93. Xiao S, Wang H, Hart J, Fleming D, Beard M. cDNA arrays and immunohistochemistry identification of CD10/CALLA expression in hepatocellular carcinoma. *Am J Pathol* 2001;159:1415–1421.
94. Johnson DE, Herndier BG, Medeiros LJ, Warnke RA, Rouse RV. The diagnostic utility of the keratin profiles of hepatocellular carcinoma and cholangiocarcinoma. *Am J Surg Pathol* 1988;12:187–197.

95. Van Eyken P, Sciot R, Brock P, Casteels-Van Daele M, Ramaekers FC, Desmet VJ. Abundant expression of cytokeratin 7 in fibrolamellar carcinoma of the liver. *Histopathology* 1990;17:101–107.
96. D'Errico A, Baccarini P, Fiorentino M, et al. Histogenesis of primary liver carcinomas: strengths and weaknesses of cytokeratin profile and albumin mRNA detection. *Hum Pathol* 1996;27:599–604.
97. Tot T. Adenocarcinomas metastatic to the liver: the value of cytokeratins 20 and 7 in the search for unknown primary tumors. *Cancer* 1999;85:171–177.
98. Leong AS, Sormunen RT, Tsui WM, Liew CT. Hep Par 1 and selected antibodies in the immunohistological distinction of hepatocellular carcinoma from cholangiocarcinoma, combined tumours and metastatic carcinoma. *Histopathology* 1998;33:318–324.
99. Miskad U, Yano Y, Nakaji M, et al. Histological study of PIVKA-II expression in hepatocellular carcinoma and adenomatous hyperplasia. *Pathol Int* 2001;51:916–922.
100. Willuda J, Honegger A, Waibel R, et al. High thermal stability is essential for tumor targeting of antibody fragments: engineering of a humanized anti-epithelial glycoprotein-2 (epithelial cell adhesion molecule) single-chain Fv fragment. *Cancer Res* 1999;59:5758–5767.
101. Yabuuchi I, Kawata S, Tamura S, et al. Aromatase activity in human hepatocellular carcinoma. Relationship with the degree of histologic differentiation. *Cancer* 1993;71:56–61.
102. Volpes R, van den Oord JJ, Desmet VJ. Integrins as differential cell lineage markers of primary liver tumors. *Am J Pathol* 1993;142:1483–1492.
103. Torii A, Nakayama A, Harada A, et al. Expression of the CD15 antigen in hepatocellular carcinoma. *Cancer* 1993;71:3864–3867.
104. Sciot R, Paterson AC, van Eyken P, Callea F, Kew MC, Desmet VJ. Transferrin receptor expression in human hepatocellular carcinoma: an immunohistochemical study of 34 cases. *Histopathology* 1988;12:53–63.
105. Haglund C, Lindgren J, Roberts PJ, Nordling S. Difference in tissue expression of tumour markers CA 19-9 and CA 50 in hepatocellular carcinoma and cholangiocarcinoma. *Br J Cancer* 1991;63:386–389.
106. Nalesnik MA, Lee RG, Carr BI. Transforming growth factor alpha (TGFalpha) in hepatocellular carcinomas and adjacent hepatic parenchyma. *Hum Pathol* 1998;29:228–234.
107. Lamas E, Le Bail B, Housset C, Boucher O, Brechot C. Localization of insulin-like growth factor-II and hepatitis B virus mRNAs and proteins in human hepatocellular carcinomas. *Lab Invest* 1991;64:98–104.
108. Ganjei P, Nadji M, Albores-Saavedra J, Morales AR. Histologic markers in primary and metastatic tumors of the liver. *Cancer* 1988;62:1994–1998.
109. Cohen C, Berson SD, Shulman G, Budgeon LR. Immunohistochemical ferritin in hepatocellular carcinoma. *Cancer* 1984;53:1931–1935.
110. Deprez C, Vangansbeke D, Fastrez R, Pasteels JL, Verhest A, Kiss R. Nuclear DNA content, proliferation index, and nuclear size determination in normal and cirrhotic liver, and in benign and malignant primary and metastatic hepatic tumors. *Am J Clin Pathol* 1993;99:558–565.
111. Erler BS, Hsu L, Truong HM, et al. Image analysis and diagnostic classification of hepatocellular carcinoma using neural networks and multivariate discriminant functions. *Lab Invest* 1994;71:446–451.
112. Ochiai T, Urata Y, Yamano T, Yamagishi H, Ashihara T. Clonal expansion in evolution of chronic hepatitis to hepatocellular carcinoma as seen at an X-chromosome locus. *Hepatology* 2000;31:615–621.
113. Wilkens L, Bredt M, Flemming P, Klempnauer J, Heinrich Kreipe H. Differentiation of multicentric origin from intra-organ metastatic spread of hepatocellular carcinomas by comparative genomic hybridization. *J Pathol* 2000;192:43–51.
114. Kubo S, Nishiguchi S, Hirohashi K, et al. Clinicopathological criteria for multicentricity of hepatocellular carcinoma and risk factors for such carcinogenesis. *Jpn J Cancer Res* 1998;89:419–426.

115. Miyagawa S, Kawasaki S, Makuuchi M. Comparison of the characteristics of hepatocellular carcinoma between hepatitis B and C viral infection: tumor multicentricity in cirrhotic liver with hepatitis C. *Hepatology* 1996;24:307–310.
116. Tannapfel A, Geissler F, Kockerling F, Katalinic A, Hauss J, Wittekind C. Apoptosis and proliferation in relation to histopathological variables and prognosis in hepatocellular carcinoma. *J Pathol* 1999;187:439–445.
117. Suehiro T, Matsumata T, Itasaka H, Yamamoto K, Kawahara N, Sugimachi K. Clinicopathologic features and prognosis of resected hepatocellular carcinomas of varied sizes with special reference to proliferating cell nuclear antigen. *Cancer* 1995;76:399–405.
118. Ito Y, Matsuura N, Sakon M, et al. Both cell proliferation and apoptosis significantly predict shortened disease-free survival in hepatocellular carcinoma. *Br J Cancer* 1999;81:747–751.
119. Yamamoto K, Takenaka K, Kajiyama K, et al. Cell proliferation and cell loss in nodule-in-nodule hepatocellular carcinoma. *Hepatogastroenterology* 1999;46:813–819.
120. Nakajima T, Moriguchi M, Mitsumoto Y, et al. Simple tumor profile chart based on cell kinetic parameters and histologic grade is useful for estimating the natural growth rate of hepatocellular carcinoma. *Hum Pathol* 2002;33:92–99.
121. Ozturk M. Genetic aspects of hepatocellular carcinogenesis. *Semin Liver Dis* 1999;19:235–242.
122. Ng IO. Prognostic significance of pathological and biological factors in hepatocellular carcinoma. *J Gastroenterol Hepatol* 1998;13:666–670.
123. Joo M, Kang YK, Kim MR, Lee HK, Jang JJ. Cyclin D1 overexpression in hepatocellular carcinoma. *Liver* 2001;21:89–95.
124. Huo TI, Wang XW, Forgues M, et al. Hepatitis B virus X mutants derived from human hepatocellular carcinoma retain the ability to abrogate p53-induced apoptosis. *Oncogene* 2001;20:3620–3628.
125. Hui AM, Li X, Makuuchi M, Takayama T, Kubota K. Over-expression and lack of retinoblastoma protein are associated with tumor progression and metastasis in hepatocellular carcinoma. *Int J Cancer* 1999;84:604–608.
126. Jeng KS, Sheen IS, Chen BF, Wu JY. Is the p53 gene mutation of prognostic value in hepatocellular carcinoma after resection? *Arch Surg* 2000;135:1329–1333.
127. Naka T, Toyota N, Kaneko T, Kaibara N. Protein expression of p53, p21WAF1, and Rb as prognostic indicators in patients with surgically treated hepatocellular carcinoma. *Anticancer Res* 1998;18:555–564.
128. Kondoh N, Wakatsuki T, Hada A, et al. Genetic and epigenetic events in human hepatocarcinogenesis. *Int J Oncol* 2001;18:1271–1278.
129. Peng XM, Peng WW, Yao JL. Codon 249 mutations of p53 gene in development of hepatocellular carcinoma. *World J Gastroenterol* 1998;4:125–127.
130. Shiota G, Kishimoto Y, Suyama A, et al. Prognostic significance of serum anti-p53 antibody in patients with hepatocellular carcinoma. *J Hepatol* 1997;27:661–668.
131. Zhao M, Zimmermann A. Liver cell dysplasia: reactivities for c-met protein, Rb protein, E- cadherin and transforming growth factor-beta 1 in comparison with hepatocellular carcinoma. *Histol Histopathol* 1998;13:657–670.
132. Azechi H, Nishida N, Fukuda Y, et al. Disruption of the p16/cyclin D1/retinoblastoma protein pathway in the majority of human hepatocellular carcinomas. *Oncology* 2001;60:346–354.
133. Cohen C, DeRose PB. Immunohistochemical p53 in hepatocellular carcinoma and liver cell dysplasia. *Mod Pathol* 1994;7:536–539.
134. Hui AM, Makuuchi M. Molecular basis of multistep hepatocarcinogenesis: genetic and epigenetic events. *Scand J Gastroenterol* 1999;34:737–742.
135. Tannapfel A, Grund D, Katalinic A, et al. Decreased expression of p27 protein is associated with advanced tumor stage in hepatocellular carcinoma. *Int J Cancer* 2000;89:350–355.
136. Inagawa S, Itabashi M, Adachi S, et al. Expression and prognostic roles of beta-catenin in hepatocellular carcinoma: correlation with tumor progression and postoperative survival. *Clin Cancer Res* 2002;8:450–456.

137. Asayama Y, Taguchi Ki K, Aishima Si S, Nishi H, Masuda K, Tsuneyoshi M. The mode of tumour progression in combined hepatocellular carcinoma and cholangiocarcinoma: an immunohistochemical analysis of E-cadherin, alpha-catenin and beta-catenin. *Liver* 2002;22:43–50.
138. Yuen MF, Wu PC, Lai VC, Lau JY, Lai CL. Expression of c-Myc, c-Fos, and c-jun in hepatocellular carcinoma. *Cancer* 2001;91:106–112.
139. Kawate S, Fukusato T, Ohwada S, Watanuki A, Morishita Y. Amplification of c-myc in hepatocellular carcinoma: correlation with clinicopathologic features, proliferative activity and p53 overexpression. *Oncology* 1999;57:157–163.
140. Miura N, Horikawa I, Nishimoto A, et al. Progressive telomere shortening and telomerase reactivation during hepatocellular carcinogenesis. *Cancer Genet Cytogenet* 1997;93:56–62.
141. Nakashio R, Kitamoto M, Nakanishi T, Takaishi H, Takahashi S, Kajiyama G. [Telomere length and telomerase activity in hepatocellular carcinoma]. *Nippon Rinsho* 1998;56:1239–1243.
142. Park Y, Choi J, Byun B, Cho C, Kim H, Kim B. Telomerase is strongly activated in hepatocellular carcinoma but not in chronic hepatitis and cirrhosis. *Exp Mol Med* 1998;30:35–40.
143. Sun BH, Zhang J, Wang BJ, et al. Analysis of in vivo patterns of caspase 3 gene expression in primary hepatocellular carcinoma and its relationship to p21(WAF1) expression and hepatic apoptosis. *World J Gastroenterol* 2000;6:356–360.
144. Kojiro M, Nakashima O. Histopathologic evaluation of hepatocellular carcinoma with special reference to small early stage tumors. *Semin Liver Dis* 1999;19:287–296.
145. Nakanuma Y, Terada T, Terasaki S, et al. 'Atypical adenomatous hyperplasia' in liver cirrhosis: low-grade hepatocellular carcinoma or borderline lesion? *Histopathology* 1990;17:27–35.
146. Tsuda H, Hirohashi S, Shimosato Y, Terada M, Hasegawa H. Clonal origin of atypical adenomatous hyperplasia of the liver and clonal identity with hepatocellular carcinoma. *Gastroenterology* 1988;95:1664–1666.
147. Farber E. Hepatocyte proliferation in stepwise development of experimental liver cell cancer. *Dig Dis Sci* 1991;36:973–978.
148. Marsh JW, Dvorchik I, Subotin M, et al. The prediction of risk of recurrence and time to recurrence of hepatocellular carcinoma after orthotopic liver transplantation: a pilot study. *Hepatology* 1997;26:444–450.
149. Mor E, Kaspa RT, Sheiner P, Schwartz M. Treatment of hepatocellular carcinoma associated with cirrhosis in the era of liver transplantation. *Ann Intern Med* 1998;129:643–653.
150. Schulte-Hermann R, Timmermann-Trosiener I, Barthel G, Bursch W. DNA synthesis, apoptosis, and phenotypic expression as determinants of growth of altered foci in rat liver during phenobarbital promotion. *Cancer Res* 1990;50:5127–5135.
151. Tannapfel A, Wittekind C. Genes involved in hepatocellular carcinoma: deregulation in cell cycling and apoptosis. *Virchows Arch* 2002;440:345–352.
152. Laurent-Puig P, Legoix P, Bluteau O, et al. Genetic alterations associated with hepatocellular carcinomas define distinct pathways of hepatocarcinogenesis. *Gastroenterology* 2001; 120:1763–1773.
153. Buendia MA. Genetics of hepatocellular carcinoma. *Semin Cancer Biol* 2000;10:185–200.
154. Dumble ML, Croager EJ, Yeoh GC, Quail EA. Generation and characterization of p53 null transformed hepatic progenitor cells: oval cells give rise to hepatocellular carcinoma. *Carcinogenesis* 2002;23:435–445.
155. Tarsetti F, Lenzi R, Salvi R, et al. Liver carcinogenesis associated with feeding of ethionine in a choline-free diet: evidence against a role of oval cells in the emergence of hepatocellular carcinoma. *Hepatology* 1993;18:596–603.
156. Wada Y, Nakashima O, Kutami R, Yamamoto O, Kojiro M. Clinicopathological study on hepatocellular carcinoma with lymphocytic infiltration. *Hepatology* 1998;27:407–414.

157. Hsu HC, Wu TT, Sheu JC, et al. Biologic significance of the detection of HBsAg and HBcAg in liver and tumor from 204 HBsAg-positive patients with primary hepatocellular carcinoma. *Hepatology* 1989;9:747–750.
158. Kawata A, Une Y, Hosokawa M, Uchino J, Kobayashi H. Tumor-infiltrating lymphocytes and prognosis of hepatocellular carcinoma. *Jpn J Clin Oncol* 1992;22:256–263.
159. Chedid A, Ryan LM, Dayal Y, Wolf BC, Falkson G. Morphology and other prognostic factors of hepatocellular carcinoma. *Arch Pathol Lab Med* 1999;123:524–528.
160. Berman MM, Libbey NP, Foster JH. Hepatocellular carcinoma. Polygonal cell type with fibrous stroma—an atypical variant with a favorable prognosis. *Cancer* 1980;46:1448–1455.
161. Hoshino H, Katada N, Nishimura D, et al. Case report: fibrolamellar hepatocellular carcinoma in a Japanese woman's case report and review of Japanese cases. *J Gastroenterol Hepatol* 1996;11:551–555.
162. Yamaguchi R, Tajika T, Kanda H, Nakanishi K, Kawanishi J. Fibrolamellar carcinoma of the liver. *Hepatogastroenterology* 1999;46:1706–1709.
163. Caballero T, Aneiros J, Lopez-Caballero J, Gomez-Morales M, Nogales F. Fibrolamellar hepatocellular carcinoma. An immunohistochemical and ultrastructural study. *Histopathology* 1985;9:445–456.
164. An T, Ghatak N, Kastner R, Kay S, Lee HM. Hyaline globules and intracellular lumina in a hepatocellular carcinoma. *Am J Clin Pathol* 1983;79:392–396.
165. Lefkowitch JH, Muschel R, Price JB, Marboe C, Braunhut S. Copper and copper-binding protein in fibrolamellar liver cell carcinoma. *Cancer* 1983;51:97–100.
166. Cheuk W, Chan J. Clear cell variant of fibrolamellar carcinoma of the liver. *Arch Pathol Lab Med* 2001;125:1235–1238.
167. Berman MA, Burnham JA, Sheahan DG. Fibrolamellar carcinoma of the liver: an immunohistochemical study of nineteen cases and a review of the literature. *Hum Pathol* 1988;19:784–794.
168. Okano A, Hajiro K, Takakuwa H, Kobashi Y. Fibrolamellar carcinoma of the liver with a mixture of ordinary hepatocellular carcinoma: a case report. *Am J Gastroenterol* 1998;93:1144,1145.
169. Nerlich AG, Majewski S, Hunzelmann N, et al. Excessive collagen formation in fibrolamellar carcinoma of the liver: a morphological and biochemical study. *Mod Pathol* 1992;5:580–585.
170. Orsatti G, Hytiroglou P, Thung SN, Ishak KG, Paronetto F. Lamellar fibrosis in the fibrolamellar variant of hepatocellular carcinoma: a role for transforming growth factor beta. *Liver* 1997;17:152–156.
171. Saul SH, Titelbaum DS, Gansler TS, et al. The fibrolamellar variant of hepatocellular carcinoma. Its association with focal nodular hyperplasia. *Cancer* 1987;60:3049–3055.
172. Hemming AW, Langer B, Sheiner P, Greig PD, Taylor BR. Aggressive surgical management of fibrolamellar hepatocellular carcinoma. *J Gastrointest Surg* 1997;1:342–346.
173. Zografos GN, Palmer S, Papastratis G, Habib NA. Aggressive surgical management of fibrolamellar hepatocellular carcinoma in puberty. *Eur J Surg Oncol* 1997;23:570–572.
174. Starzl TE, Iwatsuki S, Shaw BW Jr, Nalesnik MA, Farhi DC, Van Thiel DH. Treatment of fibrolamellar hepatoma with partial or total hepatectomy and transplantation of the liver. *Surg Gynecol Obstet* 1986;162:145–148.
175. Pinna AD, Iwatsuki S, Lee RG, et al. Treatment of fibrolamellar hepatoma with subtotal hepatectomy or transplantation. *Hepatology* 1997;26:877–883.
176. Wu PC, Lai CL, Lam KC, Lok AS, Lin HJ. Clear cell carcinoma of liver. An ultrastructural study. *Cancer* 1983;52:504–507.
177. Sasaki K, Okuda S, Takahashi M, Sasaki M. Hepatic clear cell carcinoma associated with hypoglycemia and hypercholesterolemia. *Cancer* 1981;47:820–822.
178. Emile J, Lemoine A, Azoulay D, Debuire B, Bismuth H, Reynes M. Histological, genomic and clinical heterogeneity of clear cell hepatocellular carcinoma. *Histopathology* 2001;38:225–231.

179. Orsatti G, Arnold MM, Paronetto F. DNA image cytometric analysis of primary clear cell carcinoma of the liver. *Arch Pathol Lab Med* 1994;118:1226–1229.
180. Murakata LA, Ishak KG, Nzeako UC. Clear cell carcinoma of the liver: a comparative immunohistochemical study with renal clear cell carcinoma. *Mod Pathol* 2000;13:874–881.
181. Okuda K. Hepatocellular carcinoma: clinicopathological aspects. *J Gastroenterol Hepatol* 1997;12:S314–S318.
182. Albar JP, De Miguel F, Esbrit P, Miranda R, Fernandez-Flores A, Sarasa JL. Immunohistochemical detection of parathyroid hormone-related protein in a rare variant of hepatic neoplasm (sclerosing hepatic carcinoma). *Hum Pathol* 1996;27:728–731.
183. Yamashita Y, Fan ZM, Yamamoto H, et al. Sclerosing hepatocellular carcinoma: radiologic findings. *Abdom Imaging* 1993;18:347–351.
184. Omata M, Peters RL, Tatter D. Sclerosing hepatic carcinoma: relationship to hypercalcemia. *Liver* 1981;1:33–49.
185. Papotti M, Sambataro D, Marchesa P, Negro F. A combined hepatocellular/cholangiocellular carcinoma with sarcomatoid features. *Liver* 1997;17:47–52.
186. Gil-Benso R, Martinez-Lorente A, Pellin-Perez A, et al. Characterization of a new rat cell line established from 2' AAF-induced combined hepatocellular cholangiocellular carcinoma. *In Vitro Cell Dev Biol Anim* 2001;37:17–25.
187. Akasofu M, Kawahara E, Kaji K, Nakanishi I. Sarcomatoid hepatocellular-carcinoma showing rhabdomyoblastic differentiation in the adult cirrhotic liver. *Virchows Arch* 1999; 434:511–515.
188. Sasaki A, Yokoyama S, Nakayama I, Nakashima K, Kim YI, Kitano S. Sarcomatoid hepatocellular carcinoma with osteoclast-like giant cells: case report and immunohistochemical observations. *Pathol Int* 1997;47:318–324.
189. Leger-Ravet MB, Borgonovo G, Amato A, Lemaigre G, Franco D. Carcinosarcoma of the liver with mesenchymal differentiation: a case report. *Hepatogastroenterology* 1996;43:255–259.
190. Haratake J, Horie A. An immunohistochemical study of sarcomatoid liver carcinomas. *Cancer* 1991;68:93–97.
191. Kim D, Park S, Kim H, Chun Y, Moon W, Park S. A comprehensive karyotypic analysis on a newly established sarcomatoid hepatocellular carcinoma cell line SH-J1 by comparative genomic hybridization and chromosome painting. *Cancer Genet Cytogenet* 2002;132:120–124.
192. Bortolasi L, Marchiori L, Dal Dosso I, Colombari R, Nicoli N. Hepatoblastoma in adult age: a report of two cases. *Hepatogastroenterology* 1996;43:1073–1078.
193. Altmann HW. Epithelial and mixed hepatoblastoma in the adult. Histological observations and general considerations. *Pathol Res Pract* 1992;188:16–26.
194. Ishak KG, Glunz PR. Hepatoblastoma and hepatocarcinoma in infancy and childhood. Report of 47 cases. *Cancer* 1967;20:396–422.
195. Ito E, Sato Y, Kawauchi K, et al. Type 1a glycogen storage disease with hepatoblastoma in siblings. *Cancer* 1987;59:1776–1780.
196. Giardiello FM, Offerhaus GJ, Krush AJ, et al. Risk of hepatoblastoma in familial adenomatous polyposis. *J Pediatr* 1991;119:766–768.
197. Lynch HT, Thorson AG, McComb RD, Franklin BA, Tinley ST, Lynch JF. Familial adenomatous polyposis and extracolonic cancer. *Dig Dis Sci* 2001;46:2325–2332.
198. Weinberg AG, Finegold MJ. Primary hepatic tumors of childhood. *Hum Pathol* 1983;14:512–537.
199. Stocker JT. Hepatoblastoma. *Semin Diagn Pathol* 1994;11:136–143.
200. Ding SF, Michail NE, Habib NA. Genetic changes in hepatoblastoma. *J Hepatol* 1994;20:672–675.
201. Tsuchida Y, Ikeda H, Suzuki N, et al. A case of well-differentiated, fetal-type hepatoblastoma with very low serum alpha-fetoprotein. *J Pediatr Surg* 1999;34:1762–1764.

202. Watanabe I, Yamaguchi M, Kasai M. Histologic characteristics of gonadotropin-producing hepatoblastoma: a survey of seven cases from Japan. *J Pediatr Surg* 1987;22:406–411.
203. Conran RM, Hitchcock CL, Waclawiw MA, Stocker JT, Ishak KG. Hepatoblastoma: the prognostic significance of histologic type. *Pediatr Pathol* 1992;12:167–183.
204. Joshi VV, Kaur P, Ryan B, Saad S, Walters TR. Mucoid anaplastic hepatoblastoma. A case report. *Cancer* 1984;54:2035–2039.
205. Sola Perez J, Perez-Guillermo M, Bas Bernal AB, Mercader JM. Hepatoblastoma. An attempt to apply histologic classification to aspirates obtained by fine needle aspiration cytology. *Acta Cytol* 1994;38:175–182.
206. Pollice L, Zito FA, Troia M. Hepatoblastoma: a clinico-pathologic review. *Pathologica* 1992;84:25–32.
207. Ruck P, Harms D, Kaiserling E. Neuroendocrine differentiation in hepatoblastoma. An immunohistochemical investigation. *Am J Surg Pathol* 1990;14:847–855.
208. Kasai M, Watanabe I. Histologic classification of liver-cell carcinoma in infancy and childhood and its clinical evaluation. A study of 70 cases collected in Japan. *Cancer* 1970;25:551–563.
209. Gonzalez-Crussi F. Undifferentiated small cell ("anaplastic") hepatoblastoma. *Pediatr Pathol* 1991;11:155–161.
210. Lack EE, Neave C, Vawter GF. Hepatoblastoma. A clinical and pathologic study of 54 cases. *Am J Surg Pathol* 1982;6:693–705.
211. Emura I, Ohnishi Y, Yamashita Y, Iwafuchi M. Immunohistochemical and ultrastructural study on erythropoiesis in hepatoblastoma. *Acta Pathol Jpn* 1985;35:79–86.
212. Gonzalez-Crussi F, Upton MP, Maurer HS. Hepatoblastoma. Attempt at characterization of histologic subtypes. *Am J Surg Pathol* 1982;6:599–612.
213. Manivel C, Wick MR, Abenoza P, Dehner LP. Teratoid hepatoblastoma. The nosologic dilemma of solid embryonic neoplasms of childhood. *Cancer* 1986;57:2168–2174.
214. Morinaga S, Yamaguchi M, Watanabe I, Kasai M, Ojima M, Sasano N. An immunohistochemical study of hepatoblastoma producing human chorionic gonadotropin. *Cancer* 1983;51:1647–1652.
215. Abenoza P, Manivel JC, Wick MR, Hagen K, Dehner LP. Hepatoblastoma: an immunohistochemical and ultrastructural study. *Hum Pathol* 1987;18:1025–1035.
216. Tagge EP, Tagge DU, Reyes J, et al. Resection, including transplantation, for hepatoblastoma and hepatocellular carcinoma: impact on survival. *J Pediatr Surg* 1992;27:292–296; discussion, 297.
217. Filler RM, Ehrlich PF, Greenberg ML, Babyn PS. Preoperative chemotherapy in hepatoblastoma. *Surgery* 1991;110:591–596; discussion, 596,597.
218. Saxena R, Leake JL, Shafford EA, et al. Chemotherapy effects on hepatoblastoma. A histological study. *Am J Surg Pathol* 1993;17:1266–1271.
219. Haas JE, Muczynski KA, Krailo M, et al. Histopathology and prognosis in childhood hepatoblastoma and hepatocarcinoma. *Cancer* 1989;64:1082–1095.

5 Use of Imaging Techniques to Screen for Hepatocellular Carcinoma

Michael P. Federle, MD

Contents

1. INTRODUCTION

Accurate detection, characterization, and staging of hepatocellular carcinoma (HCC) are among the most difficult challenges facing radiologists and other physicians caring for patients with chronic liver disease. Most HCCs occur within the cirrhotic liver, and the diffuse and focal abnormalities that characterize the cirrhotic liver often are difficult to differentiate by any imaging test. Nevertheless, cross-sectional imaging methods (sonography, computed tomography [CT], and magnetic resonance imaging [MRI]) are applied frequently in the evaluation and surveillance of patients with chronic liver disease, and much has been learned about the relative merits and accuracy of these tools. There are substantial variations among investigations regarding recommendations for the choice and timing of imaging studies, many of which reflect the relative geographic prevalence of HCC and the availability and expense of imaging tests, as well as the enthusiasm and expertise of the interpreting physicians. This chapter reviews the current knowledge and published recommendations for imaging surveillance of chronic liver disease and presents our approach at the University of Pittsburgh Medical Center.

From: *Current Clinical Oncology: Hepatocellular Cancer: Diagnosis and Treatment*
Edited by: B. I. Carr © Humana Press Inc., Totowa, NJ

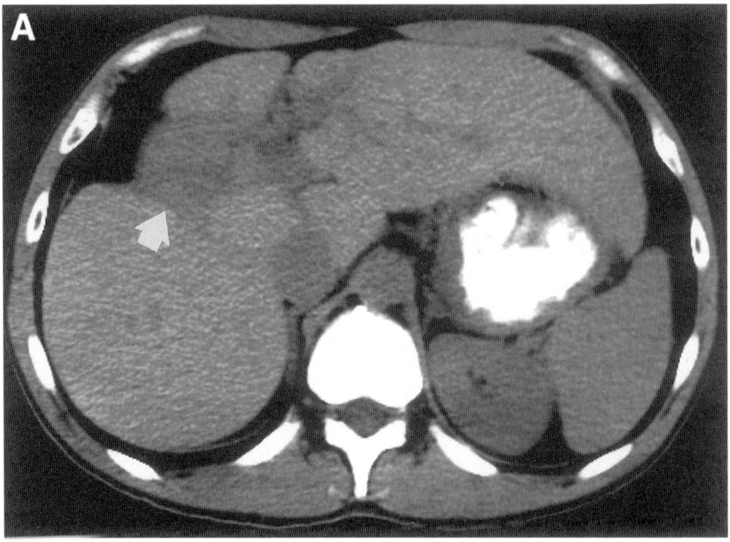

2. MONITORING THE CIRRHOTIC PATIENT

A variety of clinical and biochemical parameters are used to observe the progression of cirrhosis, including serum tests of liver function and tumor markers, such as α-fetoprotein (AFP) and protein induced by vitamin K absence or antagonist (PIVKA II). The role of imaging is to measure and characterize the morphological manifestations of cirrhosis (liver size, scarring, etc.), to evaluate the hepatic and extrahepatic vasculature, to assess the effects of portal hypertension, and to detect and characterize focal hepatic masses.

3. FOCAL LESIONS IN THE CIRRHOTIC LIVER

3.1. Fibrosis

Fibrosis is present in all cirrhotic livers but uncommonly is visualized as a discrete structure on cross-sectional imaging. Fibrosis imparts the coarse, heterogeneous echo pattern that is the typical ultrasound appearance of the cirrhotic liver. When fibrosis forms thick septa or a confluent mass, it is detectable by CT or MRI. Confluent fibrosis can be mistaken for a mass lesion *(1,2)* but has a characteristic set of features that allows confident diagnosis in most cases. On unenhanced CT, it is hypodense to liver. On contrast-enhanced CT, the fibrotic area shows progressive and prolonged enhancement and evidence of volume loss of the affected part of the liver, resulting in crowded vessels and hepatic capsular retraction (Fig. 1). MRI shows similar morphological features, including delayed

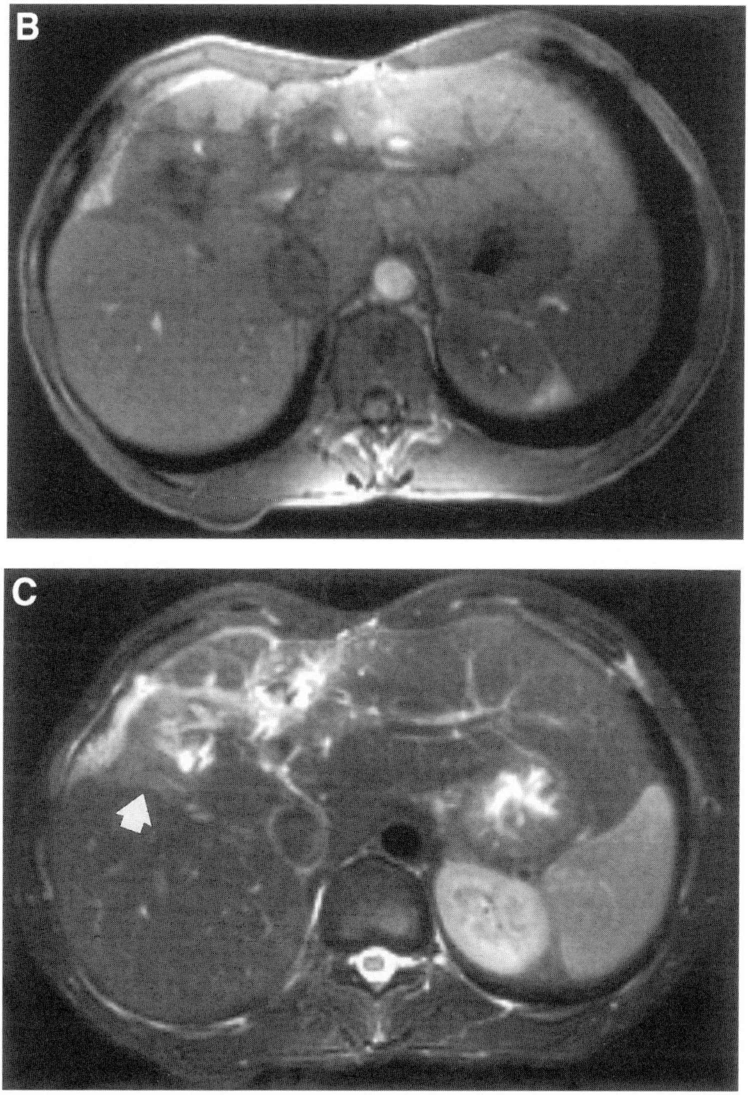

Fig. 1. (*opposite page and above*) Confluent hepatic fibrosis. **(A)** Unenhanced CT scan showing a hypodense lesion (arrow) bridging the anterior and medial segments of the liver. Note the overlying retraction of the hepatic capsule indicating volume loss of this part of the liver. The lesion was isodense to the liver (invisible) on enhanced CT scans. **(B)** T1-weighted MRI section showing the lesion as a hypointense focus. **(C)** The fibrotic lesion (arrow) is hyperintense on T2-weighted images.

persistent enhancement with intravenous gadolinium (gadopentetate dimeglumine) contrast material. More intense enhancement on arterial or portal venous phase images (CT or MRI) may make it difficult to distinguish confluent fibrosis from an infiltrative neoplasm such as HCC or cholangiocarcinoma.

3.2. Regenerating Nodules

The regenerating nodules of the cirrhotic liver include macronodular (typical in chronic hepatitis B) and micronodular (more common in other causes of cirrhosis). Most regenerating nodules are not detected as discrete masses by cross-sectional imaging because they are too small or are too similar to surrounding liver parenchyma in terms of echogenicity (ultrasound), density or attenuation (CT), or intensity (MRI).

Ultrasound may suggest a regenerating nodule as a relatively hypoechoic lesion relative to the surrounding hyperechoic fibrotic cirrhotic liver; however, ultrasound cannot accurately distinguish between regenerating nodules and malignant masses. Almost all sonographically detected focal hepatic lesions within a cirrhotic liver require further evaluation by CT or MRI, percutaneous image-guided biopsy, or a combination thereof.

CT detects regenerating nodules when they are surrounded by fibrosis (with the fibrotic bands being hypodense on unenhanced CT) or when they contain iron deposits, so-called siderotic nodules. Regenerating nodules typically are hyperdense to liver on nonenhanced CT and are isodense to liver (undetectable) on hepatic arterial and portal venous phase CT images (Fig. 2) *(3)*.

MRI detects more regenerating nodules than CT, although it, too, depicts only the larger or more siderotic nodules. Most regenerating nodules are isointense to liver on both T1- and T2-weighted images. Siderotic nodules have characteristic imaging features, including decreased signal intensity on T2-weighted pulse sequences and "blooming" (appearing larger and more prominent) on gradient echo sequences with longer echo times (Fig. 3) *(4)*.

Regenerating nodules usually enhance to the same or a lesser degree than the surrounding liver, a feature that makes them less apparent on contrast-enhanced CT or MRI examinations but that serves as a useful distinguishing feature from other focal lesions. However, some cirrhotic nodules demonstrate definite enhancement, making them impossible to distinguish from dysplastic nodules or even HCC in some cases.

3.3. Dysplastic Nodules

Sakamoto et al. *(5)* and other Japanese investigators *(6)* have proposed that HCC frequently develops from pre-existing regenerating nodules that have undergone metaplastic or dysplastic change. Analogous to a colonic adenoma evolving into a colonic carcinoma, this theory proposes that some overt HCCs

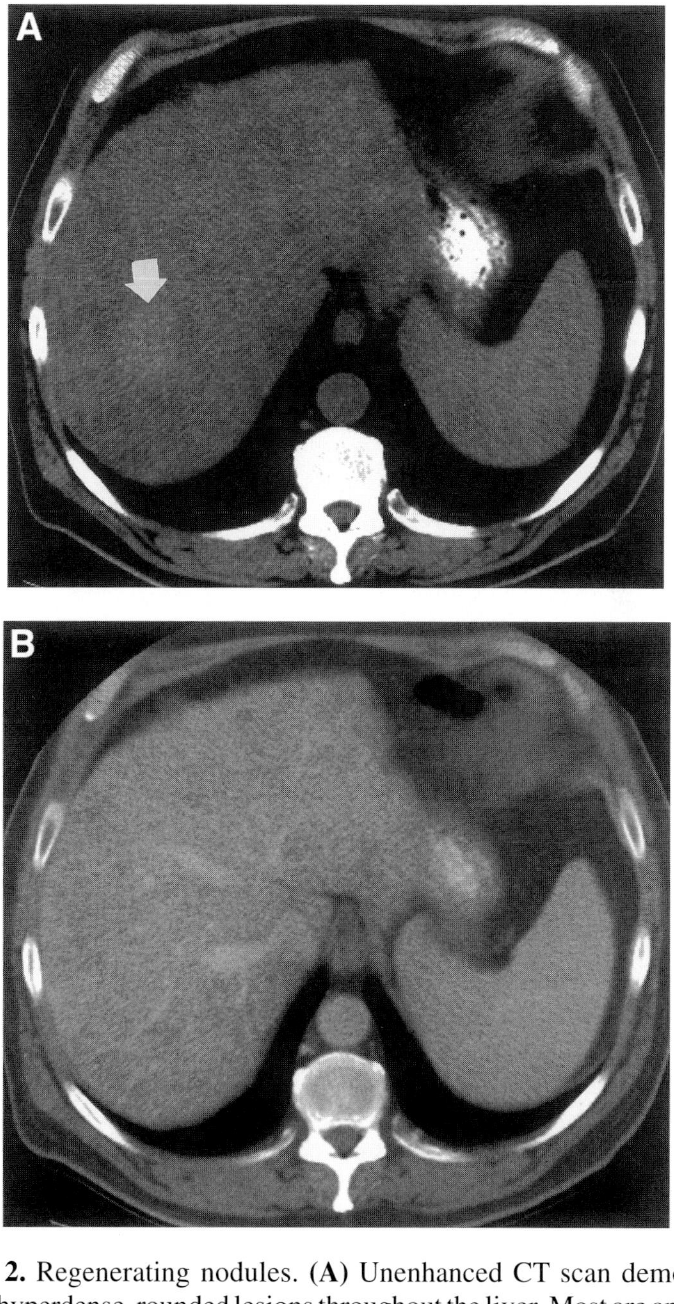

Fig. 2. Regenerating nodules. **(A)** Unenhanced CT scan demonstrating dozens of hyperdense, rounded lesions throughout the liver. Most are approx 1 cm in diameter, whereas one (arrow) is 3 cm. **(B)** Enhanced CT (portal venous phase). The nodules become isodense with the liver and can not be detected.

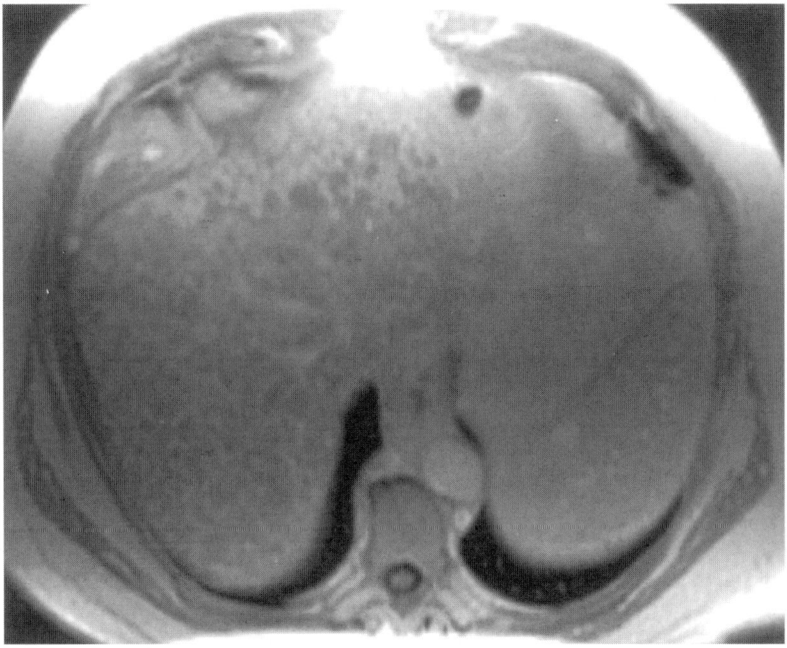

Fig. 3. Regenerating nodules. Gradient echo T1-weighted MRI scan demonstrating innumerable dark (hypointense) subcentimeter lesions representing siderotic nodules. These nodules were undetectable on CT and standard T1-weighted images.

are the end result of a multistep evolution of regenerating nodule to a low-grade then high-grade dysplastic nodule, and subsequently into HCC. Accordingly, dysplastic nodules are considered premalignant. Dysplastic nodules are found in 11–25% of explanted livers at transplantation *(7–9)*.

Unfortunately, dysplastic nodules are difficult to recognize on imaging and may have features in common with regenerating nodules or HCC. Dysplastic nodules are reported to show homogeneous low echogenicity and, on Doppler sonography, continuous afferent waveform signals that reflect their portal venous supply, rather than pulsatile arterial flow *(10)*. In our practice, we have rarely diagnosed or even correctly suggested the presence of a dysplastic nodule by sonography. Bennett et al. *(11)* detected only 1.6% of dysplastic nodules within cirrhotic livers by sonography compared with thin-section explanted liver pathological results.

Because dysplastic nodules receive predominantly portal venous flow, they usually do not demonstrate bright enhancement on arterial phase CT or MRI. Therefore, marked arterial phase enhancement should suggest HCC rather than dysplastic nodule, although well-differentiated HCCs often show substantial portal venous rather than arterial enhancement *(9,12)*. A diagnosis of dysplastic nodule can be suggested based on a CT finding of a small nodule (≤2 cm) that is nonencapsulated and hypodense to surrounding liver on enhanced CT scan. However, CT is quite limited in diagnosing dysplastic nodules, with reported sensitivity of 10–34% *(7,9)* and poor specificity as well.

MRI offers the most promise in diagnosing dysplastic nodules that are reported to demonstrate isointensity or hyperintensity on T1-weighted images and hypointensity on T2-weighed images, in sharp contrast to typical findings for HCC (Fig. 4) *(13)*. Arterial phase bright enhancement should suggest development of a focus of HCC within a dysplastic nodule. However, in an excellent study comparing MRI with explanted livers among transplantation recipients, Krinsky et al. *(8)* were able to detect only 15% of dysplastic nodules on pretransplant MRI studies. Moreover, 4 of 59 dysplastic nodules demonstrated arterial phase enhancement and were mistaken for HCC. Finally, some nondysplastic regenerating nodules were hyperintense and hypointense on T1- and T2-weighted images, respectively, further limiting the specificity of MRI for this diagnosis.

The typical CT and MRI findings that may be helpful in distinguishing among various nodular lesions in the cirrhotic liver are summarized in Table 1.

4. HEPATOCELLULAR CARCINOMA

Detection of any mass lesion is dependent on its size and the "contrast difference" between the mass and the surrounding liver. Distinguishing a small nodular HCC within the cirrhotic liver is challenging, especially because the "background" liver is usually heterogeneous because of varying amounts of fibrosis, necrosis, fat, regenerating nodules, and so forth. Almost all imaging tests rely on intravascular administration of contrast media to increase the conspicuity of mass vs liver, as well as to characterize the hemodynamic features of the mass.

Ultrasonography often is used as a screening method for high-risk patients and is repeated at frequent intervals. A small HCC may be hypoechoic, hyperechoic, or isoechoic on sonography; the latter is detectable only if set off by a peripheral halo or pseudocapsule *(10)*. Early work with "microbubble" sonographic contrast agents suggests that they are useful in demonstrating heterogeneous hypervascularity within HCC and may increase the sensitivity and specificity of sonography in diagnosing HCC *(14)*. HCC is never diagnosed by sonography alone; percutaneous biopsy, usually preceded by CT, MRI, or angiography alone or in combination, is routine. Moreover, even in the small adult, it is difficult to avoid sonographic "blind spots" in the liver because of overlying ribs or bowel gas or excessive fibrosis or fat that attenuates the ultrasound beam.

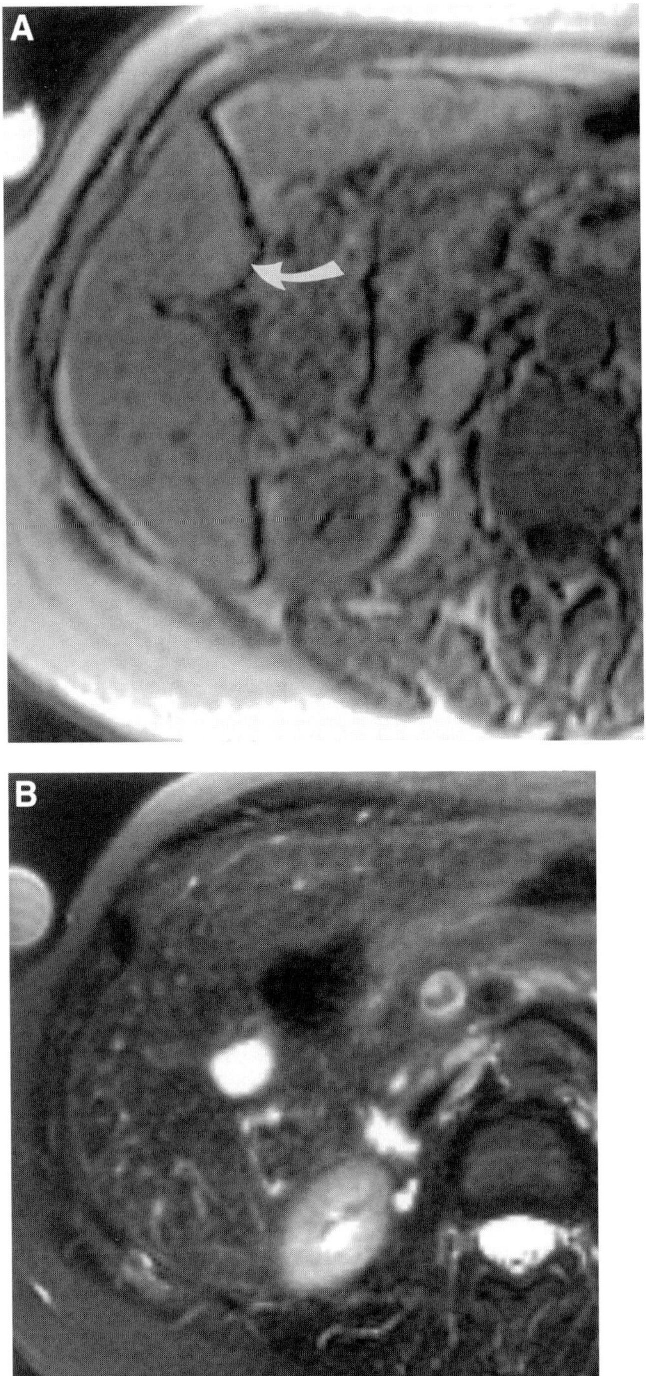
A
B

Table 1
Nodular Lesions in Cirrhosis

	CT				*MRI*			
	NC	*HAP*	*PVP*	*Delay*	*T1*	*HAP*	*PVP*	*T2*
Regenerative nodule	— or ↑	—	—	—	— or ↑	—	—	— or ↓
Dysplastic nodule	— or ↑	— or ↑	—	—	— or ↑	— or ↑	—	— or ↓
Well-differentiated HCC	— or ↓	— or ↓	↓	↓	— or ↑	— or ↑	— or ↑	↑
Moderately differentiated HCC	— or ↓	— or ↑	— or ↓	↓	— or ↓	↑	— or ↑	↑

HAP, hepatic arterial phase; PVP, portal venous phase; —, not seen (isodense, isointense); ↑, hyperdense (hyperintense) to liver; ↓, hypointense (hypointense) to liver.

In most institutions, helical CT is the mainstay in imaging surveillance of the cirrhotic liver. Helical CT technology (and newer MRI pulse sequences) allows efficient breath-held scanning through the liver before contrast administration, as well as during the arterial, portal venous, and (in special circumstances) delayed or equilibrium phases of the circulating intravenous bolus of contrast material *(15,16)*. It warrants emphasis to state that a CT or MRI scan performed without multiple phases of imaging or without the rapid intravenous bolus administration of contrast medium will miss most small (treatable) HCCs and is nearly useless as a screening test.

Helical CT allows the detection and characterization of most hepatic masses more than 2 cm in diameter. Common benign lesions, such as cysts, hemangiomas, and focal fat, should be identified with confidence (Fig. 5), and there is ample documentation of the reliability of CT findings in this setting *(17,18)*.

HCCs can have a variety of appearances on CT, but the morphological and hemodynamic characteristics of this tumor are well depicted. Large tumors are heterogeneous and often multifocal and frequently obstruct or invade intrahe-

---

Fig. 4. Dysplastic nodule. **(A)** T1-weighted MRI scan demonstrating a 1.5-cm nodule (arrow) that is slightly hyperintense to surrounding liver. **(B)** T2-weighted MRI scan showing the same lesion is slightly hypointense to liver.

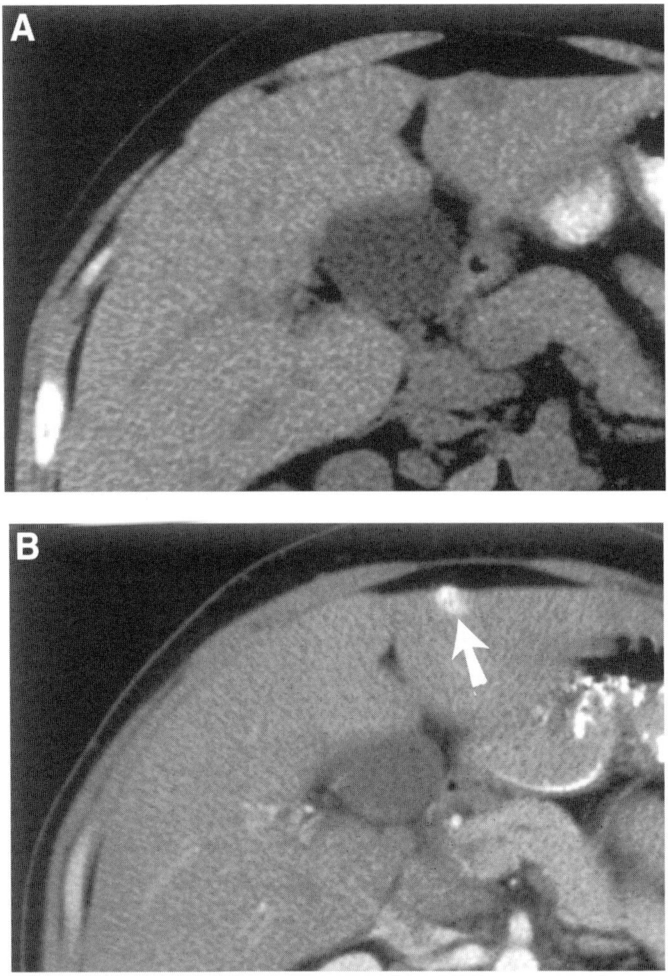

patic bile ducts or the hepatic or portal veins (Fig. 6). Large tumors such as these are relatively easy to detect and stage by CT but are not curable and, as such, represent a failure of screening.

Aggressive screening should result in detection of much smaller HCCs that often are amenable to treatment, whether for palliation or cure. Small well-differentiated HCCs still may receive predominantly portal venous flow and, therefore, appear relatively hypodense to isodense to liver on the nonenhanced and arterial phase images, and distinctly hypodense to liver on portal venous and delayed phase images (Fig. 7) *(9,12,19)*. Most HCCs, even when small, develop increased arterial flow through tumor vessels and are best detected on the arterial phase CT images as a homogeneous or slightly heterogeneous hyperdense mass

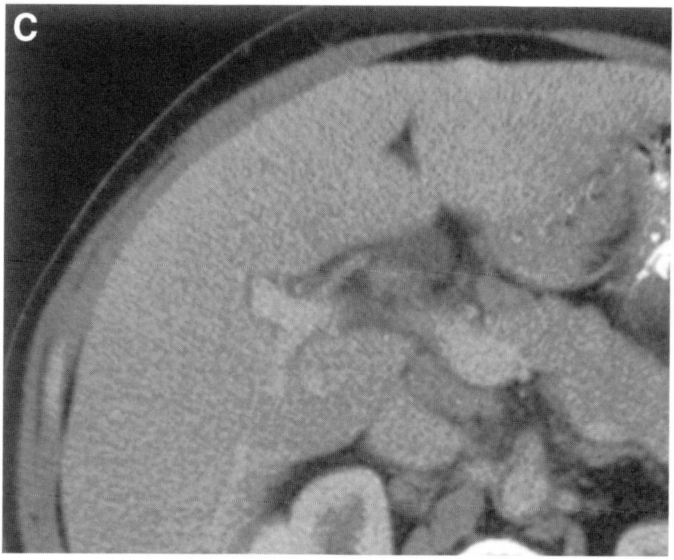

Fig. 5. (*opposite page and above*) Small cavernous hemangioma. **(A)** Unenhanced CT scan. **(B)** Arterial phase enhanced CT scan. **(C)** Portal venous phase CT scan. A 1-cm nodule (arrow) in the lateral segment is isodense with blood vessels on all three phases, identifying it as an hemangioma rather than HCC.

with rapid washout of contrast resulting in a slightly hypodense mass on portal venous or delayed images (Fig. 8). The delayed or equilibrium phase of imaging can be helpful as an added sequence; some HCC will have a capsule or small foci of fat, whereas regenerating and dysplastic nodules do not.

Caution is necessary to avoid mistaking certain perfusion abnormalities of the liver for hypervascular tumors. A small, peripheral wedge-shaped area of increased density seen only on the arterial phase of imaging is a transient hepatic attenuation difference (THAD) and is usually the result of arterioportal shunts or aberrant venous drainage *(20,21)*. Larger segmental or even lobar enhancement differences should prompt close scrutiny for portal venous occlusion or invasion that may result from HCC.

Well-differentiated HCC often contains microscopic or macroscopic deposits of fat that impart characteristic imaging features. Intralesional fat renders the HCC hyperechoic on sonography, hypodense on noncontrast CT, and hyperintense on T1-weighted MRI (Figs. 9 and 10). Some HCCs are surrounded by a complete or partial "capsule" that may be fibrotic and visible as hypodense on nonenhanced CT (and T1-weighted MRI) but becomes hyperdense on delayed enhanced CT (or T2-weighted) images.

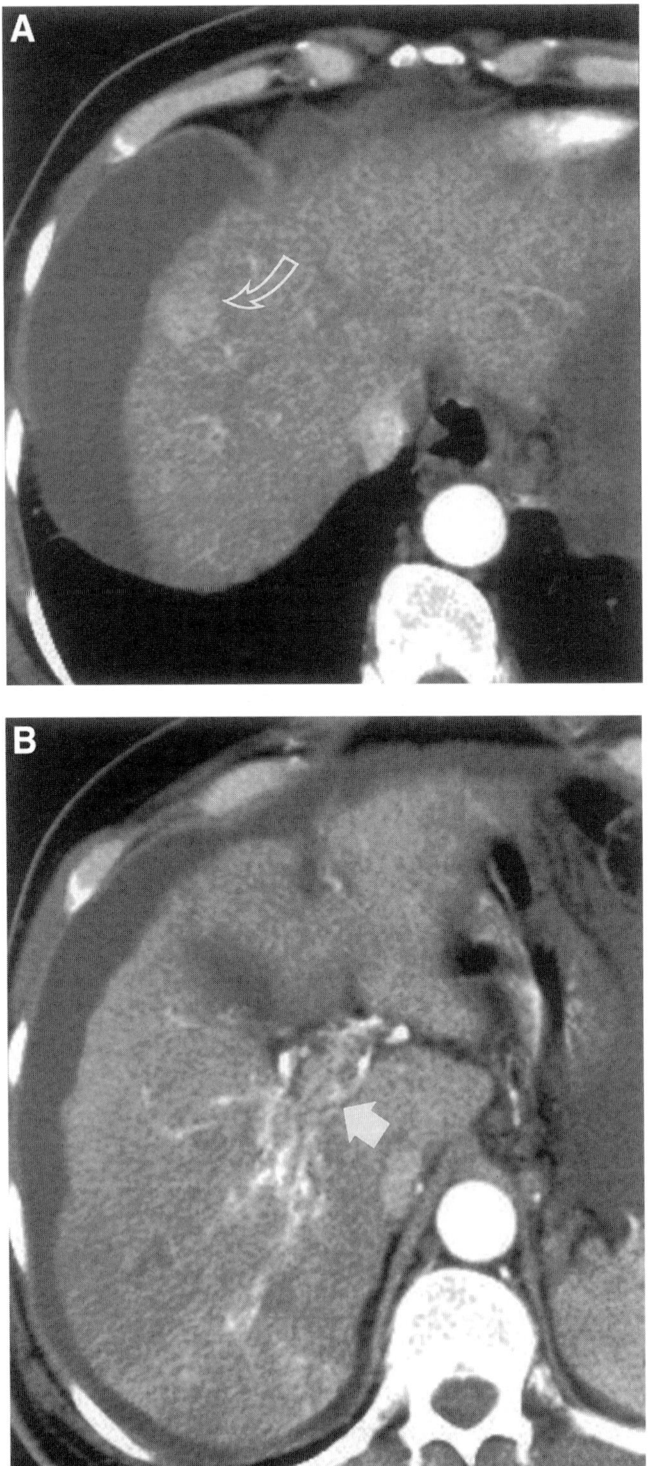
A
B

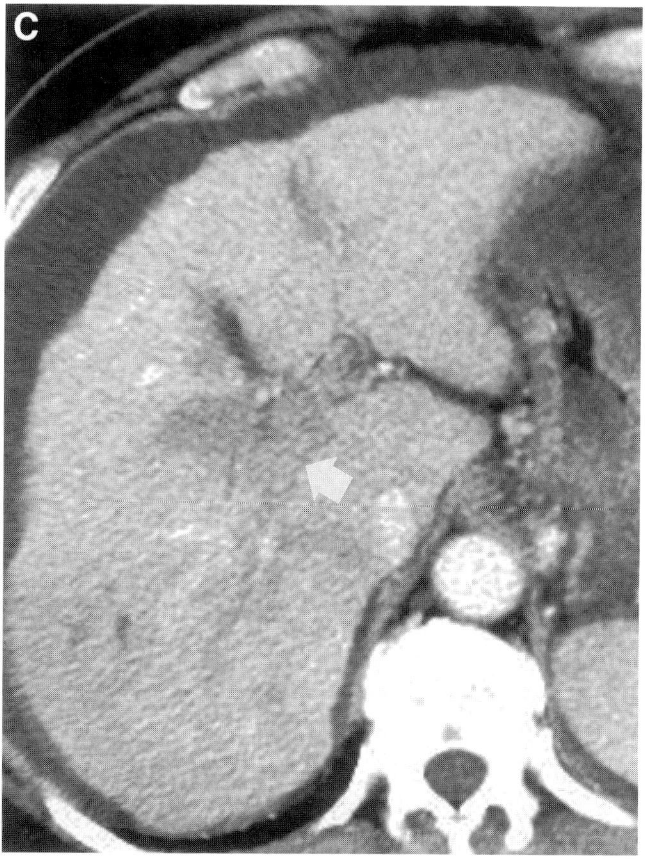

Fig. 6. Hepatocellular carcinoma (HCC). **(A)** Arterial phase CT scan showing a hypervascular 2-cm tumor (arrow). **(B)** Arterial phase CT. The tumor has invaded the portal vein with enhancing tumor thrombus evident (arrow). **(C)** Portal venous phase CT scan. The anterior and posterior branches of the right portal vein are occluded by tumor (arrow).

HCC can be variably intense on T1-weighetd MRI (35% hyperintense, 25% isointense, 40% hypointense), but almost all are hyperintense on T2-weighted images *(22)*. Multiphasic imaging after bolus administration of intravenous contrast medium is just as essential for MRI evaluation of HCC as for CT. The usual intravenous agent is gadolinium (Gd-DTPA, gadopentetate dimeglumine). Arterial, portal venous, and delayed phase imaging demonstrate the same hemodynamic tumor characteristics as detailed for CT *(16,22)*.

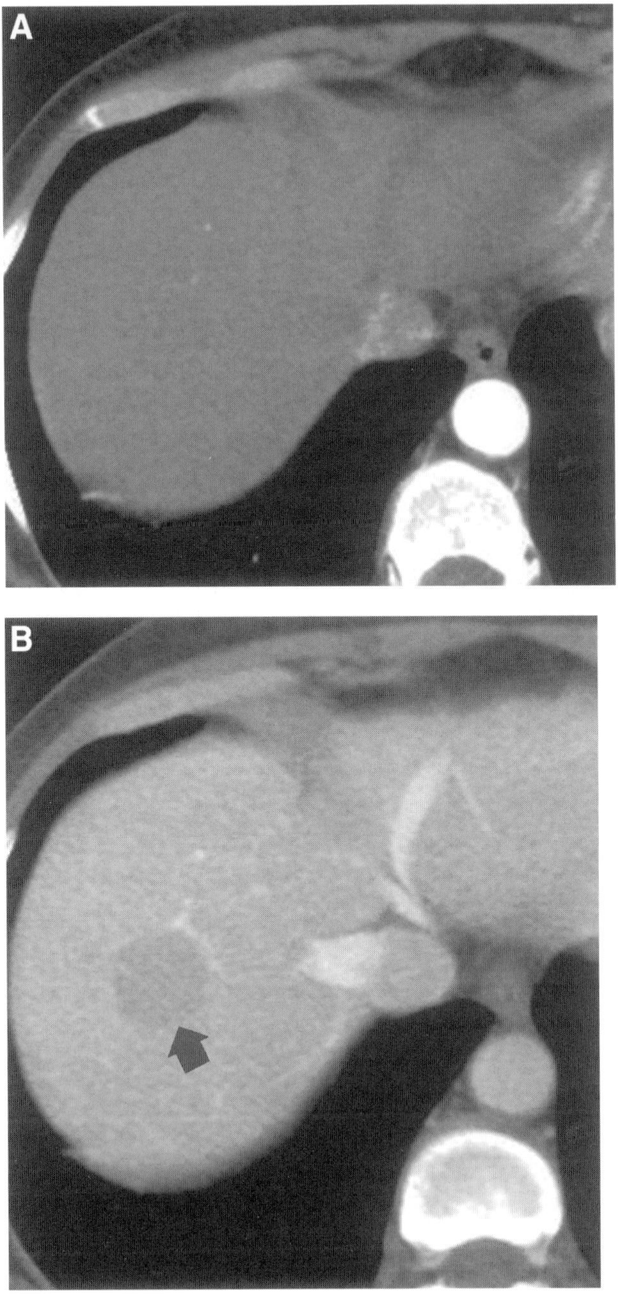

Fig. 7. Well-differentiated HCC. **(A)** Arterial phase CT scan showing no mass. **(B)** Portal venous phase CT scan showing the HCC (arrow) as hypodense to liver.

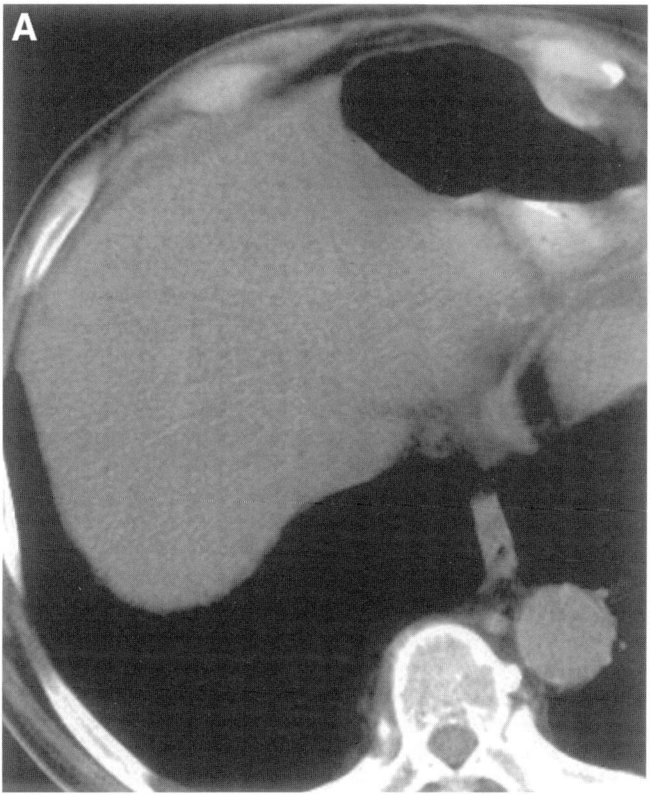

Fig. 8. (*above and page 126*) Moderately differentiated HCC. **(A)** Unenhanced CT scan. **(B)** Arterial phase CT scan. **(C)** Portal venous phase CT scan. The tumor (arrow) is nearly isodense with liver on unenhanced and portal venous phase images, but is hyperdense and visible on arterial phase images because of hypervascularity. Note the capsule around the tumor.

Liver-specific MRI contrast agents occasionally are useful in evaluation of masses within the cirrhotic liver. One class of these agents, the superparamagnetic iron oxides (ferumoxides), is phagocytized by Kupffer cells and accentuates the difference between normal liver and tissue that lacks Kupffer cells. Another class of agents, including mangafodipir (Teslascan; Amersham, Princeton, NJ), is incorporated into functioning hepatocytes and is useful in detecting nonhepatocellular masses. Unfortunately, well-differentiated HCC often contains Kupffer cells and functioning hepatocytes and may not be detected as a tumor *(23)*. Moreover, in the cirrhotic liver, scarring and inflammation may result in decreased uptake of the contrast agents. These agents may help to evaluate the histological grade of HCC, but the practical value of this is uncertain.

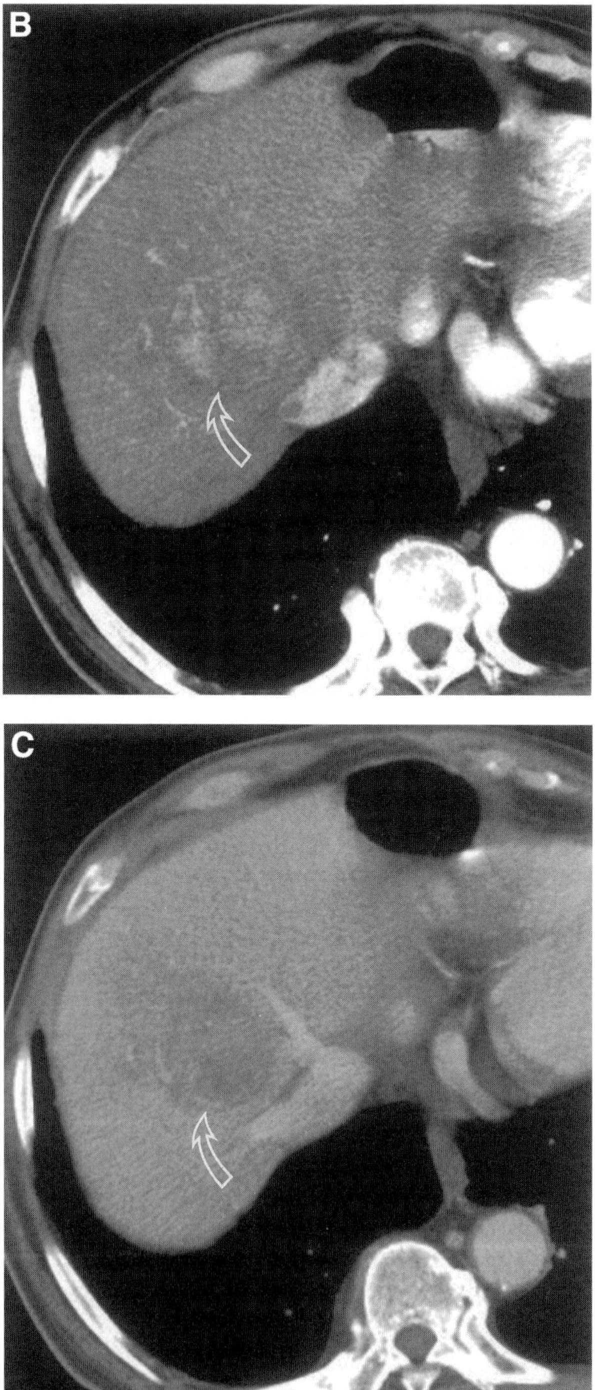
B
C

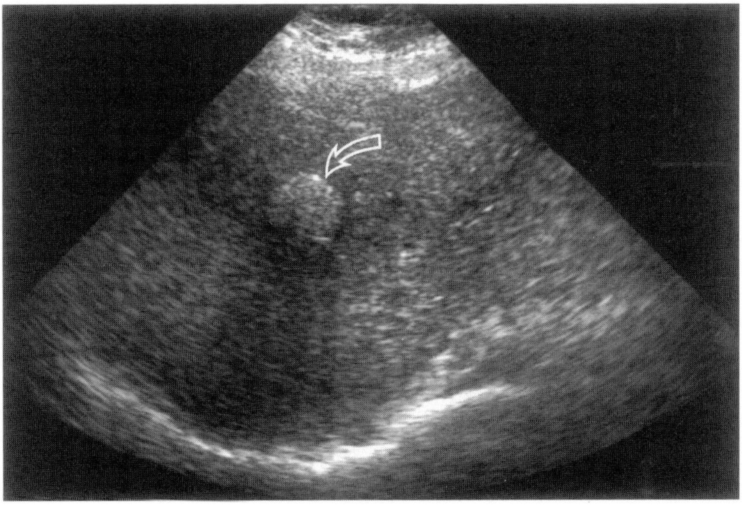

Fig. 9. Fat-containing HCC. Ultrasonography shows an echogenic mass (arrow) with "acoustic shadowing."

5. ACCURACY OF SONOGRAPHY CT AND MRI AS SCREENING METHODS

Many reports claim accuracy, sensitivity, and specificity of more than 90% for CT and MRI in diagnosis of HCC and only slightly less for sonography. Most of these are retrospective studies, report predominantly on large tumors that were known or suspected before imaging, lack a gold standard of proof, and suffer from numerous sources of bias. The most reliable reports are based on investigations comparing the imaging test with pathological examination of the explanted liver or with a combination of sophisticated imaging tests, resection, biopsy, and clinical follow-up. Several studies meet these criteria.

Bennett et al. *(11)* correlated pretransplant sonography results with explant pathological results in 200 patients. Ultrasound detected tumors in only 30% of patients; individual lesion detection sensitivity was 21%. We have had similarly poor success with ultrasound screening in Pittsburgh *(24)*.

Our team in Pittsburgh *(25)* studied 195 patients who had transplantation after single-slice helical dual-phase CT, and 32 patients (16%) were found to have HCC in the explanted liver. We were able to detect these by CT prospectively in only 19 of 32 patients (59%) and found only 23 of 63 HCCs (36%). Eighty-two percent of the HCCs in our series were smaller than 20 mm. Tumor detection rates were higher with CT performed within 60 days before transplantation; some tumors surely arose or grew in the longer intervals between scanning and transplantation.

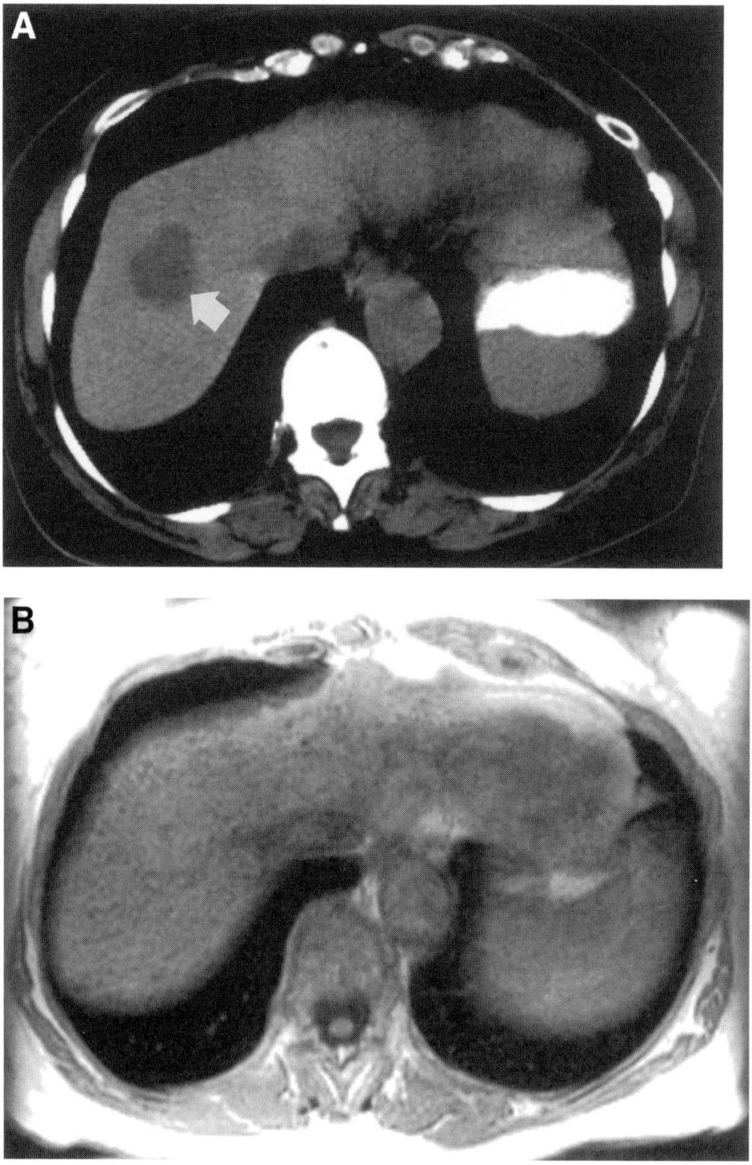

Lim et al. *(9)* studied 41 patients who underwent multiphase CT before liver transplantation; 15 of these patients had 21 HCC nodules found in the explanted liver, with a mean diameter of 19 mm. These investigators were able to detect HCC in 80% of patients (12 of 15), and they identified 15 of 21 HCC (71% sensitivity).

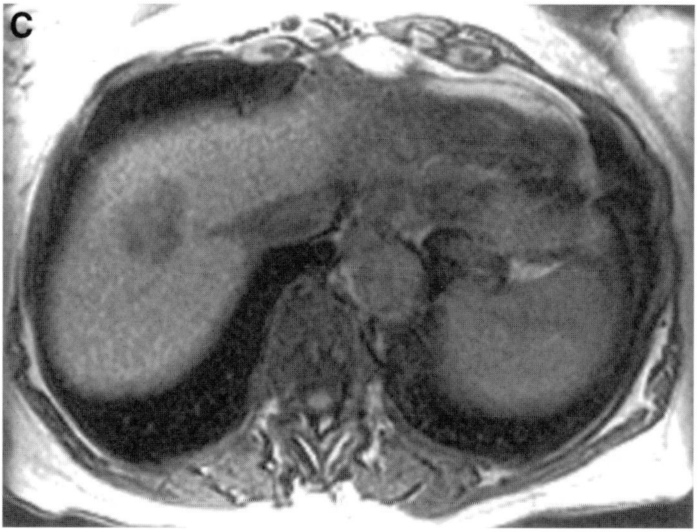

Fig. 10. (*opposite page and above*) Fat-containing HCC. **(A)** Unenhanced CT scan showing markedly hypodense mass (arrow). **(B)** In-phase T1-weighted MRI scan barely detects the mass. **(C)** Out-of-phase T1-weighted MRI scan. There is marked hypointensity indicating signal suppression and lipid content of the HCC.

Murakami et al. *(21)* studied 51 patients with 96 hypervascular HCCs using the latest generation of helical CT (multidetector or multislice CT) and multiphasic imaging that included two sets of arterial phase images. Double arterial phase imaging showed significantly greater sensitivity and specificity than either phase alone, with an overall sensitivity of 86% and positive predictive value of 92%. Only the multislice helical CT scanner is capable of acquiring images through the entire liver in as little as 6 seconds, resulting in a definite diagnostic advantage over single-slice helical and conventional (nonhelical) scanners. The double arterial phase imaging also allowed them to avoid some false-positive diagnoses resulting from arterioportal shunts. The mean size of HCCs in their series was 22 mm, and almost half of the lesions were less than 2 cm in diameter. Hypervascular HCCs clearly are imaged best during the phase of maximum tumor enhancement and minimal hepatic parenchymal enhancement, and this arterial phase may last only a few seconds. Owing to variations in tumor vascularity and patient cardiovascular status, some means of optimally timing the bolus of contrast and initiation of imaging is essential.

Krinsky et al. *(8)* performed multiphasic MRI in 71 patients who had transplantation and pathological correlation of the explanted liver with the prospective MRI interpretation. MRI enabled diagnosis of HCC in only 6 of 11 patients (54%) who had HCC and of only 10 of 19 tumors (53%). The mean size of the HCCs that were missed was 13 mm. Four patients, each with confluent hepatic fibrosis and dysplastic nodules, had a false-positive diagnosis of HCC.

Excluded from the Krinsky study and our Pittsburgh report were patients who had HCC known or suspected before MRI or transplantation. Reporting exclusively on patients with HCC who have had transplantation probably underestimates the accuracy of CT and MRI for several reasons, including the close scrutiny for small lesions in the explanted liver that otherwise may not have come to clinical attention. In addition, many patients are excluded from transplantation because CT or MRI demonstrates advanced HCC, removing them from the study population. Higher sensitivity and specificity can be achieved in patient populations that include larger tumors or those that are symptomatic or are associated with markedly elevated serum tumor markers.

6. WHY, WHEN, AND HOW TO SCREEN

It is clear that detection of curable or treatable HCC by imaging is challenging, but newer therapeutic options make this a worthwhile goal. Small HCCs are amenable to resection or various ablation techniques, such as alcohol injection or radiofrequency coagulation, and surgical treatment for smaller tumors has resulted in improved 5-year survival (Fig. 11) *(26)*. Liver transplantation is an appropriate option for patients with small tumors, with reports of a recurrence-free survival rate of 85% after transplantation in patients with early-stage HCC (one lesion <5 cm or up to three lesions ≤3 cm) *(27,28)*.

The European Association for the Study of the Liver convened a panel of experts on HCC in Barcelona in September 2000 and has published their findings and recommendations for surveillance and management of HCC *(29)*.They note that the prevalence and causes of HCC vary markedly throughout the world, but the most significant risk factor is the presence of cirrhosis, regardless of its cause. As soon as cirrhosis is established, the main predictors of HCC are male gender and increased levels of AFP. However, AFP is not a very good screening test because it has a sensitivity of 39–64%, a specificity of 76–91%, and a positive predictive value of 19–32% *(30,31)*.

The Barcelona panel recommended ultrasonography as the preferred surveillance tool, but noted that sonography is highly operator-dependent and requires specific training and interest to acquire the skills necessary to detect early HCC. The European group recommended that sonography be repeated every 6 months along with serum AFP levels. If the AFP becomes elevated or if a liver nodule is detected by sonography, they recommend helical CT (or MRI or angiography) for further evaluation.

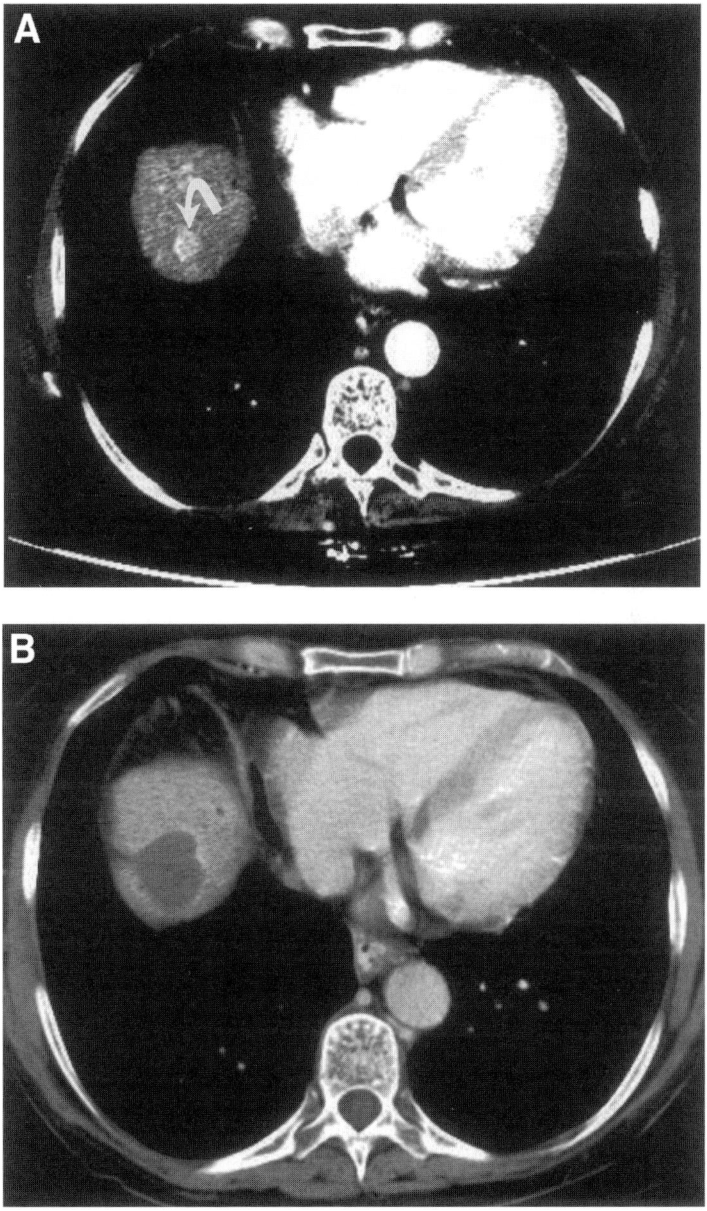

Fig. 11. Small HCC treated with radiofrequency ablation. **(A)** Arterial phase CT scan showing a 1-cm hypervascular nodule (arrow). **(B)** After RF ablation by a probe placed during surgery under ultrasound guidance, the ablation defect is shown, with no viable tumor.

Recommended intervals between surveillance tests are based, in part, on estimates of tumor growth rate. The doubling time of HCC lesions less than 2 cm has been estimated to be 2–12 months *(32–34)*. The Barcelona panel has set a goal of detecting tumors smaller than 3 cm in diameter and recommends surveillance at 6-month intervals, whereas some Japanese groups are much more aggressive, recommending serum AFP, PIVKA measurements, or both every 2 months, sonography every 3 months, and CT or MRI every 6 months *(19)*. This surveillance protocol is applied to patients with established cirrhosis; for patients with chronic hepatitis without established cirrhosis, the intervals are doubled (e.g., AFP every 4 months, sonography every 6 months, CT every 12 months). Murakami et al. *(19)* report that in Japan, this screening protocol has resulted in detection of 20–30% of the HCC nodules when smaller than 2 cm in diameter and detection of 50–60% of the HCC nodules when smaller than 5 cm.

Some modification of these screening protocols may be necessary for applicability to a North American setting for several reasons. Despite recent increases in the prevalence of chronic hepatitis in this country, the prevalence of HCC is still much lower than in Asia or southern Europe, making the disease and its manifestations less familiar to American physicians. For a surveillance program to work properly, patients must be evaluated in their own community; referral to specialized centers usually occurs only after a disease process is documented and treatment is initiated. In most North American medical settings, hepatic sonography will be an ineffective screening tool, in part because American physicians are not likely to perform the detailed dedicated sonographic analysis of the cirrhotic liver necessary to detect and distinguish focal hepatic masses. American cirrhotic patients also are more likely to be larger and to have hepatic steatosis, factors that further limit the accuracy of sonography.

MRI is less appealing as a routine screening test because it is less widely available, more expensive, and less acceptable to many patients. There are considerable technical differences between individual MRI scanners, making it difficult to apply specific imaging protocols or to obtain reproducible results from one setting to another. Nevertheless, MRI may be the single most accurate imaging test assuming optimized technique and expert interpretation.

Helical CT is likely to remain the predominant imaging method for detection and staging of HCC in North America. Technical improvements, especially the rapid emergence of multidetector row (multislice) CT have resulted in improved accuracy that rivals that of more expensive and invasive studies, such as CT catheter angiography and portography. The frequency with which CT should be used for surveillance is likely to remain controversial. I believe that the Barcelona recommendations are too restrictive in the use of CT. It is noteworthy that many Japanese investigators use CT and more invasive studies very liberally despite their enthusiasm for ultrasonography. Ultimately, the choice and timing of screening tests will depend on many factors, including the cause and stage of chronic liver disease, level of serum tumor markers, and local expertise and availability of high-quality imaging. The rapid development of innovative contrast media and improved ultrasound, CT, and MRI scanners makes it mandatory for all physicians involved in the care of patients with chronic liver disease to stay abreast of new developments and to implement these into their own practices.

REFERENCES

1. Ohtomo K, Baron RL, Dodd GD III, Federle MP. Confluent hepatic fibrosis in advanced cirrhosis: appearance at CT. *Radiology* 1993;188:31–35.
2. Ohtomo K, Baron RL, Dodd GD III, Federle MP. Confluent hepatic fibrosis in advanced cirrhosis: evaluation with MR. *Radiology* 1993;189:871–874.
3. Murakami T, Nakamura H, Hoi S, et al. CT and MRI of siderotic regenerating nodules in cirrhotic liver. *J Comput Assist Tomogr* 1992;16:578–582.
4. Ohtomo K, Stoi Y, Ohtomo Y, et al. Regenerating nodules of liver cirrhosis: MR imaging with pathologic correlation. *AJR Am J Roentgenol* 1990;154:505–507.
5. Sakamoto M, Hirohashi S, Shimosato Y. Early stages of multistep hepatocarcinogenesis: adenomatous hyperplasia and early hepatocellular carcinoma. *Hum Pathol* 1991;22:172–178.
6. Takayama T, Makuuchi M, Hirohashi S, et al. Malignant transformation of adenomatous hyperplasia to hepatocellular carcinoma. *Lancet* 1990;336:1150–1153.
7. Dodd GD III, Baron RL, Oliver JH III, Federle MP. Spectrum of imaging findings of the liver in end-stage cirrhosis. Part II: focal abnormalities. *AJR Am J Roentgenol* 1999;173:1185–1192.
8. Krinsky GA, Lee VS, Theise ND, et al. Hepatocellular carcinoma and dysplastic nodules in patients with cirrhosis: prospective diagnosis with MR imaging and explantation correlation. *Radiology* 2001;219:445–454.
9. Lim JH, Kim CK, Lee WJ, et al. Detection of hepatocellular carcinoma and dysplastic nodules in cirrhotic livers: accuracy of helical CT in transplant patients. *AJR Am J Roentgenol* 2000;175:693–698.
10. Tanaka S, Kitamura T, Fujita M, et al. Small hepatocellular carcinoma: differentiation from adenomatous hyperplastic nodule with color Doppler flow imaging. *Radiology* 1992;182: 161–165.
11. Bennett GL, Krinsky GA, Abitbol RJ, et al. Ultrasound detection of hepatocellular carcinoma and dysplastic nodules in patients with cirrhosis: correlation of pretransplant ultrasound findings and liver explant pathology in 200 patients [abstract]. *Am J Roentgenol* 2002;179:75–80.
12. Matsui O, Kadoya M, Kameyama T, et al. Benign and malignant nodules in cirrhotic livers: distinction based on blood supply. *Radiology* 1991;178:493–497.
13. Ebara M, Ohto M, Waranabe Y, et al. Diagnosis of small hepatocellular carcinoma: correlation of MR imaging and tumor histologic studies. *Radiology* 1986;159:371–377.
14. Wilson SR, Burns PN. Liver mass evaluation with ultrasound: the impact of microbubble contrast agents and pulse inversion imaging. *Semin Liver Dis* 2001;21:147–159.
15. Federle MP, Blachar A. CT evaluation of the liver: principles and techniques. *Semin Liver Dis* 2001;21:135–146.
16. Beavers KL, Semelka RC. MRI evaluation of the liver. *Semin Liver Dis* 2001;21:161–194.
17. Kim T, Federle MP, Baron RL, Peterson MS, Kawamori Y. Discrimination of small hepatic hemangiomas from hypervascular malignant tumors smaller than 3cm with three-phase helical CT. *Radiology* 2001;219:699–706.
18. Brancatelli G, Federle MP, Blachar A, Grazioli L. Hemangioma in the cirrhotic liver: diagnosis and natural history. *Radiology* 2001;219:69–74.

19. Murakami T, Mochizaki K, Nakamura H. Imaging evaluation of the cirrhotic liver. *Semin Liver Dis* 2001;21:213–224.
20. Mori K, Yoshioka H, Itai Y, et al. Arterioportal shunts in cirrhotic patients: evaluation of the difference between tumorous and nontumorous arterioportal shunts on MR imaging with superparamagnetic iron oxide. *AJR Am J Roentgenol* 2000;175:1659–1664.
21. Murakami T, Kim T, Takamura M, et al. Hypervascular hepatocellular carcinoma: detection with double arterial phase multi-detector row helical CT. *Radiology* 2001;218:763–767.
22. Kadoya M, Matsui O, Takashima T, Nonomura A. Hepatocellular carcinoma: correlation of MR imaging and histologic findings. *Radiology* 1992;183:819–825.
23. Murakami T, Baron RL, Federle MP, et al. Hepatocellular carcinoma: MR imaging with mangafodipir trisodium (Mn-DPDP). *Radiology* 1996;2000:69–77.
24. Miller WJ, Federle MP, Campbell WL. Diagnosis and staging of hepatocellular carcinoma: comparison of CT and sonography in 36 liver transplantation patients. *AJR Am J Roentgenol* 1991;157:303–306.
25. Peterson MS, Baron RL, Marsh JW Jr, et al. Pretransplant surveillance for possible hepatocellular carcinoma in patients with cirrhosis: epidemiology and CT-based tumor detection rate in 430 cases with surgical pathologic correlation. *Radiology* 2000;217:743–749.
26. Arii S, Tobe T. Results of surgical treatment. Follow-up study by liver cancer study group of Japan. In: *Primary Liver Cancer in Japan* (Tobe T, et al., eds.), Springer Verlag, Tokyo, 1992, pp. 243–255.
27. Mor E, Kaspa RT, Sheiner P, Schwartz M. Treatment of hepatocellular carcinoma associated with cirrhosis in the era of liver transplantation. *Ann Intern Med* 1998;15:129:643–653.
28. Achkar JP, Araya V, Baron RL, et al. Undetected hepatocellular carcinoma: clinical features and outcome after liver transplantation. *Liver Transpl Surg* 1998;4:477–482.
29. Bruix J, Sherman M, Llovet JM, et al. Clinical management of hepatocellular carcinoma. Conclusions of the Barcelona 2000 EASL conference. *J Hepatol* 2001;35:421–430.
30. Collier J, Sherman M. Screening for hepatocellular carcinoma. *Hepatology* 1998;27:273–378.
31. Okuda K. Early recognition of hepatocellular carcinoma. *Hepatology* 1986;6:729–738.
32. Ebara M, Ohto M, Shinagawa T, et al. Natural history of minute hepatocellular carcinoma smaller than three centimeters complicating cirrhosis: a study in 22 patients. *Gastroenterology* 1986;90:289–298.
33. Barbara L, Benzi G, Gaiani S, et al. Natural history of small untreated hepatocellular carcinoma in cirrhosis: a multivariate analysis of prognostic factors of tumor growth rate and patient survival. *Hepatology* 1992;16:132–137.
34. Kaneko S, Unoura M, Kobayashi K. Early detection of hepatocellular carcinoma. In: *Liver Cancer* (Ohuda K, Tabor E, eds.), Churchill Livingstone, New York, 1997, pp. 393–406.

6 Radiological Evaluation of Hepatocellular Carcinoma

Michael P. Federle, MD
and Michael J. Payne, MD

CONTENTS

1. INTRODUCTION

Chapter 5 discusses the rationale and techniques for screening an at-risk population for the presence of hepatocellular carcinoma (HCC). The typical appearance of small HCC on ultrasound CT, and MRI and the challenges inherent in diagnosing early HCC and distinguishing it from regenerating and dysplastic nodules, arterioportal shunts, fibrosis, and other lesions have been noted. When proper computed tomography (CT) and magnetic resonance imaging (MRI) techniques are used with expert interpretation in a well-run screening program, many HCCs should be diagnosed when they are amenable to curative treatments, including resection, ablation, and liver transplantation.

However, many patients in whom HCC develop are not enrolled in screening programs, usually because they and their physicians are unaware that they have a condition that predisposes them to hepatic cancer. It has been estimated that 15–43% of the cases of HCC in North America occur in patients without evidence of cirrhosis *(1–3)*.

In our own recent review of patients at this medical center in whom HCC developed within a noncirrhotic liver *(4)*, we reported on 39 patients, 62% of whom had no identifiable risk factor for HCC, 87% of whom had symptoms related to the tumor. These tumors were large (mean diameter: 12 cm) and were easily detectable on CT, usually as a solitary or dominant mass (Fig. 1). The tumors were well defined and had a lobulated surface. Calcified and hemorrhagic

From: *Current Clinical Oncology: Hepatocellular Cancer: Diagnosis and Treatment*
Edited by: B. I. Carr © Humana Press Inc., Totowa, NJ

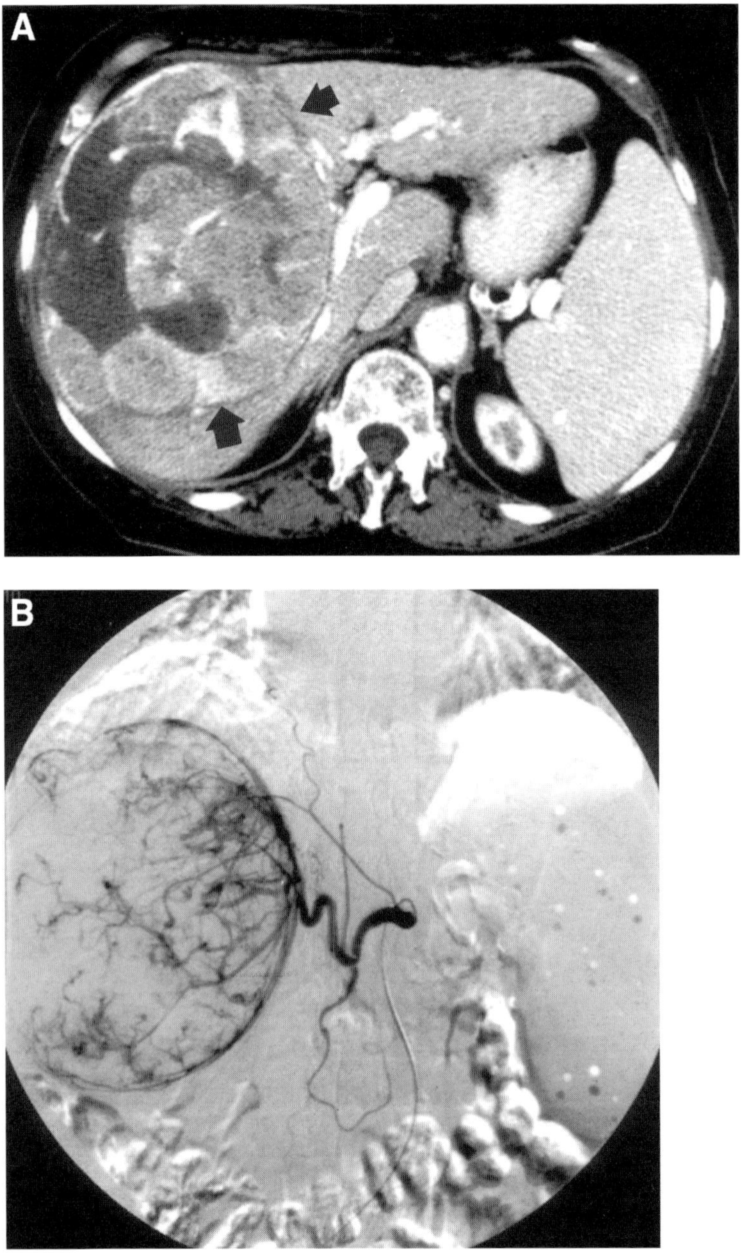

Fig. 1. HCC in a noncirrhotic liver. **(A)** Contrast-enhanced CT scan showing a huge mass (arrow) in the right lobe of liver that is encapsulated with areas of necrosis and hypervascularity. **(B)** Selective hepatic angiogram demonstrating the hypervascular encapsulated mass.

foci were evident in approx 25% and fat in 10%. Almost all tumors were heterogeneous with areas of necrosis and appeared hypodense to liver on nonenhanced CT images, heterogeneously hyperdense at arterial phase, and hypodense at portal phase imaging. Almost half the patients had CT evidence of obstruction or invasion of major intrahepatic bile ducts, portal or hepatic veins, or a combination thereof.

Winston et al. *(5)* described the MRI features of 25 patients with HCC in noncirrhotic liver, comparing these with 11 patients with HCC in cirrhotic liver. They noted that the tumors were significantly larger in the noncirrhotic group, consistent with reports from pathologists, including Yamashita et al. *(3)*. The MRI features mirror the CT findings, including heterogeneity, hypervascularity, and foci of necrosis and hemorrhage.

Some of these imaging characteristics overlap with those of fibrolamellar HCC, although we believe that most cases can be differentiated with confidence on the basis of clinical, laboratory, and imaging findings. Most patients with conventional HCC are male, older (50–70 years), and have positive serum tumor markers. However, fibrolamellar HCC typically occurs in younger patients (mean age: 27 years) with no gender predominance and appears as a large, sharply defined mass with a prominent central scar and radiating bands of fibrosis (71–95%) *(6,7)*. Other features include calcifications within the scar (40–68%); rare hemorrhage, necrosis, or fat; and frequent upper abdominal lymphadenopathy (65%; Fig. 2). On MRI, calcifications are not depicted well, but tumor heterogeneity and hypervascularity are evident, with the bulk of the tumor being hypointense to liver on T1-weighted images and hyperintense at T2-weighted images. The central scar is depicted as hypointense to surrounding tumor.

Because fibrolamellar HCC and focal nodular hyperplasia (FNH) occur in young persons without cirrhosis and often have a central fibrous scar, there may be some potential for mistaken diagnosis. However, in our experience *(8)* with 78 patients studied with multiphasic helical CT, FNH typically is a smaller (mean: 4 cm) and much more homogeneously and markedly enhancing mass and rarely (1 of 78) has calcification within its central scar. FNH, unlike fibrolamellar HCC, demonstrates little or no mass effect and rarely obstructs bile ducts or intrahepatic vessels.

HCC in the noncirrhotic liver must be distinguished from other hypervascular tumors, especially hepatocellular adenoma and metastases. Hypervascular metastases usually are encountered in a patient with a known primary tumor, such as neuroendocrine or renal cell carcinoma, and these are usually multifocal and smaller than the conventional or fibrolamellar HCC that we typically encounter. Cases of multifocal HCC would be difficult to distinguish from metastases by imaging criteria alone.

It may be difficult or impossible to distinguish hepatocellular adenoma from HCC on the basis of imaging criteria alone, but adenomas occur almost always

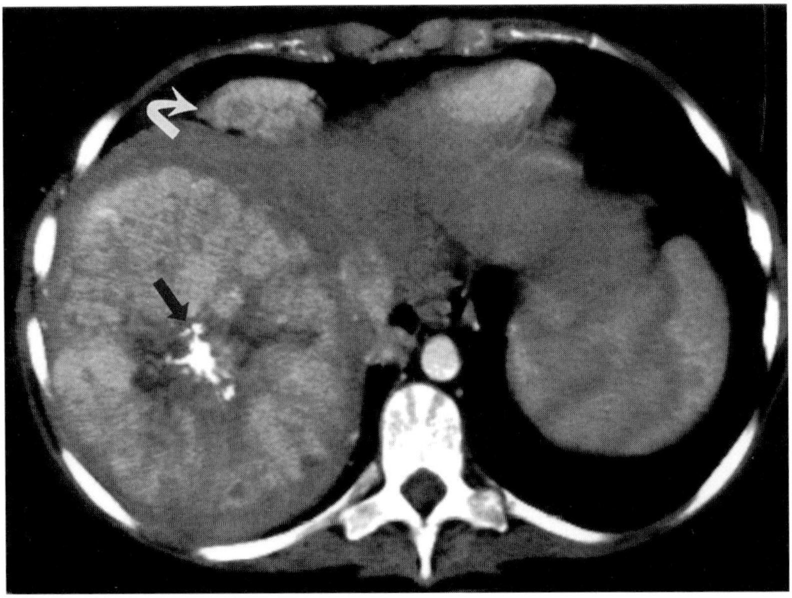

Fig. 2. Fibrolamellar HCC in a 19-year-old man. Contrast-enhanced CT scan showing a large hypervascular mass in the right lobe of liver that is heterogeneous with a large, calcified central scar (arrow). Also note the large cardiophrenic lymph node (curved arrow) representing extrahepatic spread of tumor.

in the setting of hepatic stimulation from steroids or glycogen storage disease *(9)*. Moreover, adenomas may undergo malignant transformation to HCC. For this reason, and also because large adenomas are likely to hemorrhage, these tumors are usually resected.

Much more commonly, HCC develops within a cirrhotic liver. The challenge of detecting and differentiating HCC from other focal lesions, such as regenerating nodules and fibrosis, is discussed in the prior chapter. Several cross-sectional imaging tests, including ultrasound, CT, and MRI, are capable of detecting focal masses and depicting, to a variable extent, the morphological features and hemodynamics of lesions that may aid in diagnosis, staging, and prognosis.

The size of the HCC mass and the prevalence of vascular or biliary invasion and metastases are heavily dependent on whether HCC is discovered in the course of an aggressive screening program or in a patient symptomatic with pain, jaundice, and so forth. Tumors detected during aggressive and expertly performed screening programs tend to be smaller, better differentiated, and less invasive, as discussed and illustrated in the prior chapter.

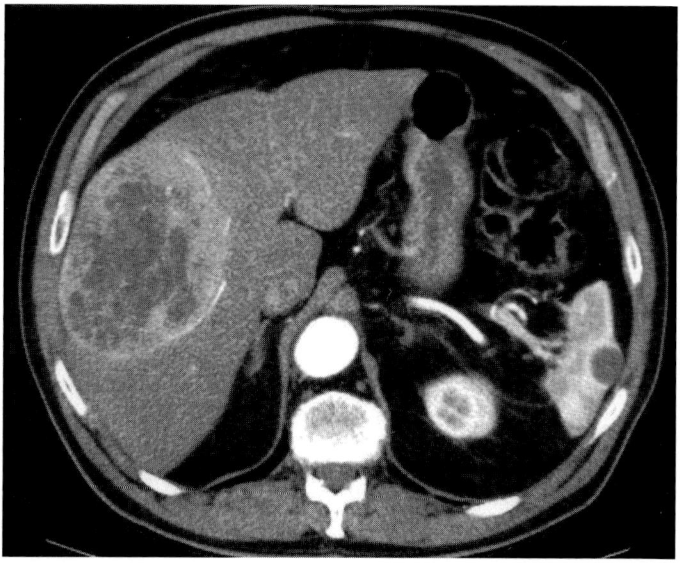

Fig. 3. HCC in a patient with chronic hepatitis but no cirrhosis. Arterial phase CT scan showing a large, spherical, hypervascular mass. The heterogeneous enhancement pattern is typical and is sometimes referred to as a mosaic pattern.

Despite improvements in imaging strategies and techniques, more than half of all patients with HCC have advanced disease at the time of first diagnosis. Therapeutic options depend on accurate staging, with attention to the size and number of the tumor(s), evidence of biliary or vascular invasion, lymphadenopathy, and distant metastases.

HCC usually is a hypervascular tumor, and many investigators have shown that the tumor is best detected and staged with multiphasic CT or MRI after intravenous bolus injection of contrast medium *(10–17)*. Most small HCC nodules are hyperdense to liver on arterial phase CT (hyperintense on MRI) and show tumor washout on portal venous phase. The signal intensity of HCC varies on MRI. An unusual feature for liver tumors is that some HCCs show high signal intensity on T1-weighted images. The cause of this is uncertain, but the presence of fat, copper, or glycoproteins has been suggested *(18)*. Other HCC nodules may be hypodense or isodense to liver parenchyma on T1-weighted images, resulting in many small lesions remaining undetected on nonenhanced MRI.

Larger (>5 cm) HCC lesions are almost always heterogenous and have at least some tumor parts that are hypervascular (hyperdense), as shown on arterial phase imaging, and are spherical masses, a combination of findings referred to as the *mosaic pattern* (Fig. 3) *(19)*. The nonenhancing components include foci of

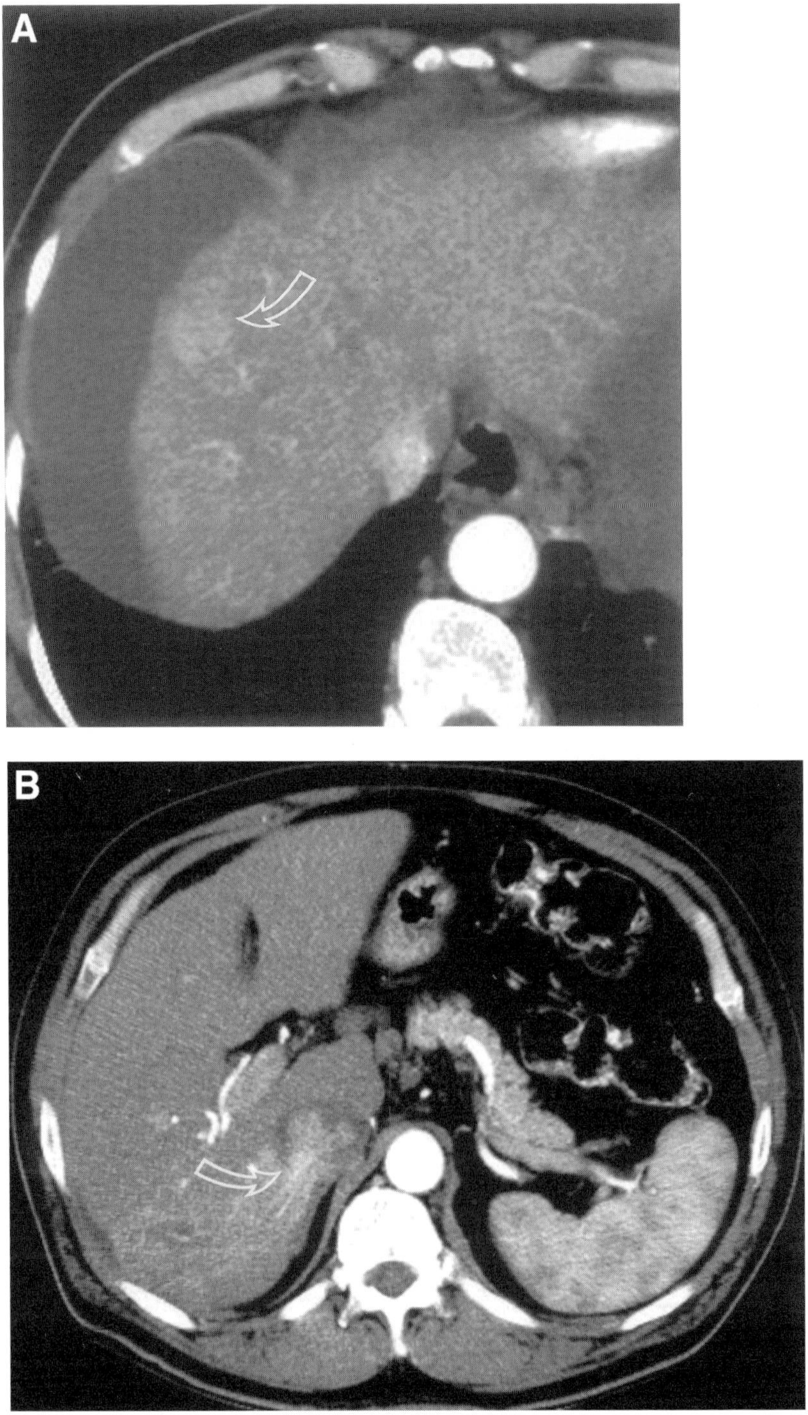
A
B

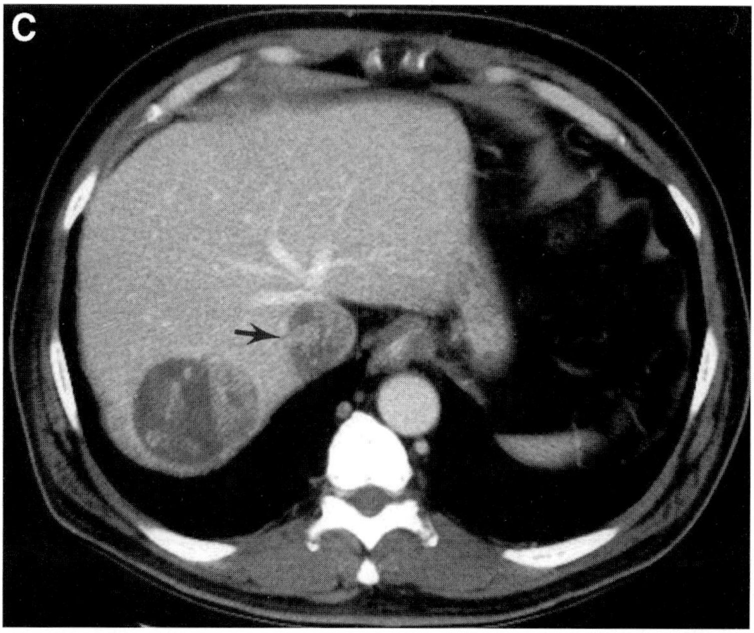

Fig. 4. (*opposite page and above*) Relatively small, but advanced stage HCC. **(A)** Nonenhanced CT scan showing a spherical mass in right lobe. Some peripheral foci in the mass are very low in density, suggesting fat within the tumor. **(B)** Arterial phase CT scan (lower anatomic level) showing streaky enhancement of tumor extending into the inferior vena cava (arrow). **(C)** Portal venous phase CT scan. Washout of contrast from the HCC shows the hypodense mass within the right lobe as well as within the IVC (arrow).

necrosis and hemorrhage. Fibrous septations and a capsule also may be present in a minority of patients. The addition of arterial phase imaging to nonenhanced and portal venous phase imaging will depict some 30% more tumor nodules, and in approx 10% of patients with HCC, it will be the only method to show tumors *(10,11,20)*.

Portal venous invasion by HCC is a common phenomenon and renders the patient unsuitable for surgery or cure (Fig. 4). We have documented portal venous invasion in 33% of HCC patients by multiphasic CT. It is important to distinguish bland thrombus, which may occur in cirrhosis with portal hypertension, from tumor thrombus. Enlargement of the vein (>23 mm) or evidence of tumor enhancement or neovascularity within the thrombus establishes malignant involvement *(21)*.

Hepatic venous invasion is less frequent, although not rare, and is a source of pulmonary metastases (Fig. 5). Extrahepatic metastases are found, in decreasing

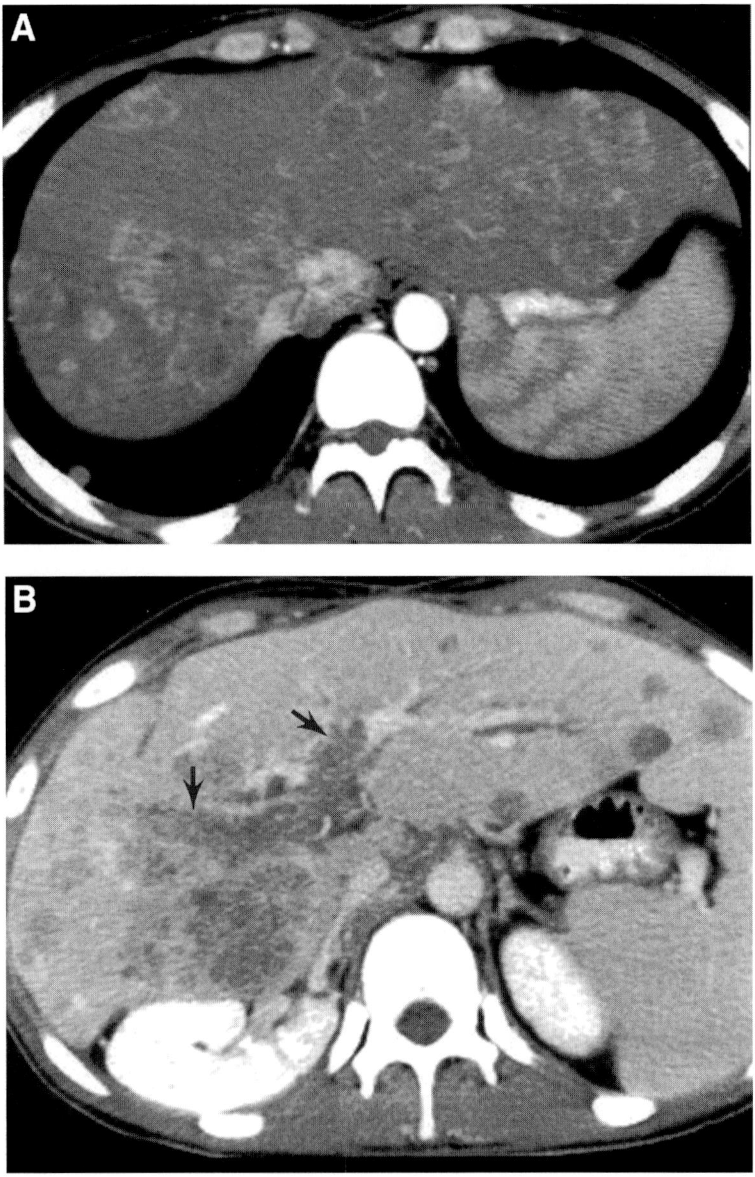

frequency, in the lungs, spleen and reticuloendothelial system, adrenals, bones, and gastrointestinal tract.

Biliary obstruction occurs and intraductal tumor masses are encountered uncommonly (Fig. 6). Biliary obstruction frequently leads to a sudden deterioration of liver function and may further limit therapeutic options, including transarterial chemoembolization. Determining the level of biliary obstruction

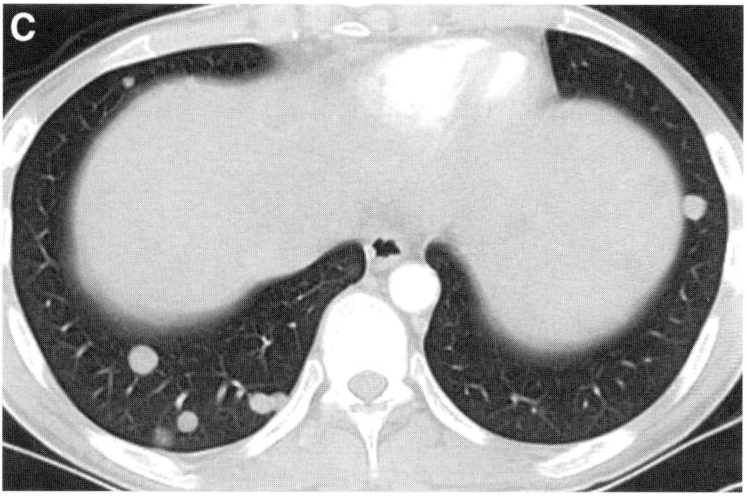

Fig. 5. (*opposite page and above*) HCC in a 20-year-old man with extensive metastases. **(A)** Arterial phase CT scan showing a multifocal tumor throughout the liver with the tumor nodules demonstrating heterogeneous or ring enhancement. Heterogeneous enhancement within the hepatic veins and IVC suggests tumor invasion. **(B)** Portal venous phase CT scan showing multifocal tumor. There is invasion of the right and left portal vein branches (arrows). **(C)** CT scan photographed at "lung windows" shows multiple pulmonary metastases.

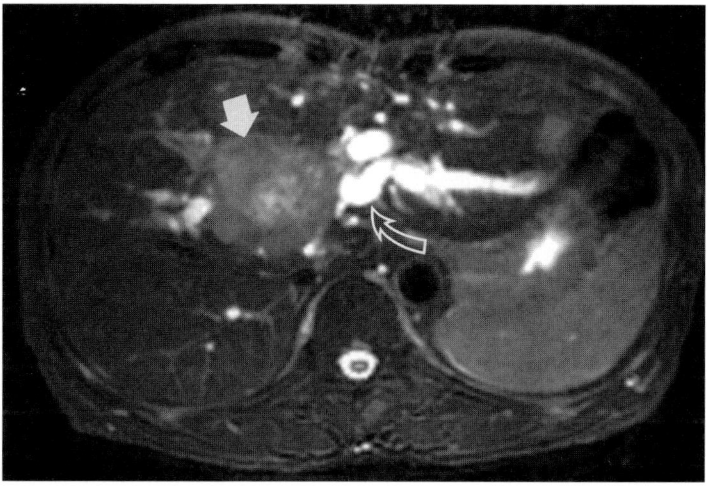

Fig. 6. HCC with biliary obstruction. T2-weighted MRI scan showing a heterogeneous mass (arrow) in segment 4 (medial segment) causing obstruction and dilation of the left intrahepatic bile ducts. (curved arrow).

with the aid of CT or MRI can help to indicate whether percutaneous transhepatic or endoscopic biliary stenting may be of value.

Diagnosing lymphatic spread of HCC is problematic. Most patients with cirrhosis of any cause will have pathologically enlarged nodes in the cardiophrenic, porta hepatis, and porto caval groups as a result of benign reactive hyperplasia. Unless we see definite hypervascularity of these nodes, we are reluctant to diagnose nodal metastases.

REFERENCES

1. Okuda K. Hepatocellular carcinoma. *J Hepatol* 2000;32:225–237.
2. Nzeako UC, Goodman ZD, Ihsak KG. Hepatocellular carcinoma in cirrhotic and noncirrhotic livers: a clinico-histopathologic study of 804 North American patients. *Anat Path* 1996; 105:67–75.
3. Yamashita Y, Takahashi M, Baba Y, et al. Hepatocellular carcinoma with or without cirrhosis: a comparison of CT and angiographic presentation in the United States and Japan. *Abdom Imaging* 1995,18:168–175.
4. Brancatelli G, Federle MP, Grazioli L. Hepatocellular carcinoma in noncirrhotic liver: CT, clinical and pathologic findings in 39 US residents. *Radiology* 2002;222:89–94.
5. Winston CB, Schwartz LH, Fong Y, Blumgart LH, Panicek DM. Hepatocellular carcinoma: MR imaging findings in cirrhotic and noncirrhotic livers. *Radiology* 1999;210:75–79.
6. Ichikawa T, Federle MP, Grazioli L, et al. Fibrolamellar hepatocellular carcinoma: imaging and pathologic findings in 31 recent cases. *Radiology* 1999;213:352–361.
7. Brandt D, Johnson CD, Stephens DH, Weiland LH. Imaging of fibrolamellar carcinoma. *AJR Am J Roentgenol* 1988;151:295–298.
8. Brancatelli G, Federle MP, Grazioli L, et al. Focal nodular hyperplasia: CT findings with emphasis on multiphasic helical CT in 78 patients. *Radiology* 2001;219:61–68.
9. Ichikawa T, Federle MP, Grazioli L, Nalesnick M. Hepatocellular adenoma: multiphasic CT and histopathologic findings in 25 patients. *Radiology* 2000;214:861–868.
10. Laghi A, Iannacone R, Rossi P, et al. Hepatocellular carcinoma: detection with triple-phase multi-detector row helical CT in patients with chronic hepatitis. *Radiology* 2003;226: 543–549.
11. Ichikawa T, Kitamura T, Nakajima H, et al. Hypervascular hepatocellular carcinoma: can double arterial phase imaging with multidetector CT improve tumor depiction in the cirrhotic liver. *Am J Roentgenol* 2002;179:751–758.
12. Kim T, Murakami T, Hori M, et al. Small hypervascular hepatocellular carcinoma revealed by double arterial phase CT performed with single breath-hold scanning and automatic bolus tracking. *Am J Roentgenol* 2002;178:899–904.
13. Kim T, Federle MP, Baron RL, Peterson MS, Kawamori Y. Discrimination of small hepatic hemangiomas from hypervascular malignant tumors smaller than 3 cm with three-phase helical CT. *Radiology* 2001;219:699–706.
14. Baron RL, Oliver JH, Dodd GD, et al. Hepatocellular carcinoma: evaluation with biphasic, contrast-enhanced, helical CT. *Radiology* 1996;199:505–511.
15. Kanematsu M, Semelka RC, Matsuo M, et al. Gadolinium-enhanced MR imaging of the liver: optimizing imaging delay for hepatic arterial and portal venous phases: a prospective randomized study in patients with chronic liver disease. *Radiology* 2002;225:407–415.
16. Kang BK, Lim JH, Kim SH, et al. Preoperative depiction of hepatocellular carcinoma: ferumoxides-enhanced MR imaging versus triple-phase helical CT. *Radiology* 2003; 226:79–85.

17. Shimizu A, Ito K, Koike S, et al. Cirrhosis or chronic hepatitis: evaluation of small (<2 cm) early-enhancing hepatic lesions with serial contrast-enhanced dynamic MR imaging. *Radiology* 2003;226:550–555.
18. Ebara M, Fukuda H, Kojima Y, et al. Small hepatocellular carcinoma: relationship of signal intensity to histopathologic findings and metal content of the tumor and surrounding hepatic parenchyma. *Radiology* 1999;210:81–88.
19. Stevens WR, Gulino SP, Batts KP, Stephens DH, Johnson CD. Mosaic pattern of hepatocellular carcinoma: histologic basis for a characteristic CT appearance. *J Comput Assist Tomogr* 1996;20:337–342.
20. Oliver JH, Baron RL, Federle MP, Rochette HE Jr. Detecting hepatocellular carcinoma: value of unenhanced or arterial phase CT imaging or both used in conjunction with conventional portal venous phase contrast-enhanced CT imaging. *Am J Roentgenol* 1996;167:71–77.
21. Tublin ME, Dodd GD, Baron RL. Benign and malignant portal vein thrombosis: differentiation by CT characteristics. *AJR Am J Roentgenol* 1997;168:719–723.

7 Percutaneous Ethanol and Acetic Acid Ablation of Hepatocellular Carcinoma

Vibhu Kapoor, MD *and F. Leland Thaete,* MD

CONTENTS

1. INTRODUCTION

Hepatocellular carcinoma (HCC) is the most common primary hepatic tumor. Globally, HCC is one of the most common malignant visceral tumors *(1,2)*, with more than 350,000 cases reported every year *(1)*. Annual incidence rate in North and South America for HCC is 2–4 cases per 100,000 persons *(1)*. The worldwide distribution of HCC is closely linked to the prevalence of hepatitis B infection. There is a 200-fold increased risk of HCC in adults who become hepatitis B virus (HBV) carriers during infancy as a result of vertical transmission from the infected mother *(3)*. HCC in this population frequently occurs without coincident cirrhosis (in approx 50% cases) and at a younger age—often between 20 and 40 years *(1)*. In contrast, cirrhosis is present in 85–90% cases of HCC in the Western population (low-incidence region), where HBV is not prevalent. The most common associations with HCC in this region are alcohol and chronic infection with hepatitis C virus (HCV) *(1)*; rarely does it occur before age 60 years *(1)*. Males

From: *Current Clinical Oncology: Hepatocellular Cancer: Diagnosis and Treatment*
Edited by: B. I. Carr © Humana Press Inc., Totowa, NJ

outnumber females in the distribution of HCC in both the high- and low-incidence regions; the male/female ratio is 8:1 in the high-incidence population and 2:1 to 3:1 in the low-incidence population *(1,2)*.

During the past decade, marked advances have been made in hepatic imaging, allowing detection of HCC in the preclinical stage *(4–11)*. Surgery, long regarded as the only procedure with a chance for a cure, remains the treatment of choice for HCC, with a 50% 5-year survival rate after surgical resection of small, asymptomatic nodules *(12)*. However, many alternative and innovative therapies have been proposed *(13–22)*, because a substantial number of these patients are not suitable candidates for surgery because of poor liver function, advanced age, concomitant diseases, multifocal unresectable disease, patient refusal, and so forth. There are two primary techniques for nonsurgical treatment of HCC: transcatheter intra-arterial administration of chemotherapeutic or embolic agents and percutaneous tumor ablation with chemicals (ethanol or acetic acid) or thermal devices (such as radiofrequency electrode needle). Although the intra-arterial technique is used primarily for hypervascular lesions, percutaneous tumor ablation can be used for treatment of both hypo- and hypervascular HCC. Various combinations of surgical and nonsurgical methods also have been used *(23,24)*. Some selected patients with poor liver function resulting from advanced cirrhosis and localized unresectable HCC are candidates for orthotopic liver transplantation (more recently, living-related liver transplantation), but potential recipients far outnumber donors. In some countries, such as Japan, liver transplantation is not allowed *(25)*.

2. PERCUTANEOUS ETHANOL PLUS ACETIC ACID INJECTION

Sugiura et al. *(26)* described percutaneous ethanol ablation of hepatic tumors as early as 1983. Following their description, Livraghi et al. *(27)* reported treatment of small hepatic and abdominal tumors by percutaneous ethanol injection in 1986, and Ohnishi et al. *(28)* reported their description of treatment of small HCC with acetic acid a decade later. Although major advances have been made in treatment of HCC since then, the basic principle of percutaneous tumor ablation remains unchanged *(29–32)*. As compared with surgical resection, percutaneous alcohol or acetic acid ablation has the ability to destroy tumor tissue while preserving the surrounding liver tissue and, therefore, retaining hepatic function. Both alcohol and acetic acid are readily available in injectable (liquid) form, are inexpensive, nonviscous, rapidly cytotoxic, and effective. Absolute (>95%) alcohol is used for percutaneous treatment of HCC; however, some studies have shown that 50% acetic acid may give better results than alcohol with less local recurrence and improved 1- and 2-year survival rates *(33)*.

It has been reported that ethanol and acetic acid preferentially diffuse into HCC because of its softer consistency as compared with surrounding cirrhotic liver *(25)*. However in our experience, HCC may be firmer than the surrounding cirrhotic liver. Ethanol and acetic acid kill tumor cells as well as normal hepatocytes by direct cytotoxic effects, causing necrosis of the treated region *(33,34)*. They diffuse rapidly into cells, causing cellular dehydration and protein denaturation with resultant coagulation necrosis. This is followed by a fibrotic reaction, thrombosis, and occlusion of small vessels *(27,34)*. Investigators of Asian hepatoma suggest that encapsulated HCC has a fibrous capsule and fibrous septa within the mass of tumor, with the frequency of the capsule and septum formation increasing with the size of the tumor *(35–37)*. Immunohistochemical analysis has shown that the fibrous capsule consists of at least type I, III, and IV collagen *(37)*. Fibrous capsule and septa occur in approx 50% of tumors between 1.5 and 2.0 cm and in approx 70% of tumors between 2.0 and 3.0 cm *(36)*. Ethanol cannot penetrate the fibrous septum of such tumors; however, acetic acid is able to penetrate the septum mainly because of its low pH, which induces swelling of the fibers of the septum and promotes dissociation of intermolecular crosslinks containing aldimine bonds of collagen *(17)*. Because of this property of acetic acid as compared with alcohol, lesser volumes and fewer of treatments are required with percutaneous acetic acid ablation.

3. PATIENT SELECTION

Patients for percutaneous alcohol or acetic acid ablation of HCC can be categorized into: (a) patients electing to undergo percutaneous chemical ablation over other therapeutic options, and (b) patients who are poor candidates for other, nonablative therapies such as surgery or transcatheter intra-arterial therapy. The latter group includes patients with inoperable HCC from metastatic disease, high surgical risk, advanced age, and proven recurrence of tumor after previous resection *(25,30)*. Patients in whom transcatheter intra-arterial therapy is not feasible include those with hypovascular lesions, occlusion of hepatic artery related to previous intraarterial embolization, poor tumor opacification on selective hepatic angiograms, technical failure of superselective catheterization, and poor liver function *(16)*.

The inclusion criteria for the elective group of patients includes all the following: (a) tumor size 3 cm or smaller (some authors describe treatment of lesions up to 5 cm *[34]*); (b) three or fewer lesions (some centers will treat up to four lesions *[33,34]*; the number of treatment sessions increases with the increase in the number of lesions being treated, and it becomes impractical to treat more than three or four lesions); (c) no extrahepatic spread of disease on routine imaging; (d) no portal vein thrombosis; (e) Child–Pugh class A or B liver cirrhosis *(25)*; (f) biopsy-proven tumor or patients with ultrasound and computed tomography (CT) findings of HCC with persistently elevated α-fetoprotein (AFP) levels *(30)*; and (g) age younger than 75 years *(25)*. Exclusion criteria for treatment include irreversible coagulopathy *(34)* and failure to satisfy any of the above criteria. The number and size of tumor nodules and the absence of portal vein thrombosis usually is established by ultrasound, color Doppler sonography, and helical CT. Extrahepatic disease as well as the other criteria outlined here are ascertained by a careful clinical history, abdominal and chest CT, bone scintigraphy, and laboratory tests.

4. TECHNIQUE OF PERCUTANEOUS ALCOHOL PLUS ACETIC ACID ABLATION

4.1. Preprocedural Imaging Workup

Preprocedural imaging workup varies between different institutions. However, conventional sonography and unenhanced and biphasic contrast-enhanced CT scan are the standard practice before percutaneous chemical ablation for HCC. It is also preferable to have histopathological confirmation. Color Doppler examination *(22,31)*, arteriography *(22)*, and CO_2-enhanced sonography *(22)* have been reported variously in the preprocedural workup. Numerous studies on intraarterial CO_2 microbubbles-enhanced ultrasound angiography for diagnosis and follow-up of hepatoma have been reported from Asia. One such study *(10)* compared the sensitivity of detection of small hypervascular HCC using intraarterial CO_2 microbubbles-enhanced ultrasound angiography with conventional angiography, digital subtraction angiography, and CT with iodized oil. In this study, ultrasound angiography was the most sensitive (86%) method for detecting small HCC (especially those less than 1 cm); it helped determine vascularity in angiographically undetectable tumors as well as assisted in determining the therapeutic strategy such as transarterial chemotherapy, percutaneous ethanol injection, or surgical resection *(10)*. This technique is limited by its ability to image a single tomographical section during a single procedure and, therefore, is not practical as a screening tool for HCC because it would be very time consuming *(10)*. However, another recent study *(22)* emphasized that CO_2-enhanced sonography may be more sensitive than contrast-enhanced CT (100% sensitivity with CO_2-enhanced sonography as compared with 97% with contrast-enhanced CT) in the detection of HCC and for evaluating residual tumor (100% sensitivity with CO_2-enhanced sonography as compared with 91% with contrast-enhanced CT) after treatment. Doppler sonography and unenhanced and biphasic contrast-enhanced CT are the standard preprocedural imaging performed at our institution.

4.2. Guidance

To achieve complete tumor necrosis, homogenous diffusion of alcohol throughout the lesion is essential. Thus, ability to place the needle precisely at multiple locations within the tumor and careful monitoring of the injected alcohol are important for successful ablation of the tumor.

Percutaneous ethanol ablation has been performed using ultrasound *(16,17,22,23,25–27,29–31,33,34)* and CT guidance *(16,23,34,38,39)*. Recent advances, such as intraarterial CO_2-enhanced sonography, have been added to the armament for guiding percutaneous ethanol ablation of HCC *(22)*. At our center, ultrasonography is used to target tumor lesions detected on CT for percutaneous chemical ablation (Fig. 1A,B).

The major advantages of ultrasonography as compared with CT are real-time monitoring of the procedure, precise placement of the needle within the lesion, and faster procedure time. Ethanol and acetic acid can be visualized under real-time perfusing into the lesion (because of the presence of microbubbles), and the injection can be stopped instantly if the microbubbles are seen to extend outside the lesion beyond the desired cytotoxic margin (Fig. 1C). However, microbubbles that are seen clearly during early injection (an advantage) may progress to obscure the lesion, later making it difficult to evaluate the extent of untreated tumor (a disadvantage). Another important limitation of conventional sonography on subsequent treatment sessions is the inability to distinguish necrotic areas produced by percutaneous ethanol injection from similar-appearing areas of residual tumor *(22,40)*. There are some early reports from Asian centers suggesting that CO_2-enhanced sonography may be a more sensitive technique for detecting viable regions of treated HCC than conventional sonography, CT, and digital subtraction arteriography *(10,22,41)*.

CT guidance is reserved for lesions not clearly discernible or safely accessible by ultrasound *(16,22)*, such as those deep within the cirrhotic liver and surface lesions, including those at the liver dome (Fig. 2A,B). Absolute alcohol has very low CT attenuation values (approx –240 HU) and is well-seen on CT, thereby permitting accurate evaluation of extent of treatment (Fig. 2C). One other advantage of CT over ultrasound is that persistent nodularity on a contrast-enhanced CT obtained immediately after percutaneous alcohol ablation indicates residual or untreated tumor *(38)*, which can be targeted preferentially in subsequent sessions. The drawbacks of CT guidance are that the procedure time is longer and real-time monitoring of intravasation of alcohol or acetic acid is not possible. If acetic acid or alcohol are seen by ultrasound to escape into bile ducts, the injection must be stopped immediately, which is not possible with CT guidance. In one report, this was suggested to have contributed to liver failure, resulting in death of a patient after CT-guided percutaneous acetic acid ablation *(16)*.

4.3. Treatment Schedule

The treatment schedule may be: (a) multisession one or more per week for multiple sessions, depending on lesion volume, patient compliance, and response to treatment or (b) single-session treatment with multiple injections of alcohol at several points within the tumor. This may need general anesthesia and can be performed for multiple small lesions or a single tumor up to 5 cm *(30)*. Conscious

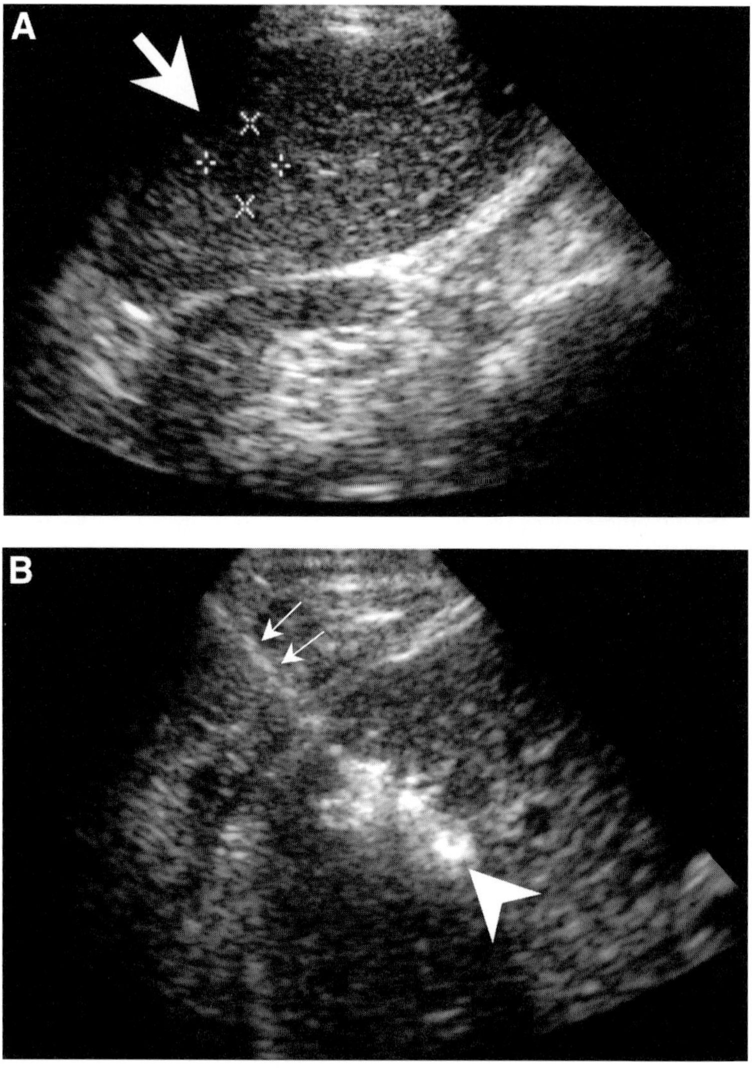

sedation is the preferred method for pain control at our center. Transient pain on injection of superficial lesions (close to liver capsule) is more intense than injection into lesions inside the liver, and this may preclude using single-session high-dose injections for surface nodules. As a general rule, we avoid injecting subcapsular tumor or lesions abutting the surface of the liver because of a significant risk of chemical peritonitis, tumor rupture, and hemorrhage.

It was suggested initially by Ohnishi et al. *(17)* that small HCC nodules could not be treated successfully with acetic acid in a single session because it takes several hours to 1 day for the acid to dissolve collagen. However, Liang et al. *(16)*

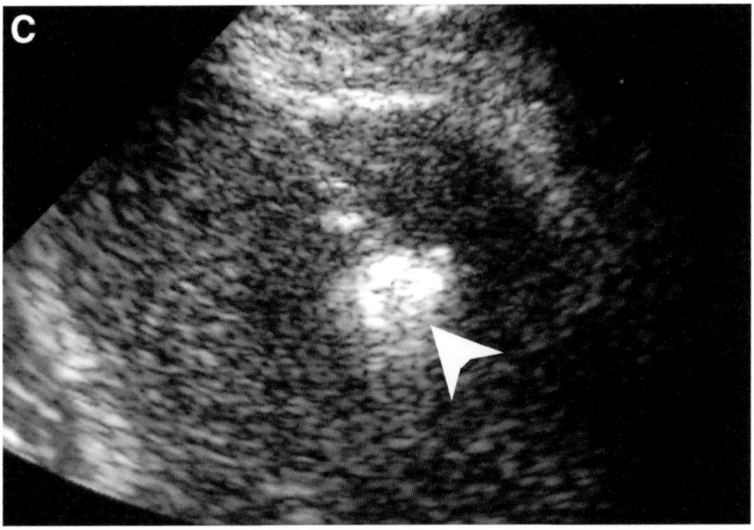

Fig. 1. (*opposite page and above*) **(A)** A man with cirrhosis and a 1-cm hypoechoic HCC in the right lobe of the liver (arrow). **(B)** Percutaneous alcohol (95%) ablation with a 21-gage spinal needle (double arrows). As alcohol is injected, it obscures the lesion. **(C)** At the end of the injection, the lesion is uniformly hyperechoic (arrow head). The needle track is still visible.

described a single high-dose percutaneous acetic acid technique that was effective for treatment of small HCC.

4.4. Sedation

Percutaneous ethanol ablation can be performed in the outpatient clinic without sedation or local anesthesia *(25,30,42)*, with the use of conscious sedation (preferred at our institution) or general anesthesia. The decision of the type of sedation depends on the practice at the institution where the procedure is being performed, patient compliance, the number of lesions being treated, multisession vs single-session treatment, and severity of pain during preceding treatment

Fig. 2. (A) (*pages 154 and 155*) Enhanced CT scan at the level of the liver in a man with cirrhosis and a 2.5-cm peripherally enhancing/faintly enhancing HCC in segment VI of liver (arrow). **(B)** CT-guided placement of a 21-gage spinal needle into the tumor (arrow). **(C)** After injection of absolute alcohol into the lesion, it is replaced by a low attenuation zone having a central region of –200 HU (long arrow). **(D)** A 2-year follow-up enhanced CT scan shows a small scar in the region of the treated tumor (arrowhead). There has been an interval progression of the cirrhosis with development of ascites.

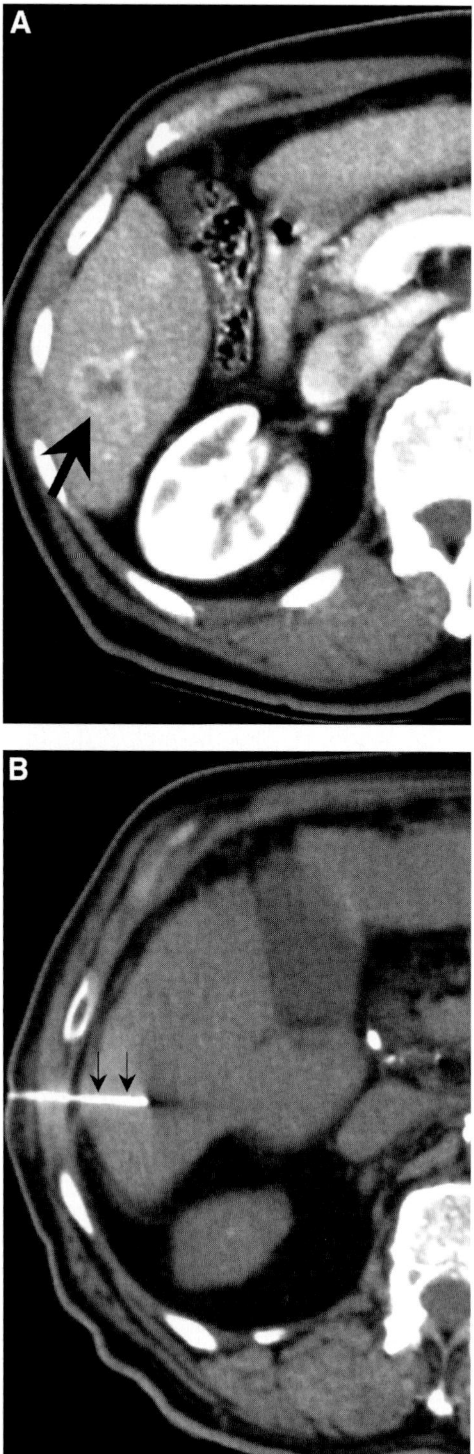

Fig. 2.

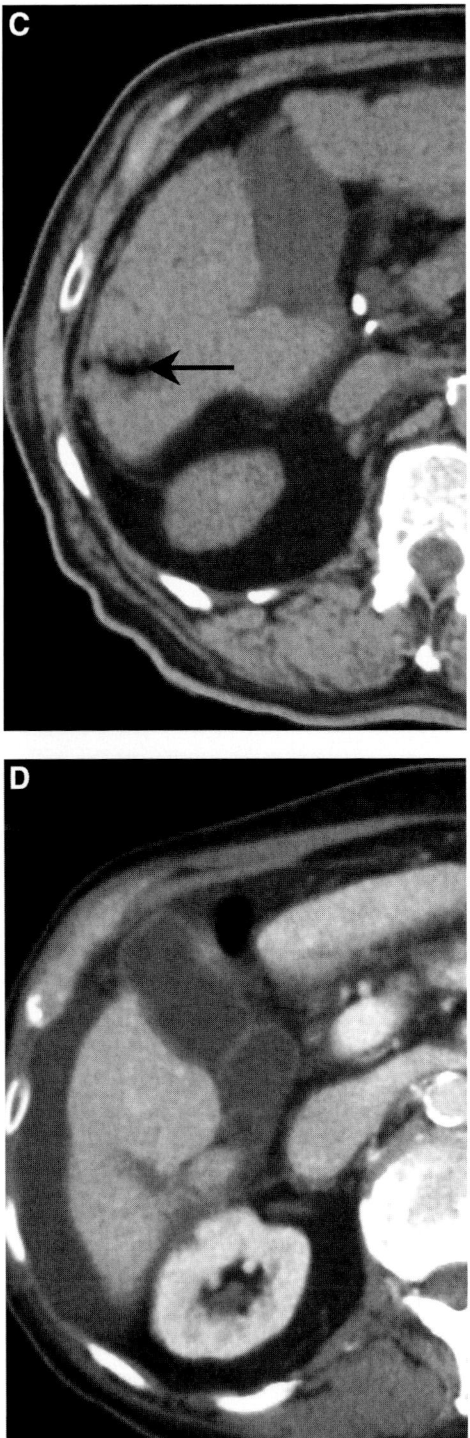

Fig. 2.

sessions. It has been noted that the pain usually decreases with subsequent treatment sessions because of the local neurotoxic effect of the ablative agent.

4.5. Equipment

For ultrasound-guided procedures, a convex or linear array transducer are used with 5.0 MHz for superficial lesions (i.e., the nearest margin of the tumor is less than 3 cm from the skin surface), or with a 2.5- to 3.5-MHz transducer for all other deeper lesions and a lateral attachable needle guidance system *(22,32)*. For color Doppler imaging, transducers with insonating frequencies of 3.5 MHz (for superficial lesions) or 2.8 MHz (for deeper lesions) are used *(32)*. We usually use 2.5- to 5.0-MHz curved and, occasionally, linear array probes depending on patient size, beam penetrability, and lesion location. CT-guided procedures can be carried out under any commercially available CT scanner; however, CT fluoroscopy facilitates the procedure and minimizes time to complete the injections.

Numerous needles are available for delivery of alcohol into the tumor, such as a 22-gage noncutting needle (Spinal Needle; Becton-Dickinson, Rutherford, NJ); a 21- or 22-gage skinny needle (Hatsuko Co., Tokyo, Japan); a 21-gage, multiple-side-hole needle (Ethanoject; TSK, Tokyo, Japan); and a 21-gage needle with a closed conical tip and three terminal side holes (PEIT needle; Hakko, Tokyo, Japan). A multiple-side-hole needle with a closed conical tip has been advocated, because the tip of the needle can be positioned at the deepest portion of the tumor and alcohol can be injected without the risk of injecting it into the distal nonneoplastic hepatic parenchyma. However, using meticulous technique any of the above-mentioned needles could be used safely.

4.6. Agent for Ablation

4.6.1. Alcohol

If multiple sessions are planned, a total dose required for cytotoxicity of the tumor and a tumor-free margin can be fractionated into doses ranging from 1 to 12 mL of 95% ethyl alcohol. Other investigators may administer the entire dose in single-session treatments. The volume of alcohol used during each session obviously must be greater with single-session treatments. In a study by Livraghi et al. *(30)*, the mean volume of alcohol injected during single-session treatments was 75 mL, with the maximum volume of alcohol administered being 165 mL. The patients for the single-session treatment were premedicated with intravenous fructose diphosphate and glutathione 30 minutes before the procedure, which quickened the rate of metabolism of alcohol and helped in neutralizing its toxic effect.

As a general guideline, the total volume of ethanol injected for each lesion is calculated by the equation given below:

$$V = 4/3\pi\ (r + 0.5)^3,$$

where V is the total volume of ethanol in milliliters (mL) and r is the radius of each tumor in centimeters (cm). A factor of 0.5 cm is added to the radius to provide a safety margin so as to include a cuff of non-neoplastic hepatic tissue, ensuring that all tumor cells are killed.

4.6.2. Acetic Acid

The hepatocyte-necrosing capability of acetic acid at concentrations of 15% approaches that of absolute alcohol, and the killing effect plateaus at approx 50% *(16)*. Fifty percent acetic acid generally is recommended for percutaneous treatment of HCC, although concentrations as low as15% have been used *(28,43)*. The volume of acetic acid at these concentrations required for treatment is approximately one-third of the volume required for tumor ablation using ethanol *(17)*. Therefore, the total volume of acetic acid required for each lesion would be:

$$V = 1/3\{4/3\pi\ (r + 0.5)^3\},$$

where V is the total volume of acetic acid in milliliters (mL) and r is the radius of each tumor in centimeters (cm). This volume may be injected in a single session or fractionated into multiple sessions.

4.7. Injection

The deepest portions of the lesion are injected first, followed by the more central portions, and the superficial portion is injected last. The rational of this sequence of injections is to prevent more superficial injections from obscuring the deeper segments of the lesion when using ultrasonography for guidance (Fig. 1C). It is also likely that by using this technique, there is more even distribution of alcohol or acetic acid throughout the lesion when compared with injecting at a single spot or with random needle placement. With CT guidance, 95% alcohol can be seen easily within the lesion, because it has attenuation of approx –240 HU. Injection is stopped when homogenous perfusion of the lesion is observed, when a strong resistance to injection is felt *(17)*, or when alcohol is seen to intravasate outside the lesion despite repeated repositioning of the needle. The needle is left *in situ* for 30 seconds after completion of the procedure to avoid peritoneal spill of alcohol or acetic acid that may cause pain. Alternatively, a mixture of Gelfoam powder (Pharmacia and Upjohn, Kalamazoo, MI) and saline can be injected into the liver as the needle is withdrawn to prevent leakage of alcohol or acetic acid. The injection is discontinued if the patient reports severe pain with either alcohol or acetic acid at any time, even if the volume of injection is less than that initially intended.

4.8. Complications

The major complications reported during percutaneous ethanol and acetic acid ablation are peritoneal or subcapsular hemorrhage, hemobilia, liver abscess, cholangitis, pneumothorax, pleural effusion, infarction and necrosis of the injected segment of the liver, hepatic decompensation, arterioportal or arterio-venous shunts (which may aggravate portal hypertension), portal vein thrombosis, bile duct injury with formation of strictures or bilomas, and needle-track seeding *(16,29,30,44–47)*. The risk of needle-track implantation is related to the number of needle punctures of the lesions *(16)*, and use of a single-session (high-dose) technique may decrease this risk. The overall rate of major complications has been reported as 1.7%, with a mortality rate of 0.1% *(30)*, with inherent risk increasing with the number of punctures.

Minor complications may occur, such as pain in the right hypochondrium, epigastric region, or radiating to the right shoulder, that may necessitate sedation or analgesia during a treatment sessions or even may require premature termination of the procedure. Transient pain on injection of superficial lesions close to liver capsule usually is more intense than that accompanying injection into lesions inside the liver, and this may preclude using single session high-dose injections for surface nodules. At our institution, we avoid injecting subcapsular tumor or lesions abutting the surface of the liver because of a significant risk of chemical peritonitis, tumor rupture, and hemorrhage. Because fractionated doses are administered over multiple sessions, pain tolerance generally increases because of the local neurotoxic effect of prior injections. Mild-to-moderate elevation in body temperature from tumor necrosis usually returns to normal in 3–5 days. Subjective perception of intoxication with ethanol ablation usually is transient and resolves within minutes to hours. Abnormal hepatic function test results (e.g., elevation of liver enzymes from baseline) may be seen, but usually resolve within several days. Increasing the number of punctures increases the risk of major and minor complications.

4.9. Follow-Up

Conventional ultrasonography, color or power Doppler sonography, contrast-enhanced color and power Doppler sonography with intravenous contrast material, intra-arterial CO_2-enhanced sonography, spiral CT, magnetic resonance imaging (MRI), and AFP assay have been evaluated and compared for assessing viable portions of HCC after transcatheter arterial chemoembolization or percutaneous ethanol ablation or after radiofrequency ablation of malignant liver tumors *(31,32,48,49)*. Although a histopathological gold standard would be ideal for follow-up, it often is difficult and sometimes is impractical to achieve.

Short-term follow-up at 1–3 months may be obtained with noninvasive studies, such as gray-scale and color Doppler sonography. On conventional gray-scale sonography, it is not always possible to distinguish necrotic areas produced by percutaneous ethanol injection from similar-appearing areas of residual tumor *(22,40)*. Color Doppler is useful to observe tumors that show intratumoral flow before treatment; residual tumor can be confidently assumed if Doppler signal persists after treatment, and further dosing may need to be administered *(31)*. Usefulness of color Doppler can be limited, because not all HCCs have distinct intratumoral flow *(31)*, and specificity of lack of flow in treated tumors is limited.

More costly examinations such as CT or MRI may be performed at greater intervals and are more comprehensive toward evaluating for possible extrahepatic disease. Multiple studies over progressive time may be necessary to distinguish necrosis from residual or recurrent tumor. On spiral CT, the lesion is considered to be completely necrotic with no residual tumor when it appears as an area of low attenuation with no enhancement on both the arterial and portal venous phases (Fig. 1E). Incomplete tumor necrosis is considered when enhancing areas within the tumor are observed in the arterial or the portal venous phase. On MRI, untreated HCCs usually are hypointense to liver on T1-weighted sequences, of variable intensity (hypointense, isointense, or hyperintense to liver) on T2-weighted sequences, and show some degree of enhancement after gadolinium administration. After percutaneous alcohol ablation, uniform low signal intensity of these lesions on T2-weighted sequences with lack of enhancement is highly suggestive of successful therapy *(50)*. Residual tumor usually shows high signal intensity on T2-weighted images with corresponding areas of enhancement on gadolinium-enhanced images. However, some investigators have found MRI, even with use of contrast enhancement, to lack specificity because of the variability of signal intensity of these treated lesions on T2-weighted images *(51)*.

Contrast-enhanced helical CT *(49)* and intra-arterial CO_2-enhanced sonography *(22)* are perhaps the most sensitive tests available for detection of residual or new lesions after percutaneous treatment of malignant liver tumors. Some studies have shown that CO_2-enhanced sonography is a more sensitive technique for detecting viable regions of treated HCC than conventional sonography, CT, and digital subtraction arteriography *(10,22,41)*.

5. RESULTS OF PERCUTANEOUS ABLATION TECHNIQUE

The prognosis of patients with HCC is dependent on several factors, such as tumor size and number of lesions, stage of cirrhosis (Child's class A, B, or C), age of patient, surgical resectability, and portal vein involvement. The 3- to 5-year survival rates in a study by Livraghi et al. *(30)* for patients with Child's class A, B, or C cirrhosis and a single tumor measuring 5 cm or smaller was 47–79%, 29–63%, and 0–12%, respectively. The 3- to 5-year survival in the same group of patients with Child's class A cirrhosis was 36–68%, 30–53%, and 0–16% for multiple lesions, single lesions larger than 5 cm, and for advanced HCC, respectively. The mean 5-year survival rate in the same study *(30)* for tumor size 5 cm or smaller was 48%. Of note, patients with Child's class C cirrhosis with HCC usually died of progression of cirrhosis, whereas patients with Child's class A cirrhosis died of tumor progression *(30)*.

Survival rate or new lesion rates in patients who undergo surgical resection for HCC are similar to those treated with percutaneous alcohol ablation *(29,30,44)*. The similar survival rates probably reflect perioperative mortality from surgery and almost negligible early mortality and liver damage from percutaneous alcohol ablation. Percutaneous chemical ablation is especially useful in patients who are not suitable candidates for surgery or chemoembolization. When compared with transcatheter arterial chemoembolization, a single transcatheter arterial chemoembolization combined with percutaneous ethanol ablation is more effective than repeated transcatheter arterial chemoembolization *(24)*. The mean 5-year survival rates in patients with HCCs with a diameter of 5 cm or smaller undergoing surgical resection, percutaneous ethanol ablation, transcatheter arterial chemoembolization, segmental transcatheter arterial chemoembolization, or orthotopic liver transplantation are 49, 48, 14, 44, and 70%, respectively *(30)*.

The reported rate of local recurrence of HCC in patients treated with percutaneous alcohol ablation is approx 37%, as compared with 8% with acetic acid *(17)*, during an approx 2-year follow-up; the 1-year survival rates were 83 and 100% for alcohol and acetic acid, respectively. The recurrence of tumor distant from the injection site is the same for both acetic acid and alcohol and probably relates to intrahepatic metastases or multiple metachronous or synchronous tumors not detected by earlier imaging *(17)*. Although new tumor recurrence may be related to the insertion of a needle into the tumor and chemical injection that may promote migration of malignant cells *(45)*, it is more likely that hepatocarcinogenesis, as a continuum process from regenerative nodule to adenomatous hyperplasia to finally HCC *(52)*, may be ongoing throughout the cirrhotic liver, predisposing to development of multiple HCCs.

6. CONCLUSIONS

Based on the current data available, percutaneous chemical ablation with alcohol or acetic acid is an excellent treatment option for patients considered to have inoperable HCC or for patients with operable albeit adverse prognostic factors such as advanced age, Child class B or C cirrhosis, prior surgical resection with recurrence, and other significant debilitating diseases. Optimal patients for this type of treatment would include those with a single tumor, 5 cm or smaller with normal liver or Child's class A cirrhosis.

REFERENCES

1. Crawford JM. The liver and the biliary tract. In: *Pathologic Basis of Disease*, 6th ed. (Cotran RS, Kumar V, Collins T, eds.), WB Saunders, Philadelphia, 1999, pp. 888–891.
2. del Pilar Fernandez M, Redvanley RD. Primary hepatic malignant neoplasms. *Radiol Clin North Am* 1998;36:333–348.
3. Beasley RP. Hepatitis B virus, the major etiology of hepatocellular carcinoma. *Cancer* 1988;61:1942–1956.

4. Baron RL, Oliver JH III, Dodd GD III, et al. Hepatocellular carcinoma: evaluation with biphasic, contrast-enhanced helical CT. *Radiology* 1996;199:505–511.
5. Oliver JH III, Baron RL, Federle MP, et al. Detecting hepatocellular carcinoma: value of unenhanced or arterial phase CT imaging or both used in conjunction with conventional portal venous phase contrast-enhanced CT imaging. *Am J Roentgenol* 1996;167:71–77.
6. Kanematsu M, Oliver JH III, Baron RL, et al. Hepatocellular carcinoma: the role of biphasic contrast-enhanced CT versus CT during arterial portography. *Radiology* 1997;205:75–80.
7. Kanematsu M, Hoshi H, Murakami T, et al. Detection of hepatocellular carcinoma in patient with cirrhosis: MR imaging versus angiographically assisted helical CT. *Am J Roentgenol* 1997;169:1507–1515.
8. Murakami T, Baron RL, Peterson MS, et al. Hepatocellular carcinoma: MR imaging with mangoafodipir trisodium (MnDPDP). *Radiology* 1996;200:69–77.
9. Shimamoto K, Sakuma S, Ishigaki T. Hepatocellular carcinoma: evaluation with color Doppler US and MR imaging. *Radiology* 1992;182:149–153.
10. Kudo M, Tomita S, Tochio H, et al. Small hepatocellular carcinoma: diagnosis with US angiography with intraarterial CO_2 microbubbles. *Radiology* 1992;182:155–160.
11. Kudo M, Tomita S, Tochio H, et al. Sonography with intraarterial infusion of carbon dioxide microbubbles (sonographic angiography): value in differential diagnosis of hepatic tumors. *Am J Roentgenol* 1992;158:65–74.
12. Makuuchi M, Kosuge T, Takayama T, et al. Surgery for small liver cancers. *Semin Surg Oncol* 1993;9:298–304.
13. Takayasu K, Shima Y, Muramatsu Y, et al. Hepatocellular carcinoma: treatment with intraarterial iodized oil with and without chemotherapeutic agents. *Radiology* 1987;162:345–351.
14. Nakamura H, Hashimoto T, Oi H, Sawada S. Transcatheter oily chemoembolization of hepatocellular carcinoma. *Radiology* 1989;170:783–786.
15. Sironi S, Cobelli F, Livraghi Y, et al. Small hepatocellular carcinoma treated with percutaneous ethanol injection: unenhanced and gadolinium-enhanced MR imaging follow-up. *Radiology* 1994;192:407–412.
16. Liang HL, Yang FC, Pan HB, et al. Small hepatocellular carcinoma: safety and efficacy of single high-dose percutaneous acetic acid injection for treatment. *Radiology* 2000;214: 769–774.
17. Ohnishi K, Yoshioka H, Ito S, Fujiwara K. Prospective randomized controlled trial comparing percutaneous acetic acid injection and percutaneous ethanol injection for small hepatocellular carcinoma. *Hepatology* 1998;27:67–72.
18. Yamada R, Sato M, Kawabata M, Nakatsuka H, Nakamura K, Takashima S. Hepatic artery embolization in 120 patients with unresectable hepatoma. *Radiology* 1983;148:397–401.
19. Matsui O, Kadoya M, Yoshikawa J, et al. Small hepatocellular carcinoma: treatment with subsegmental transcatheter arterial embolization. *Radiology* 1993;188:79–83.
20. Dodd GD III, Frank M , Aribandi M, Chopra S, Chintapalli KN. Radiofrequency thermal ablation: computer analysis of the size of the thermal injury created by overlapping ablations. *Am J Roentgenol* 2001;177:777–782.
21. Cioni D, Lencioni R, Rossi S, et al. Radiofrequency thermal ablation of hepatocellular carcinoma: using contrast-enhanced harmonic power Doppler sonography to assess treatment outcome. *Am J Roentgenol* 2001;177:783–788.
22. Numata K, Tanaka K, Kiba T, et al. Nonresectable hepatocellular carcinoma: improved percutaneous ethanol injection therapy guided by CO_2-enhanced sonography. *Am J Roentgenol* 2001;177:789–798.
23. Hanson PS, Soulen MC. Tumor ablation: a review of techniques and outcomes. *Suppl Applied Radiol* 2001;30:70–81.
24. Bartolozzi C, Lencioni R, Caramella D, et al. Treatment of large HCC: transcatheter arterial chemoembolization combined with percutaneous ethanol injection versus repeated transcatheter arterial chemoembolization. *Radiology* 1995;197:812–818.

25. Livraghi T, Bolondi L, Lazzaroni S, et al. Percutaneous ethanol injection in the treatment of hepatocellular carcinoma in cirrhosis. *Cancer* 1992;69:925–929.
26. Sugiura N, Takara K, Ohto M, Okuda K, Hirooka N. Percutaneous intratumoral injection of ethanol under ultrasound imaging for treatment of small hepatocellular carcinoma. *Acta Hepatol Jpn* 1983;24:920–923.
27. Livraghi T, Festi D, Monti F, Salmi A, Vettori C. US-guided percutaneous alcohol injection of small hepatic and abdominal tumors. *Radiology* 1986;161:309–312.
28. Ohnishi K, Chin N, Ito S. Percutaneous acetic acid injection therapy for hepatocellular carcinoma less than 3 cm in diameter [in Japanese]. *Acta Hepatol Jpn* 1993;34:504–516.
29. Ebara M, Ohto M, Sugiura N, et al. Percutaneous ethanol injection for the treatment of small hepatocellular carcinoma: study of 95 patients. *J Gastroenterol Hepatol* 1990;5:616–626.
30. Livraghi T, Giorgio A, Marin G, et al. Hepatocellular carcinoma and cirrhosis in 746 patients: long-term results of percutaneous ethanol injection. *Radiology* 1995;197:101–108.
31. Lencioni R, Caramella D, Bartolozzi C. Hepatocellular carcinoma: use of color Doppler US to evaluate response to treatment with percutaneous ethanol injection. *Radiology* 1995;194: 113–118.
32. Bartolozzi C, Lencioni Ricci P, Paolicchi A, Rossi A, Passariello R. Hepatocellular carcinoma treatment with percutaneous ethanol injection: Evaluation with contrast-enhanced color Doppler US. *Radiology* 1998;209:387–393.
33. Ohnishi K, Yoshioka H, Ito S, Fujiwara K. Prospective randomized controlled trial comparing percutaneous acetic acid injection and percutaneous ethanol injection for small hepatocellular carcinoma. *Hepatology* 1998;27:67–72.
34. Lee MJ, Mueller PR, Dawson SL, et al. Percutaneous ethanol injection for the treatment of hepatic tumors: indications, mechanism of action, technique and efficacy. *Am J Roentgenol* 1995;164:215–220.
35. Okuda K, Musha H, Nakajima J, et al. Clinicopathological features of encapsulated hepatocellular carcinoma: a study of 26 cases. *Cancer* 1977;40:1240–1245.
36. Nakajima O. Pathological study on early hepatocellular carcinoma—a study of capsule and septum formation [in Japanese]. *Acta Hepatol Jpn* 1989;30:28–34.
37. Torimura T, Mechanism of the fibrous capsular formation surrounding hepatocellular carcinoma—immunohistochemical analysis [in Japanese]. *Acta Hepatol Jpn* 1989;30:1596–1605.
38. Joseph FB, Baumgartner DA, Bernardiino ME. Hepatocellular carcinoma: CT appearance after percutaneous ethanol ablation therapy. *Radiology* 1993;186:553–556.
39. Revandly RD, Chezmar JL. Percutaneous ethanol ablation therapy of malignant hepatic tumors using CT guidance. *Semin Intervent Radiol* 1993;10:82–87.
40. Lencioni R, Caramella D, Bartolozzi C. Response of hepatocellular carcinoma to percutaneous ethanol injection: CT and MR evaluation. *J Comput Assist Tomogr* 1993;17:723–729.
41. Hashimoto M., Watanabe O, Hirano Y, Kato K, Watarai J. Use of carbon dioxide microbubble-enhanced sonographic angiography for transcatheter arterial chemoembolization of hepatocellular carcinoma. *Am J Roentgenol* 1997;169:1307–1310.
42. Livraghi T, Vettori C, Lazzaroni S. Liver metastases: results of percutaneous ethanol injection in 14 patients. *Radiology* 1991;179:709–712.
43. Ohnishi K, Ohyama N, Ito S, Fujiwara K. Ultrasound guided intratumor injection of acetic acid for the treatment of small hepatocellular carcinoma. *Radiology* 1994;193:747–752.
44. Shiina S, Tagawa K, Niwa Y, et al. Percutaneous ethanol injection therapy for hepatocellular carcinoma: results in 146 patients. *Am J Roentgenol* 1993;160:1023–1028.
45. Cedrone A, Rapaccini GL, Pompili M, Grattagliano A, Aliotta A, Trombino C. Neoplastic seeding complicating percutaneous ethanol injection for treatment of hepatocellular carcinoma. *Radiology* 1992;183:787,788.
46. Ishii H, Okada S, Okusaka T, Yoshimori M. Needle track implantation of hepatocellular carcinoma after ethanol injection. *Cancer* 1998;82:1638–1642.

47. Zerbey A, Mueller PR, Dawson S, Hoover HC Jr. Pleural seeding from hepatocellular carcinoma: a complication of percutaneous alcohol ablation. *Radiology* 1994;193:81,82.
48. Sumi S, Yamashita Y, Mitsuzaki K, et al. Power Doppler sonography assessment of tumor recurrence after chemoembolization therapy for hepatocellular carcinoma. *Am J Roentgenol* 1999;172:67–71.
49. Solbiati L, Goldberg SN, Ierace T, Dellanoce M, Livraghi T, Gazella GS. Radio-frequency ablation of hepatic metastases: postprocedural assessment with a US microbubble contrast agent—early experience. *Radiology* 1999;211:643–649.
50. Sironi S, Cobelli FD, Livraghi T, et al. Small hepatocellular carcinoma treated with percutaneous ethanol injection: unenhanced and gadolinium-enhanced MR imaging follow-up. *Radiology* 1994;192:407–412.
51. Nagel HS, Bernardino ME. Contrast enhanced MR imaging of hepatic lesions treated with percutaneous ethanol ablation therapy. *Radiology* 1993;189:265–270.
52. Takayama T, Makuuchi M, Hirohashi S, et al. Malignant transformation of adenomatous hyperplasia to hepatocellular carcinoma. *Lancet* 1990;336:1150–1153.

8 Radiofrequency Ablation of Hepatocellular Carcinoma

Martin Goodman, MD
and David A. Geller, MD

CONTENTS

1. INTRODUCTION

Hepatocellular carcinoma (HCC) is a major problem worldwide, with an estimated 1 million new cases diagnosed annually. Major risk factors are infections with hepatitis B virus (HBV) or hepatitis C virus (HCV). In Asia, the risk is as high as 30–65 per 100,000 persons per year, whereas in the United States, the incidence is 2 per 100,000 persons per year *(1)*. Although cirrhosis is not present in all cases, it has been estimated to be present 70–90% of the time *(2–5)*. The annual conversion rate of cirrhosis to HCC is 3–6% *(6)*. Therefore, any surgical therapy must consider not only the cancer but also the underlying liver function and reserve. It is often the degree of liver dysfunction or reserve that will determine the optimal treatment. Only 10–15% of patients with HCC are eligible for hepatic resection *(7–9)*. At present, surgical resection or liver transplantation offers the only chance for cure in the small subset of patients eligible. Contraindications to resection include extrahepatic involvement; multifocal, bilobar disease; inadequate hepatic reserve; or overall poor clinical condition of the patient.

From: *Current Clinical Oncology: Hepatocellular Cancer: Diagnosis and Treatment*
Edited by: B. I. Carr © Humana Press Inc., Totowa, NJ

Many treatment options exist in an attempt to palliate patients with unresectable HCC. They include intra-arterial chemotherapy, ethanol injection, chemoembolization, cryotherapy, radiofrequency (RF) ablation, and systemic chemotherapy. This chapter reviews the current status of radiofrequency ablation (RFA) in the treatment of HCC.

2. RFA BACKGROUND AND METHODS

2.1. RFA Historical Background

In 1891, d'Arsonval discovered that RF waves at an alternating electrical current (>10 kHz) could pass through living tissue without pain or neuromuscular excitation *(7,10,11)*. The resistance of the tissue to the rapidly alternating current would produce heat. This discovery helped develop the application of electrocautery in surgery. The first to use this technology was Beer *(12)* in 1908, who used RF coagulation to destroy urinary bladder tumors. Cushing and Bovie *(13)* later applied RF ablation to intracranial tumors. Lounsberry et al. *(14)* in 1961 studied the histological changes of the liver after RFA in animal models. He found that RF caused local tissue destruction with uniform necrosis. There was a demarcation line between normal cells and necrotic cells. Cooling from the circulation prevented thrombosis of adjacent blood vessels.

In the early 1990s, two independent groups of investigators proposed that RFA can be an effective method for destroying unresectable malignant liver tumors *(15,16)*. Both groups found that RF lesions had a well-demarcated area of necrosis without any viable tumor cells present. Subsequent animal and human trials have suggested that RF is safe and effective in the treatment of liver tumors *(17–19)*. Since these early reports, RFA technology has been used to ablate ectopic foci in cardiac arrhythmias and seizure disorders, sympathectomy for pain control, menorrhagia, osteoid osteomas, as well as lung, brain, kidney, breast, pancreas, and prostate tumors.

2.2. Mechanism of Ablation

RF thermal ablation is defined as thermal injury resulting from frictional heat generated by the ionic agitation of particles within tissue after the application of alternating current *(20)*. The electrode transmits alternating current within the RF range (200–1200 MHz), resulting in frictional heat in the surrounding tissue that causes cellular destruction and tissue necrosis *(21)*. The heat generated around the electrode is dissipated rapidly within a short distance from the electrode. To increase the volume of ablated tissue, the shape, size, and position of the electrode is altered *(22)*. If the current generated is too high or is applied too rapidly, the ablated area will be irregular or small. If the temperature of the tissue surrounding the electrode reaches 110°C, rapid desiccation will occur, causing tissue adherence to the electrode. This will then act as an insulator and will impede further flow of the current. The optimal temperature for coagulation of liver tissue to occur is 80–100°C, with a minimum of 50°C *(23,24)*. An understanding of the physics is essential to achieve an effective ablation.

2.3. RFA Equipment

Three different RFA systems currently are available with Food and Drug Administration approval for biomedical devices. RITA Medical Systems (Mountain View, CA) offers the Starburst XL electrode that is a 14-gage insulated needle with nine retractable-curved electrodes capable of generating a 3- to 5-cm ablation (www.ritamedical.com). The generator has a maximal 150-watt power output operating at 460 kHz frequency. Four of the electrodes are hollow and measure the temperature of the surrounding tissue. The generator is started at 25 watts and is slowly increased over a few minutes. After the temperature reaches approx 100°C, the electrodes are fully deployed. The temperature is maintained as a constant by adjusting the watts applied over a certain interval. Recently, the company has developed a Starburst XLi electrode that uses hypertonic saline infusion and is marketed to provide up to a 7-cm ablation zone, although clinical reports with this device are not yet available.

RadioTherapeutics Corporation (Sunnyvale, CA) was recently acquired by Boston Scientific Corporation. They offer a family of LeVeen RFA electrodes capable of achieving ablations of 2–4 cm (www.radiotherapeutics.com). The electrodes currently available have 10 (2.0, 3.0, 3.5 cm) or 12 (4.0 cm) retractable curved tines with length options of 12, 15, or 25 cm (for laparoscopic approach). The generators used are a 100-watt box with the 2- to 3.5-cm electrodes and a 200-watt box for the 4.0-cm electrode. The main difference between the RadioTherapeutics and RITA systems is that RadioTherapeutics uses tissue impedance as feedback monitoring, whereas RITA relies on temperature. The power is increased gradually over a 10- to 15-minute period until the impedance rises to more than 200 ohms, achieving roll-off. A second phase of thermal ablation is used for each deployment.

Radionics (Burlington, VT) was acquired by Tyco Healthcare and is the third company offering an RF ablation system. Their design is the Cool-tip 17-gage hollow needle RFA electrode that can record the temperature of the surrounding tissue (www.radionics.com). The power generator is a 200-watt box using a 480-kHz alternating current and can display temperature as well as tissue impedance. Internal channels allow chilled water to perfuse the needle. The cooled needle prevents charring around the electrode tip and keeps resistance low to produce a larger ablation zone *(7,25–27)*. The Cool-tip needles are available as a single electrode achieving 2- to 4-cm ablations, or a cluster of three single electrodes in a triangular pattern to achieve larger ablations. Similar to the other companies, the electrodes vary in length from 10 to 25 cm.

2.4. Evaluation and Patient Selection

Metastatic colorectal cancer and HCC make up the majority of hepatic tumors that undergo RFA. It is important to point out that surgical resection remains the gold standard in any patient harboring HCC or a metastatic tumor that is amenable to resection. Unfortunately, concurrent cirrhosis often limits the ability of the patient to tolerate a major resection, and these patients should be considered for liver transplantation if they meet listing criteria (*see* Chapter 10). RFA is reserved for those patients who are deemed unresectable either based on tumor size, number, location, or inadequate hepatic reserve. RFA also has been used as a bridge in patients with cirrhosis in whom a small HCC develops while awaiting a liver transplantation *(28,29)*. RFA also can be used to expand the operative indication in a subset of patients who have a resectable lesion in one lobe and a deep lesion in the contralateral lobe. Patients at risk for HCC are screened using α-fetoprotein (AFP) and des-γ-carboxyprothrombin serum tumor markers, as well as radiographic imaging with a triphasic computed tomography (CT) scan or contrast magnetic resonance imaging (MRI).

Absolute contraindications to RFA include the presence of extrahepatic disease, life expectancy less than 6 months, altered mental status, active infection, or tumor abutting a major hepatic duct (Table 1). Although there is not uniform agreement in the literature, relative contraindications include lesions larger than 5 cm (especially in a cirrhotic liver), more than four lesions, severe pulmonary or cardiac disease, and refractory coagulopathy. Tumors larger than 5 cm require overlapping fields with the current electrode technology and are associated with increased risk of abscess formation *(30)*.

2.5. Procedure

With each case, the goal is to thermally ablate the entire lesion and a 1-cm rim of normal liver at the tumor margin *(31)*. The route of RFA electrode delivery can be either percutaneous, laparoscopic, or open. The percutaneous approach is carried out either in the radiology suite or in the operating room. Because of the pain associated with the procedure, sedation and intravenous narcotics are required for the awake, percutaneous approach. For laparoscopic or open RFA cases, the procedure is performed under general anesthesia. Obviously, minimally invasive approaches (percutaneous or laparoscopic) are preferable for the patient. Several factors must be taken into consideration in deciding the best strategy for each patient. These include number of lesions, size, and location. For example, a lesion extending to the liver capsule in the left lobe or caudal side of the right lobe actually may be in close proximity to the stomach or colon. Percutaneous targeting risks thermal injury to these organs and is better handled by the laparoscopic or open approach. A history of multiple prior abdominal operations with adhesions may preclude adequate laparoscopy and may require an open

Table 1
Contraindications for RFA

Absolute contraindications	*Relative contraindications*
Extrahepatic disease	Lesions more than 5 cm, especially in cirrhotic patients
Life expectancy less than 6 months	More than four lesions
Altered mental status	Severe pulmonary or cardiac disease
Active infection	Refractory coagulopathy
Tumor abutting a major hepatic duct	

approach. A lesion high in the dome of the right lobe also can be challenging. By percutaneous route, the electrode must traverse the lung and diaphragm, risking pneumothorax or bleed. By laparoscopic approach, the high lesions can be difficult to reach.

At our institution, the RFA equipment of choice is the RadioTherapeutics system. To be eligible for a percutaneous approach, we prefer a solitary, intrahepatic tumor smaller than 3 cm and readily visualized on ultrasound. When there are multiple lesions or the tumor is not safely accessible by percutaneous route, the laparoscopic approach is preferred unless the patient is undergoing another procedure such as resection that requires a laparotomy. If the procedure is being performed percutaneously or laparoscopically, a sheathed needle is used to puncture the skin. The needle is removed, leaving the sheath for passage of the RFA electrode. This minimizes the theoretical risk of tumor seeding along the needle track in the abdominal wall *(32)*.

Regardless of the approach, ultrasound guidance is used to place the needle electrode into the tumor. It requires careful positioning to avoid leaving any viable tumor behind. If the lesion is too large to be targeted completely with one deployment, then the deep margin is ablated first, followed by electrode withdrawal to achieve the superficial margin. As soon as the ablation is initiated, gas in the tissue obscures visualization beyond the deep margin. During the procedure, the area of ablation develops a zone of increased echogenicity and microbubbles *(33)*. There is conflicting evidence regarding whether ultrasound immediately after ablation can assess the adequacy of the treatment. Some studies have shown that this does not give an accurate assessment of the tumor margins *(34,35)*. Recently, Cioni et al. *(36)* evaluated the use of a contrast-enhanced harmonic power Doppler ultrasound vs biphasic helical CT scan in evaluating postablation lesions in 50 patients with HCC. Using a microbubble contrast agent, they found that the Doppler ultrasound had similar results in evaluating the thermal zone of destruction compared with CT. During laparoscopy or laparotomy, vascular inflow occlusion with a Pringle maneuver can be performed to facilitate achieving a larger zone of ablation by decreasing the heat sink of the adjacent blood vessels *(37,38)*. For follow-up, it is our practice to obtain CT scans at 3 and 6 months after the RFA, although some groups recommend a follow-up scan as early as 1 month after RFA *(39,40)*. Depending on the level of concern, we then obtain subsequent scans every 6 months (or more frequently) for 2 years. Rising tumor markers or scans showing contrast enhancement at the periphery of the ablation zone suggest recurrence.

2.6. Complications

The complications associated with RFA are minor compared with the potential problems reported with cryosurgery *(41)*. Transient liver dysfunction with increased liver function tests is seen in all patients and reflects tissue necrosis with transaminase release. Hemorrhage, biliary stricture or leak, subcapsular hematoma, or cholecystitis are rare. Abscess formation within the RFA site has been reported in 3–15% of cases. We have seen 2 cases of delayed liver abscesses in 60 consecutive ablations (3.3%). The first occurred 5 weeks after ablation in a patient with a 5.5-cm lesion with pre-existing peripheral bile duct dilatation. (In retrospect, the patient may have had underlying cholangitis at the time of RFA with delayed seeding of what is normally a sterile cavity.) The second was an abscess detected 4 months after ablation in a patient receiving adjuvant chemotherapy who experienced neutropenia. Both were successfully managed by drainage procedures. Approximately 20–30% of patients will exhibit an ablation syndrome with fever and flulike symptoms that are usually self-limited. Fever persisting beyond 72 hours or higher than 39°C requires further evaluation. Major complications or death occur rarely.

Complications associated with RFA include liver dysfunction or failure, hemorrhage, abscess formation, bile leak, bile duct stricture, subcapsular hematoma, needle track seeding, burn at grounding pad site, cholecystitis, febrile syndrome, pneumonia, and myocardial infarction.

Table 2 outlines the morbidity and mortality in 13 RFA series reported from 1998 through 2001. Focusing on HCC, Curley et al. *(42)* undertook a prospective study evaluating RFA of 149 HCC tumor nodules in 110 patients with cirrhosis. Child's classification at the time of RFA treatment was Child's A in 50 patients (45.4%), Child's B in 31 patients (28.2%), and Child's C in 29 patients (26.4%). Percutaneous approach was performed in 76 patients (69.1%), whereas 31 patients (28.2%) were treated at laparotomy, and 3 patients (2.7%) were treated with laparoscopy. There were no deaths within 90 days of the treatment. Complications occurred in 14 patients (12.7%). Treatment-related complications occurred in 4 patients (8%) with Child's A, 2 patients (6.5%) with Child's B, and 8 patients (27.6%) with Child's C cirrhosis. The complication rates were similar regardless of the RFA approach used and included hemorrhage, subcapsular hematoma, wound hematoma, ascites, hydropneumothorax, pleural effusion, and ventricular fibrillation.

Buscarini et al. *(43)* evaluated 88 patients with HCC and cirrhosis. Percutaneous RFA was used in all cases, accounting for 101 total tumor ablations. Fifty-six patients had Child's A cirrhosis (65%), 29 patients had Child's B cirrhosis (34%), and 1 patient had Child's C cirrhosis (1%). Two patients (2.3%) experienced subcapsular hematoma. There were 14 (15.9%) minor complications requiring oral analgesics. Nicoli et al. *(44)* reviewed their experience of 79 patients with recurrent HCC treated with RFA. Two patients (2%) died as a result of the procedure. Both patients experienced sepsis, one from a colonic perforation, and one from an unknown source. One patient (1.2%) experienced ascites and another (1.2%) experienced liver insufficiency. They had a 20% minor complication rate.

Tumor seeding along the needle track was reported in 4 of 32 patients (12.5%) undergoing percutaneous RFA for HCC by the Barcelona Clinic Liver Cancer Group *(32)*. They used the cooled-tip single electrode system from Radionics. Seeding occurred outside the hepatic capsule in three patients and in the paracolic gutter in one patient at 4–18 months after RFA. Presence of subcapsular location that precluded ablation of the needle track or poor degree of differentiation were independent variables predicting tumor seeding. Although tumor track seeding is a serious complication, it is interesting that it has not been reported in other series with hundreds of cumulative patients. It is unclear whether the increased risk of seeding in the current study was related to the antecedent liver biopsy in 84% of cases, or whether the saline cooled-tip design predisposes to such an event compared with the retractable arrays with the RITA or RadioTherapeutics devices.

3. RESULTS

It is unknown whether RFA is comparable with resection because long-term follow-up (5 years) is not yet available. There are numerous studies in the literature that look at outcomes and local recurrences after RFA (Table 2). In the largest reported series of 110 cirrhotic patients undergoing RFA for HCC, the recurrence rate was 49%, with a median follow-up of 19 months *(42)*. Fifty-three of the 54 recurrences were diagnosed within 12 months of the initial RFA treatment. Interestingly, the local failure rate at the RFA site was only 4%, and all of these occurred in tumors larger than 4 cm. All local recurrences were evident within 6 months of ablation. Hepatic recurrences not involving the RFA site were detected in 37 patients (34%), and extrahepatic spread was identified in 13 cases (12%). Sites of extrahepatic metastases were lung (nine patients), bone (two patients), adrenal gland (one patient), or peritoneum (one patient). Of the 37 patients who had a recurrence in the liver, 14 underwent a second RFA

Table 2
Morbidity, Mortality, and Recurrence From RFA

Study	*No. patients*	*No. lesions*	*Morbidity and mortality*	*Median follow-up (months)*	*Recurrence at RFA site*	*Distant recurrence*
Buscarini, 2001 *(43)*	88 (100%)	101	2.3% morbidity, 0 mortality, 2 subcapsular hematoma	34	12 (11.8%)	Liver, 29 (33.0%)
Nicoli, 2001 *(44)*	79 (100%)	86	2.5% morbidity, 2.5% mortality, 1 ascites, 1 liver failure, 2 deaths from sepsis	NA	NA	NA
Bowles, 2001 *(45)*	76 (33%)	328	19.7% morbidity, 1.3% mortality, 3 bile leaks, 2 bile duct stricture, 1 bleeding, 2 grounding pad burns, 2 wound infections, 5 myoglobinuria, 1 death liver failure	15	30 (9%)	NA
Chung, 2001 *(48)*	27 (15%)	85	3.7% morbidity, 0 mortality, 1 delayed bleeding	14	4 (4.7%)	16 (59%)
Bilchik, 2000 *(41)*	68 (13.2%)	181	8.8% morbidity, 1.5% mortality, 1 bile duct stricture, 3 abscesses, 1 bleeding, 1 diaphragmatic necrosis	12	5 (2.8%)	28 (41%)
Curley, 2000 *(42)*	110 (100%)	149	8% morbidity, 0 mortality, 1 delayed bleeding, 4 ascites, 2 pleural effusions,	19	4 (3.6%)	Liver, 37 (33.6%); extrahepatic, 13 (11.8%)

			1 persistent fever, 1 V-fib			
Goldberg, 2000 *(46)*	22 (18%)	23	4.5% morbidity, 0 mortality, 1 grounding pad burn	NA	NA	NA
Siperstein, 2000 *(47)*	43 (6.1%)	181	NA	12	22 (12.2%)	NA
Wood, 2000 *(49)*	84 (13%)	231	9.5% morbidity, 3.6% mortality, 1 grounding pad burn, 1 delayed bleeding, 3 abscesses, 1 liver, insufficiency, 1 heart attack, 3 deaths	9	15 (6.5%)	33 (39.3%)
Elias, 2000 *(50)*	21 (0)	33	23.8% morbidity, 0 mortality, 1 bile leak, 4 liver insufficiencies	17.3	1 (3.1%)	Liver, 7 (21%); extrahepatic, 8 (24%)
Goletti, 2000 *(51)*	7 (100%)	10	NA	6	0	Liver, 2 (28.6%)
Cuschieri, 1999 *(52)*	10 (20%)	32	0 morbidity, 10% mortality, 1 death liver failure, hepatorenal	13	0	Liver, 1 (10%)
Pearson, 1999 *(53)*	92 (37%)	138	3.3% morbidity, 0 mortality, 1 delayed bleeding, 2 abscess	15	3 (2.2%)	NA
Curley, 1999 *(54)*	123 (39%)	169	2.4% morbidity, 0 mortality, 2 abscesses 1 delayed bleeding	15	3 (1.8%)	Liver, 27 (21.9%); extrahepatic, 7 (5.7%)
Rossi, 1998 *(55)*	37 (62%)	40	2.7% morbidity, 0 mortality, 1 capsular necrosis	11	HCC, 1 (4.2%); Other, 1 (6.3%) 5 (21.7%);	Liver, extrahepatic, 0; liver, 5 (35.7%); extrahepatic 7 (50%)

treatment. Twelve of the 14 patients had no evidence of any new disease with a median follow-up of 6 months. The survival data from this study showed that 28 patients (25.4%) died of recurrent disease, 26 patients (23.6%) were alive but had recurrent disease, 53 patients (48.2%) are alive and disease-free, and 3 patients (2.7%) died of other causes. Serum AFP levels were elevated in 79 patients (71.8%) before surgery. All 79 patients had lower AFP levels 1 month after RFA, but 26 of these did not return to the normal range.

Bowles et al. *(45)* evaluated 76 patients who underwent 99 operations on 328 tumors. The tumors were HCC in 33% and metastatic disease in 67% of the patients. With a median follow-up of 15 months, local recurrence was identified in 9% of the ablated tumors. The recurrence rate was higher in metastatic tumors compared with HCC. Higher recurrence rates were statistically significant in patients with vascular invasion ($p < 0.001$), size >4 cm ($p < 0.001$), and larger total volume ablated ($p < 0.001$). There was no correlation with recurrence regarding age, sex, Child's classification, number of tumors, or the occurrence of complications. Tumor markers were elevated in 76% of patients before surgery and declined in all but four patients after surgery. At the time of writing, 30 patients (39.4%) were alive without recurrence, 19 patients (25%) were alive with recurrence, 23 patients (30.3%) died of cancer, and 4 patients (5.3%) died free of disease.

Pulvirenti et al. *(29)* reported the largest series evaluating RFA of HCC before liver transplantation. Fourteen cirrhotic patients on the waiting list for a liver transplant underwent 18 RFA treatments of 16 HCC tumors. The median interval between RFA and transplantation was 8 months (range: 2–24 months), with a median tumor diameter of 3.5 cm (range: 1.7–6.0 cm). There were no deaths or major complications associated with the RFA. At time of writing, all patients were alive and disease free, with a mean posttransplant follow-up of 16 months. Ten of 14 patients (71%) had complete tumor necrosis on pretransplant CT scans and pathological analysis after explant. The remaining four patients had residual disease noted on CT scan as well as on pathological evaluation. Tumor satellites smaller than 1 cm were noted in 8 explants (57%), with a mean of two nodules (range: 1–5) per patient.

Goldstein et al. *(28)* reported on 23 patients who underwent 24 RFA procedures for biopsy-proven HCC while waiting on the liver transplant list. Ten of the RFA procedures were laparoscopic, and 14 were open. Lesions ranged in size from 1.5 to 5.0 cm. Seven patients with eight treated HCC lesions received liver transplants at a mean interval of 7 months from RFA. Seven of the eight treated lesions showed no viable tumor in the explanted liver. All patients were alive and disease-free with a mean posttransplant follow-up of 8 months.

4. CONCLUSIONS

RFA currently is used to treat patients with unresectable HCC or metastatic liver tumors. Although long-term follow-up is still pending, the early results are encouraging when compared with the limited options available for these patients. Major complications occur in less than 10% of cases in most series, with minimal to no mortality. Although randomized trials are lacking, application of RFA to treat patients with early HCC while awaiting liver transplant seems promising. In general, RFA is best applied to tumors smaller than 5 cm. Local recurrences at the RFA site have been documented to occur in 2–12% of cases and usually can be diagnosed by follow-up imaging studies. However, recurrences elsewhere in the liver or at extrahepatic sites will occur in 20–60% of cases, depending on the length of follow-up, and suggest that trials with a multimethod approach may be warranted.

REFERENCES

1. Mor E, Kaspa RT, Sheiner P, Schwartz M. Treatment of hepatocellular carcinoma associated with cirrhosis in the era of liver transplantation. *Ann Intern Med* 1998;129:643–653.
2. Nerenstone SR, Ihde DC, Friedman MA. Clinical trials in primary hepatocellular carcinoma: current status and future directions. *Cancer Treat Rev* 1988;15:1–31.
3. Okuda K. Hepatocellular carcinoma: recent progress. *Hepatology* 1992;15:948–963.
4. Ikeda K, Saitoh S, Koida I, et al. A multivariate analysis of risk factors or hepatocellular carcinogenesis: a prospective observation of 795 patients with viral and alcoholic cirrhosis. *Hepatology* 1993;18:47–53.
5. Colombo M, de Franchis R, Del Ninno E, et al. Hepatocellular carcinoma in Italian patients with cirrhosis. *N Engl J Med* 1991;325:675–680.
6. Colombo M. Hepatocellular carcinoma: an overview. In: *Viral Hepatitis and Liver Disease* (Rizzeto M, Purcell RH, Gerin JL, Verme G, eds.), Springer-Verlag, New York, 1994, pp. 479–483.
7. McGahan JP, Dodd GD III. Radiofrequency ablation of liver: current status. *Am J Roentgenol* 2001;176:3–14.
8. Tsuzuki T, Sugioka A, Ueda M. Hepatic resection for hepatocellular carcinoma. *Surgery* 1990;107:511–520.
9. Choi TK, Lai ECS, Fan ST, et al. Results of surgical resection for hepatocellular carcinoma. *Hepatogastroenterology* 1990;37:172–175.
10. d'Arsonval MA. Action physiologique des courants alternatifs. *CR Soc Biol* 1891; 43:283–286.
11. Siperstein AE, Gitomirski A. History and technological aspects of radiofrequency thermoablation. *Cancer J* 2000;6(suppl 4):s293–s303.
12. Beer E. Removal of neoplasms of the urinary bladder: a new method employing high frequency (oudin) currents through a cauterizing cystoscope. *JAMA* 1910;54:1768,1769.
13. Cushing H, Bovie WT. Electro-surgery as an aid to the removal of intracranial tumors. *Surg Gynecol Obstet* 1928;47:751–784.
14. Lounsberry W, Goldschmint V, Linke CA, et al. The early histologic changes following electrocoagulation. *J Urol* 1961;86:321–329.

15. McGahan JP, Browning PD, Brock JM, Tesluk H. Hepatic ablation using radiofrequency electrocautery. *Invest Radiol* 1990;25:267–270.
16. Rossi S, Fornari F, Pathies C, Buscarini L. Thermal lesions induced by 480 KHz localized current field in guinea pig and pig liver. *Tumori* 1990;76:54–57.
17. Rossi S, Fornari F, Buscarini L. Percutaneous ultrasound-guided radiofrequency electrocautery for the treatment of small hepatocellular carcinoma. *J Intervent Radiol* 1993;8:97–103.
18. Rossi S, Di Stasi M, Buscarini L, et al. Percutaneous radiofrequency interstitial thermal ablation in the treatment of small hepatocellular carcinoma. *Cancer J Scientific Am* 1995;1:73–81.
19. McGahan JP, Brock JM, Tesluk H, et al. Hepatic ablation with use of radiofrequency electrocautery in the animal model. *J Vasc Interv Radiol* 1992;3:291–297.
20. Chamberlain RS, Fong Y. Radiofrequency thermal ablation of liver tumors. In: *Surgery of the Liver and Biliary Tract*, 3rd ed. (Blumgart LH, Fong Y, eds.), WB Saunders, Philadelphia, 2000, pp. 1589–1595.
21. Scudamore C. Volumetric radiofrequency ablation: technical considerations. *Cancer J* 2000;6(suppl 4):s316–s318.
22. Goldberg SN, Gazelle GS, Dawson SL, Rittman WJ, Mueller PR, Rosenthal DI. Tissue ablation with radiofrequency: effect of probe size, gauge, duration, and temperature on lesion volume. *Acad Radiol* 1995;2:399–404.
23. Haines DE. The biophysics of radiofrequency catheter ablation the heart: the importance of temperature monitoring. *Pacing Clin Electrophysiol* 1993;16:586–591.
24. McGahan JP, Gu WZ, Brock JMP, et al. Hepatic ablation using bipolar radiofrequency electrocautery. *Acad Radiol* 1996;3:418–422.
25. Goldberg SN, Gazelle GS, Solbiati L, Rittman WJ, Mueller PR. Radiofrequency tissue ablation: increased lesion diameter with a perfusion electrode. *Acad Radiol* 1996;3:636–644.
26. Lorentzen T, Christensen NE, Nolsle CP, Torp-Pedersen ST. Radiofrequency tissue ablation with cooled needle in vitro: ultrasonography, dose response, and lesion temperature. *Acad Radiol* 1997;4:292–297.
27. Livraghi T, Goldberg SN, Monti F, et al. Saline-enhanced radio-frequency tissue ablation the treatment of liver metastases. *Radiology* 1997;202:205–210.
28. Goldstein RM, Orr DW, Meyer RL, Derrick GC, Westmoreland MV, Levy MF, et al. Treatment of hepatomas in cirrhotic patients with radiofrequency thermal ablation. *Transplantation* 2000;69(8 suppl):S137.
29. Pulvirenti A, Garbagnati F, Regalia E, et al. Experience with radiofrequency ablation of small hepatocellular carcinomas before liver transplantation. *Trans Proc* 2001;33:1516,1517.
30. Goldberg SN, Gazelle GS, Halpern EF, et al. Radiofrequency tissue ablation: importance of local temperature along the electrode tip exposure in determining lesion shape and size. *Acad Radiol* 1996;3:212–218.
31. Cady B, Jenkins RL, Steele GD Jr, et al. Surgical margin in hepatic resection for colorectal metastasis: a critical and improvable determination of outcome. *Ann Surg* 1998;227:566–571.
32. Llovet JM, Milana R, Bru C, Bianchi L, et al. Increased risk of tumor seeding after percutaneous radiofrequency ablation for single hepatocellular carcinoma. *Hepatology* 2001;33:1124–1129.
33. Solbiati L, Goldberg SN, Ierance T, et al. Radiofrequency ablation of hepatic metastases: postprocedural assessment with a US microbubble contrast agent—early experience. *Radiology* 1999;221:643–649.
34. Rossi S, Di Stasi M, Buscarini E, et al. Percutaneous RF interstitial thermal ablation in the treatment of hepatic cancer. *Am J Roentgenol* 1996;167:759–768.
35. Solbiati L. New applications of ultrasonography: interventional ultrasound. *Eur J Radiol* 1998;27:S200–S206.
36. Cioni D, Lencioni R, Rossi S, et al. Radiofrequency thermal ablation of hepatocellular carcinoma: using contrast-enhanced harmonic power Doppler sonography to assess treatment outcome. *Am J Roentgenol* 2001;177:783–788.

37. Delva E, Camus Y, Nordlinger B, et al. Vascular occlusions for liver resection. *Ann Surg* 1989;209:297–304.
38. Curley SA, Davidson BS, Fleming RYD, et al. Laparoscopically guided bipolar radiofrequency ablation of areas of porcine liver. *Surg Endoscopy* 1997;11:729–733.
39. Dromain C, De Baere TJ, Elias D, Ducre M, Sabourin J, Vanel D. Follow-up imaging of liver tumors treated using percutaneous radio frequency therapy with helical CT and MRI imaging. *Radiology* 1999;219:382.
40. Choi H, Loyer EM, DuBrow RA, et al. Radiofrequency ablation of liver tumors: assessment of therapeutic response and complications. *Radiographics* 2001;21:S41–S54.
41. Bilchik AJ, Wood TF, Allegra D, et al. Cryosurgical ablation and radiofrequency ablation for unresectable hepatic malignant neoplasms. *Arch Surg* 2000;135:657–664.
42. Curley SA, Izzo F, Ellis LM, Vauthey JN, Vallone P. Radiofrequency ablation of hepatocellular cancer in 110 patients with cirrhosis. *Ann Surg* 2000;232:381–391.
43. Buscarini L, Buscarini E, Di Stasi M, Vallisa D, Quaretti P, Rocca A. Percutaneous radiofrequency ablation of small hepatocellular carcinoma: long-term results. *Eur Radiol* 2001;11:914–921.
44. Nicoli N, Casaril A, Marchiori L, Mangiante G, Hasheminia AR. Treatment of recurrent hepatocellular carcinoma by radiofrequency ablation. *J Hepatobiliary Panc Surg* 2001;8: 417–421.
45. Bowles BJ, Machi J, Limm WML, et al. Safety and efficacy of radiofrequency thermal ablation in advanced liver tumors. *Arch Surg* 2001;136:864–869.
46. Goldberg SN, Gazelle GS, Compton CC, Mueller PR, Tanabe KK. Treatment of intrahepatic malignancy with radiofrequency ablation. *Cancer* 2000;88:2452–2463.
47. Siperstein A, Garland A, Engle K, et al. Local recurrence after laparoscopic radiofrequency thermal ablation of hepatic tumors. *Ann Surg Oncol* 2000;7:106–113.
48. Chung MH, Wood TF, Tsioulias GJ, Rose DM, Bilchik AJ. Laparoscopic radiofrequency ablation of unresectable hepatic malignancies. *Surg Endosc* 2001;15:1020–1026.
49. Wood TF, Rose DM, Chung M, Allegra DP, Foshag LJ, Bilchik AJ. Radiofrequency ablation of 231 unresectable hepatic tumors: indications, limitations, and complications. *Ann Surg Oncol* 2000;7:593–600.
50. Elias D, Goharin A, Otmany E, et al. Usefulness of intraoperative radiofrequency thermoablation of liver tumours associated or not with hepatectomy. *Eur J Surg Oncol* 2000;26:763–769.
51. Goletti O, Lencioni R, Armillotta N, et al. Laparoscopic radiofrequency thermal ablation of hepatocarcinoma: preliminary experience. *Surg Laparosc Endosc Percutan Tech* 2000;10:284–290.
52. Cuschieri A, Bracken J, Boni L. Initial experience with laparoscopic ultrasound-guided radiofrequency thermal ablation of hepatic tumours. *Endoscopy* 1999;31:318–321.
53. Pearson AS, Izzo F, Fleming RYD, et al. Intraoperative radiofrequency ablation or cryoablation for hepatic malignancies. *Am J Surg* 1999;178:592–599.
54. Curley SA, Izzo F, Delrio P, et al. Radiofrequency ablation of unresectable primary and metastatic hepatic malignancies. *Ann Surg* 1999;230:1–8.
55. Rossi S, Buscarini L, Garbagnati F, et al. Percutaneous treatment of small hepatic tumors by an expandable RF needle electrode. *Am J Roentgenol* 1998;170:1015–1022

9 Hepatic Resection for Hepatocellular Carcinoma

Katsuhiko Yanaga, MD, PhD,
Sadayuki Okudaira, MD, PhD,
Takashi Kanematsu, MD, PhD,
and J. Wallis Marsh, MD

Contents

1. INTRODUCTION

Hepatocellular carcinoma (HCC) is one of the most common tumors worldwide, with an estimated incidence of new cases ranging between 500,000 and 1 million annually. Historically, hepatic resection, either partial or total, has been considered to be the mainstay of surgical therapy. Liver transplantation, although known to have superior outcomes in patients with advanced concomitant cirrhosis, often is not feasible because the availability of hepatic allografts cannot meet demand; therefore, liver transplantation can be applied to only a small

From: *Current Clinical Oncology: Hepatocellular Cancer: Diagnosis and Treatment*
Edited by: B. I. Carr © Humana Press Inc., Totowa, NJ

percentage of patients with HCC. To date, considerable knowledge and experience have been accumulated in resectional treatment for HCC, particularly in industrialized countries with a high incidence of viral hepatitis, and include: patient selection, improved preoperative diagnosis of tumor size and location in relation to intrahepatic vasculature, refined techniques for parenchymal dissection, improved understanding of the oncological behavior of HCC, and the influence of hepatic parenchymal inflammation on recurrence.

This chapter describes the current indications for and outcomes of resectional treatment for HCC, including extrahepatic metastatic lesions.

2. PREOPERATIVE EVALUATION

The accurate preoperative assessment of hepatic reserve as well as tumor size and distribution are extremely important factors when considering surgery for HCC and include some or all of the following: radiological diagnostic tests (computed tomography [CT], ultrasound, magnetic resonance imaging [MRI], angiography); viral serological markers (hepatitis B virus [HBV], hepatitis C virus [HCV]); tumor markers (α-fetoprotein [AFP], AFP subtype lectin 3 [L3], protein induced by vitamin K absence or antagonist [PIVKA]); assessment of cardiac disease, diabetes mellitus, ascites, icterus, nutrition; and assessment of hepatic reserve (indocyanine green retention rate).

Among the radiological diagnostic tests, helical, triphasic CT is the standard study; ultrasonography is sensitive for small, early HCCs but is inherently subjective. Angiography gives accurate information on the anatomical characteristics of the inflow vessels (hepatic artery and portal vein), although this information most often can be obtained during surgery. MRI allows for an objective assessment of the intrahepatic vasculature, especially the hepatic veins as they relate to the tumor(s). Magnetic resonance cholangiography (MRC) gives information on the intrahepatic biliary tree without the need for invasive studies such as endoscopic retrograde cholangiography (ERC) or percutaneous transhepatic cholangiography (PTC); however, the resolution of MRC does not produce the fine detail of the other two.

Screening for hepatitis B and C should be performed. If results for hepatitis B surface antigen (HBsAg) are positive, results for hepatitis B surface antibody (HBsAb), hepatitis B core antibody (HBcAb), hepatitis B e antigen (HBeAg), and hepatitis B e antibody (HBeAb) as well as blood HBV DNA should be obtained. If HCVAb results are positive, the quantitative viral load is assessed by blood HCV RNA, and HCV serotyping is performed.

3. STRATEGY FOR HEPATIC RESECTION

Because HCC usually develops in a cirrhotic or fibrotic liver, patient selection is of utmost importance. Preoperative selection criteria based on hepatic reserve consists of Child–Pugh classification and indocyanine dye retention rate at 15 minutes (ICG R15) *(1–3)*. Generally, patients should be in Child–Pugh class A or B, and the ICG R15 should be less than 35%. A value of less than 25 ng/mL for the lidocaine metabolism test with monoethylglycinexylidide (MEGX) also has been associated with safe hepatic resection *(4)*. Liver scintigraphy with 99m galactosyl-human serum albumin allows an assessment of hepatic reserve based on the selective uptake by asialoglycoprotein receptors on hepatocytes, which can be performed even in icteric patients *(5)*.Galactose elimination capacity also has been reported to predict complications and survival after hepatic resection *(6)*.

Of these studies, ICG R15 is the most frequently used determinant for the extent of hepatic resection and is used as follows: <15% for trisegmentectomy, <20% for lobectomy and anterior segmentectomy, <25% for posterior or medial segmentectomy, <30% for lateral segmentectomy, and <35% for subsegmentectomy or less.

To prevent postoperative hepatic failure, the preservation of hepatic parenchyma through the use of anatomical segmental or subsegmental resection as well as the judicious use of limited hepatic resection for small HCCs is advocated *(1,2)*.

The spread of HCC takes place primarily through the bloodstream, first via the portal vein to cause intrahepatic metastases and later to extrahepatic organs such as the lung, bone, and adrenal glands. During the late phase of hepatic resection for HCC, tumor cells have been documented in the portal vein in 23% of patients whose tumor diameter exceeds 5 cm with macroscopic or microscopic vein invasion, or both *(7)*. Therefore, inflow vessels should be occluded before hepatic mobilization or parenchymal dissection to minimize tumor cell dislodgment and spread *(8)*.

For resection of fibrotic or cirrhotic livers, conventional hilar dissection with separate control of the hepatic artery, portal vein, and bile duct of the segment or lobe to be resected often results in intractable ascites as a result of lymphorrhea. For this reason, hepatic inflow control is best achieved by *en masse* ligation and division of the Glisson's pedicle of the hepatic segment or lobe that harbors HCC *(8–10)*.

When the HCC to be resected is located in the anterosuperior or posterosuperior subsegment, a thoracoabdominal or transdiaphragmatic approach may be required *(11,12)*. For resection of large HCCs, conventional inflow control and hepatic mobilization may be difficult or even dangerous. In such circumstances, it is best to start the transection of the hepatic parenchyma and control inflow vessels and hepatic veins as they are encountered during the parenchymal dissection *(13,14)*.

For hepatic lobotomy or trisegmentectomy, residual liver size is an important determinant of early outcome *(15,16)*. Therefore, selected patients considered for extensive hepatic resection may benefit from preoperative portal vein embolization to induce compensatory hypertrophy of the unaffected liver *(17)*.

In cirrhotic patients, upper gastrointestinal endoscopy should be performed to evaluate esophagogastric varices before resectional therapy. In patients with a history of variceal hemorrhage and in those with large varices, endoscopic injection sclerotherapy or variceal ligation should be performed *(18,19)*. In selected patients with nonadvanced HCC, concomitant devascularization procedures may be performed during laparotomy *(19)*.

The significance of preoperative transarterial chemotherapy does not seem to improve the outcome of hepatic resection for HCC *(20,21)*. However, selected patients may become operable by preoperative systemic chemoimmunotherapy that includes interferon *(22)*.

4. PERIOPERATIVE MANAGEMENT

Although the liver is a sterile organ, infectious complications are not uncommon after liver resection *(23)*. Preoperative nasopharyngeal culture or decontamination by mupirocin ointment is recommended. For prophylactic purposes, patients without obvious bacterial contamination are covered during surgery with broad-spectrum antibiotics intravenously.

During surgery, ultrasonography is first performed to confirm the size and location of the tumor(s) and to identify their relationship to the intrahepatic vasculature; this allows determination of the hepatic resection plane *(24,25)*. During hepatic parenchymal transection, central venous pressure is preferably maintained at less than 5 cm H_2O to minimize blood loss *(26)*. For diaphragmatic invasion, combined resection of the diaphragm is a safe technique that can give long-term survival comparable with those without such invasion *(27,28)*.

After surgery, intravenous fluid of 5% glucose with electrolyte composition of quarter normal saline is given sparingly to maintain a low central venous pressure. Hypovolemia is corrected by intravenous colloids rather than crystalloids to avoid tissue and liver edema. Generally, the nasogastric tube can be removed on the first postoperative day, and oral intake is resumed the next day to minimize bacterial translocation through the intestine *(29,30)*. For uncomplicated patients, the drains are removed by the fifth postoperative day. For patients with persistent bile leakage with or without signs of infection, the drains should be left in place until this subsides. Daily irrigation of the cavity and antibiotic therapy may be required.

If signs of infection develop after the abdominal drains have been removal, CT with contrast is performed to rule out abscesses. If the tissue around the fluid collection exhibits enhancement, or if the fluid contains air-fluid levels or air bubbles, the fluid is drained percutaneously under ultrasound or CT guidance. Early recognition of intraperitoneal septic complications is important because uncontrolled infection among patients with cirrhosis can lead to hepatic failure *(23)*.

Table 1
Comparison of Early and Late Outcomes Among Eastern and Western Populations

Author	*Study years*	*No. of patients*	*No. with cirrhosis*	*Percent with cirrhosis*	*Mortality (%)*	*3-Year survival*	*3-Year disease-free survival*	*5-Year survival*	*5-Year disease-free survival*
Eastern experience									
Takenaka	1985–1993	280	146	(52%)	[6 (2%)][a]	70%	41%	50%	29%
Makuuchi	1990–1998	367	N/A		3 (0.8%)[b]	73%	32%	47%	13%
Hsia	1991–1996	168	79	(47%)	[3 (1.8%)]	70%	49%	59%	40%
Poon	1994–1999	241	104	(43%)	6(2.5%)	62%	38%	49%	25%
Hanazaki	1983–2000	386	171	(44%)	27 (7%)	51%	37%	34%	23%
Present authors	1991–2001	137	56	(41%)	10 (7.3%)[c]	70%	35%	55%	22%
Western experience									
Fong	1991–1999	1540			7 (4.5%)	54%	—	37%	—
Grazi[d]	1992–2001	157	157	100%	3 (1.3%)	72%	49%	50%	28%

[a] 30-day operative mortality.
[b] None of 193 since October 1994.
[c] One of 61 (1.6%) since January 1996.
[d] Cirrhotic patients only.

5. MORTALITY AND MORBIDITY OF HEPATIC RESECTION FOR HCC

Early and late outcomes for both Eastern and Western populations, respectively, are shown in Table 1 *(2,3,31–35)*.

Improved patient selection, better understanding of intrahepatic vascular anatomy, and reduced intraoperative blood loss are clinically relevant factors responsible for the improvement in outcomes during the past one to two decades *(18,36)*.

Complications of hepatic resection include intraperitoneal hemorrhage, gastrointestinal bleeding, atelectasis, pleural effusion, ascites, wound infection, intraperitoneal septic complications such as subphrenic abscess, and liver failure. Mortality after hepatic resection for HCC usually is the result of liver failure caused directly by excessive resection or indirectly after infectious or hemorrhagic complications, or both. As soon as progressive hyperbilirubinemia with a ratio of direct-to-indirect serum bilirubin of 2:1 and hyperammonemia with poor synthetic function are observed, liver failure is usually fatal without urgent liver replacement.

6. ONCOLOGICAL OUTCOME: PROGNOSTIC FACTORS

Prognostic factors of HCC after hepatic resection are listed in Table 2. Disease recurrence is related to advanced cancer stages as determined by tumor size and number, vascular invasion, and growth pattern.

As previously stated, because HCC usually coexists with diseased hepatic parenchyma, major hepatic resections are associated with the risk of developing liver failure. For this reason, obtaining a wide resection margin often is inadvisable *(1)*. The significance of the resection margin as a prognostic factor remains controversial *(18,32,36)*. Although the histological margin seems to be an important determinant of local recurrence, the gross surgical margin does not seem to be crucial *(37)*. For HCCs located below the diaphragmatic dome, combined resection of the liver with diaphragm is safe and gives survival comparable with those without diaphragmatic involvement, probably because histological invasion is unusual *(27,28)*.

Gross portal vein tumor thrombosis is associated with poor prognosis *(38)*. Technically, however, removal of extensive tumor thrombi such as those extending into or beyond the portal bifurcation can be performed with acceptable mortality, which can lead to long-term survival in selected patients *(39–43)*. Extensive portal vein tumor thrombi often show invasion of the portal vein wall, for which resection rather than simple thrombectomy should be considered *(42)*. The clinical significance of portal thromboembolectomy for portal decompression with the resultant prevention of variceal bleeding has yet to be determined.

Biliary tumor thrombosis is a rare complication of HCC that usually does not invade the bile duct wall *(44,45)*. With appropriate management of jaundice, if present, hepatic resection with thrombectomy through a choledochotomy gives long-term survival comparable with that of conventional resection.

7. EFFECT OF NONCANCEROUS HEPATIC PARENCHYMA ON RECURRENCE

Active inflammatory and proliferative hepatitic activity of the noncancerous hepatic parenchyma seems to play a major role in intrahepatic recurrence *(46–49)*. Further, fibrosis or cirrhosis seems to be associated with poor survival beyond 5 years after surgery *(50)*.

Table 2
Prognostic Factors of HCC After Hepatic Resection

Tumor or patient characteristics	*Risk of recurrence*
Clinical factors	
Preoperative liver function status	Child–Pugh A < B or C
Sex	Male > female
Age	Young < old
Underlying liver disease	Hepatitis B < C
Diabetes mellitus	Yes > no
Rupture	Yes > no
Operative	
Number of tumors	Multiple > single
Size of tumors	Large > small
Surgical manipulation of tumors	Yes > minimal
Anatomical resection	Yes < no
Perioperative blood transfusion	Yes > no
Postoperative factors	
Interval to recurrence	Before or at 1 year > after 1 year
Concurrent extrahepatic recurrence	Yes > no
Type of treatment for recurrence	Transarterial oily chemoembolization > re-resection
Pathological HCC factors	
Microvascular invasion	Yes > no
Satellite nodules	Yes > no
pTNM stage	III or IV > I or II
Nuclear grade	3 > 1 or 2
Fibrolamellar HCC	Yes < no
DNA ploidy	Diploid < aneuploid with multiple G0 or G1 peaks
Mitotic count	High > low
Proliferative activity	High > low
Noncancerous parenchyma	
Inflammation in the liver remnant	Yes > minimal
Liver cirrhosis or fibrosis	Yes > no
Laboratory	
Preoperative blood values	
Serum AFP	More than 400 ng/mL > less than 10 ng/mL
Serum VEGF	More than > equal to or less than 500 pg/mL
Serum IL-10	More than >, equal to, or less than 12 pg/mL
VEGF IL-10	

Abbreviations: HCC, hepatocellular carcinoma; AFP, α-fetoprotein; VGEF, vascular endothelial growth factor; IL, interleukin.

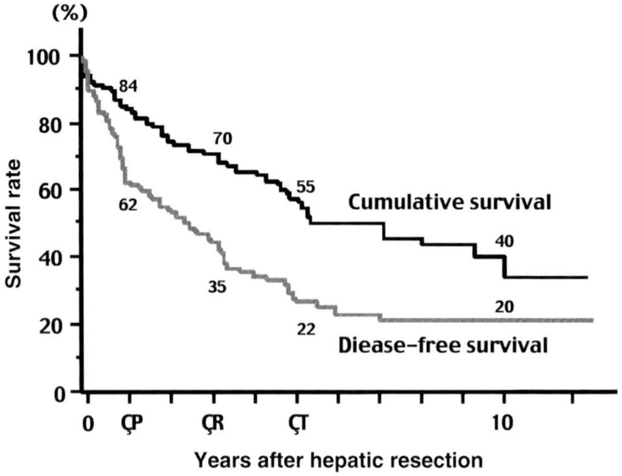

Fig. 1. Cumulative and disease-free survival (in years) after liver resection for hepatocellular carcinoma.

8. SIGNIFICANCE OF PALLIATIVE HEPATIC RESECTION

Because the survival for patients with unresectable HCC is limited and can be associated with tumor rupture, palliative hepatic resection in combination with other therapeutic methods such as intraoperative treatment of residual HCCs have been advocated to prolong survival *(51–53)*. After rupture, HCC is best treated by transarterial embolization followed by elective hepatic resection *(54,55)*. For cases of intraabdominal HCC rupture, peritoneal dissemination frequently follows successful resection *(55,56)*. Many other clinical, histological, oncologic, viral, and laboratory parameters also have been correlated with recurrence of HCC *(57–66)*.

9. PREVENTION AND TREATMENT OF RECURRENCE AFTER RESECTION

The cumulative and disease-free survival of patients who underwent hepatic resection for HCC between June 1991 and December 2001 at the Department of Surgery II, Nagasaki University Hospital, Japan, are shown in Fig. 1.

The high incidence of recurrent HCC after hepatic resection is a universal phenomenon for which better treatment methods are required (Fig. 2). As shown in Fig. 3, the most common site of recurrence in this series was the remnant liver, which accounted for 88% of recurrence, followed by lung and bone.

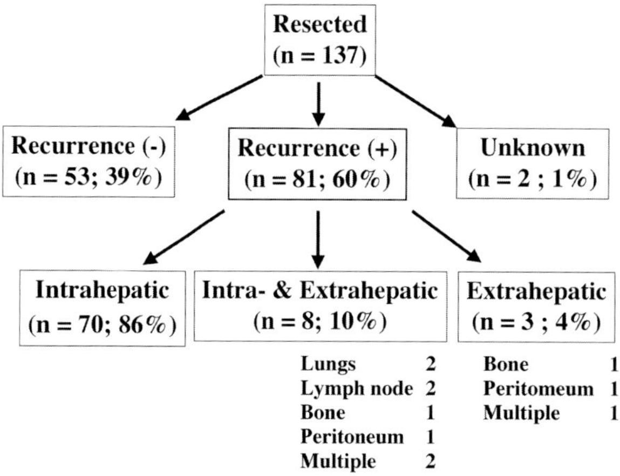

Fig. 2. Outcome of 137 patients who underwent resection for hepatocellular carcinoma showing incidence of recurrence and sites of recurrence.

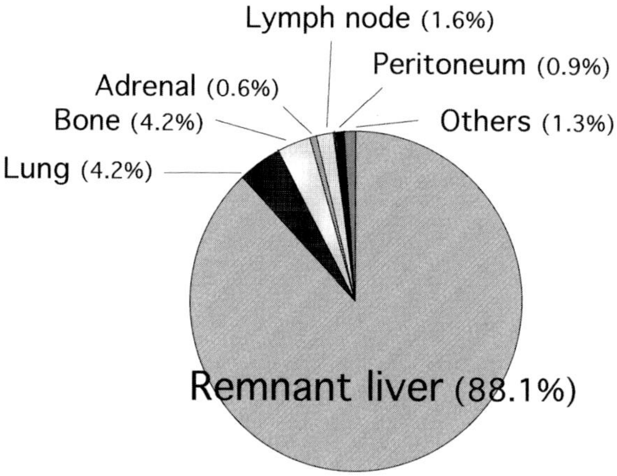

Fig. 3. Sites and frequency of recurrence of hepatocellular carcinoma after liver resection.

9.1. Prevention of Recurrent HCC After Hepatic Resection

Systemic or selective chemotherapy after hepatic resection of HCC has been associated with a deterioration of long-term prognosis in patients with cirrhosis *(67)*. Adoptive immunotherapy with autologous lymphocytes activated in vitro with recombinant interleukin-2 and antibody to CD3 *(68)* or long-term postoperative interferon therapy may reduce the incidence of recurrent HCC *(68–71)*. Adjuvant therapy with acyclic retinoid and iodine-131-laveled lipiodol has been reported to decrease the incidence of recurrent HCC after hepatic resection *(72,73)*.

9.2. Treatment of Recurrent HCC

9.2.1. Remnant Liver

Recurrence in the remnant liver accounts for 75–100% of the recurrences after hepatic resection worldwide, the cause of which may be either intrahepatic recurrence or metachronous, multicentric HCC *(18,38,74)*. Current therapeutic methods consist of repeat hepatic resection, transarterial chemoembolization or lipiodolization, and percutaneous needle-ablative therapy; of these, repeat resection seems to be the most effective *(74–77)*. Patients with metachronous, multicentric HCCs seem to have a better survival compared with those with intrahepatic recurrence *(77)*.

9.2.2. Resection of Metastatic HCC

Generally, the response rate of advanced HCC to systemic chemotherapy is low *(38)*. For selected patients with a solitary lung metastasis, 5-year survival as high as 67% has been reported *(78)*. Long-term survival after resection of extrahepatic recurrence such as peritoneal metastases or metastasis to the adrenal gland also has been reported *(77)*. Because the response rate to systemic chemotherapy is low, aggressive surgical treatment may be an effective option in selected patients with extrahepatic recurrent disease *(38)*.

REFERENCES

1. Kanematsu T, Takenaka K, Matsumata T, Furuta T, Sugimachi K, Inokuchi K. Limited hepatic resection effective for selected cirrhotic patients with primary liver cancer. *Ann Surg* 1984;199:51–56.
2. Hsia CY, Lui WY, Chau GY, King KL, Loong CC, Wu CW. Perioperative safety and prognosis in hepatocellular carcinoma patients with impaired liver function. *J Am Coll Surg* 2000;190:574–579.
3. Makuuchi M, Takayama T, Kubota K, et al. Hepatic resection for hepatocellular carcinoma—Japanese experience. *Hepatogastroenterology* 1998;45(suppl 3):1267–1274.
4. Ercolani G, Grazi GL, Calliva R, et al. The lidocaine (MEGX) test as an index of hepatic function: its clinical usefulness in liver surgery. *Surgery* 2000;127:464–471.
5. Kim YK, Nakano H, Yamaguchi M, et al. Prediction of postoperative decompensated liver function by technetium-99m galactosyl-human serum albumin liver scintigraphy in patients with hepatocellular carcinoma complicating chronic liver disease. *Br J Surg* 1997;84: 793–796.
6. Redaelli CA, Dufour JF, Wagner M, et al. Preoperative galactose elimination capacity predicts complications and survival after hepatic resection. *Ann Surg* 2002;235:77–85.
7. Yamanaka N, Okamoto E, Fujihara S, et al. Do the tumor cells of hepatocellular carcinomas dislodge into the portal venous stream during hepatic resection? *Cancer* 1992;70:2263–2267.
8. Yamamoto M, Takasaki K, Ohtsubo T, Katsuragawa H, Fukuda C, Katagiri S. Effectiveness of systematized hepatectomy with Glisson's pedicle transection at the hepatic hilus for small nodular hepatocellular carcinoma: retrospective analysis. *Surgery* 2001;130:443–448.
9. Okamoto E, Yamanaka N, Toyosaka A, Tanaka N, Yabuki K. Current status of hepatic resection in the treatment of hepatocellular carcinoma. In: *Neoplasms of the Liver* (Okuda K, Ishak KG, eds.), Springer-Verlag, Tokyo, 1987, pp. 353–365.

10. Takasaki K, Kobayashi S, Tanaka S, Saito A, Yamamoto M, Hanyu F. Highly anatomically systematized hepatic resection with Glissonean sheath code transection at the hepatic hilus. *Int Surg* 1990;75:73–77.
11. Lumsden AB, Colborn GL, Sreeram S, Skandalakis LJ. The surgical anatomy and technique of the thoracoabdominal incision. *Surg Clin North Am* 1993;73:633–644.
12. Takenaka K, Fujiwara Y, Gion T, et al. A thoracoabdominal hepatectomy and a transdiaphragmatic hepatectomy for patients with cirrhosis and hepatocellular carcinoma. *Arch Surg* 1998;133:80–83.
13. Yanaga K, Kawahara N, Taketomi A, et al. Retrograde right hepatic trisegmentectomy. *Surgery* 1996;119:592–595.
14. Liu CL, Fan ST, Lo CM, Tung-Ping Poon R, Wong J. Anterior approach for major right hepatic resection for large hepatocellular carcinoma. *Ann Surg* 2000;232:25–31.
15. Okamoto E, Kyo A, Yamanaka N, Tanaka N, Kuwata K. Prediction of the safe limits of hepatectomy by combined volumetric and functional measurements in patients with impaired hepatic function. *Surgery* 1984;95:586–592.
16. Yamanaka N, Okamoto E, Oriyama T, et al. A prediction scoring system to select the surgical treatment of liver cancer: further refinement based on 10 years of use. *Ann Surg* 1994; 219:342–346.
17. Kubota K, Makuuchi M, Kusaka K, et al. Measurement of liver volume and hepatic functional reserve as a guide to decision-making in resectional surgery for hepatic tumors. *Hepatology* 1997;26:1176–1181.
18. Nagasue N. Liver resection for hepatocellular carcinoma: indications, techniques, complications, and prognostic factors. *J Hepatobiliary Pancreat Surg* 1998;5:7–13.
19. Higashi H, Matsumata T, Utsunomiya T, Koyanagi N, Hashizume M, Sugimachi K. Successful treatment of early hepatocellular carcinoma and concomitant esophageal varices. *World J Surg* 1993;17:398–402.
20. Wu CC, Ho YZ, Ho WL, Wu TC, Liu TJ, P'eng FK. Preoperative transcatheter arterial chemoembolization for resectable large hepatocellular carcinoma: a reappraisal. *Br J Surg* 1995;82:122–126.
21. Yamasaki S, Hasegawa H, Kinoshita H, et al. A prospective randomized trial of the preventive effect of pre-operative transcatheter arterial embolization against recurrence of hepatocellular carcinoma. *Jpn J Cancer Res* 1996;87:206–211.
22. Yamasaki S, Hasegawa H, Kinoshita H, et al. A prospective randomized trial of the preventive effect of pre-operative transcatheter arterial embolization against recurrence of hepatocellular carcinoma. *Jpn J Cancer Res* 1996;87:206–211.
23. Yanaga K, Kanematsu T, Takenaka K, Sugimachi K. Intraperitoneal septic complications after hepatectomy. *Ann Surg* 1986;203:148–152.
24. Makuuchi M, Hasegawa H, Yamazaki S, Takayasu K, Moriyama N. The use of operative ultrasound as an aid to liver resection in patients with hepatocellular carcinoma. *World J Surg* 1987;11:615–621.
25. Rifkin MD, Rosato FE, Branch HM, et al. Intraoperative ultrasound of the liver. An important adjunctive tool for decision making in the operating room. *Ann Surg* 1987;205:466–472.
26. Jones RM, Moulton CE, Hardy KJ. Central venous pressure and its effect on blood loss during liver resection. *Br J Surg* 1998;85:1058–1060.
27. Lau WY, Leung KL, Leung TW, Liew CT, Chan M, Li AK. Resection of hepatocellular carcinoma with diaphragmatic invasion. *Br J Surg* 1995;82:264–266.
28. Leung KF, Chui AK, Leung KL, Lai PB, Liew CT, Lau WY. Clinicopathological study of hepatocellular carcinoma with diaphragmatic involvement. *Br J Surg* 2001;88:681,682.
29. Wang X, Andersson R, Soltesz V, Bengmark S. Bacterial translocation after major hepatectomy in patients and rats. *Arch Surg* 1992;127:1101–1106.

30. Mochizuki H, Togo S, Tanaka K, Endo I, Shimada H. Early enteral nutrition after hepatectomy to prevent postoperative infection. *Hepatogastroenterology* 2000;47:1407–1410.
31. Takenaka K, KawaharaN, Yamamoto K, et al. Results of 280 liver resections for hepatocellular carcinoma. *Arch Surg* 1996;131:71–76.
32. Hanazaki K, Kajikawa S, Shimozawa N, et al. Survival and recurrence after hepatic resection of 386 consecutive patients with hepatocellular carcinoma. *J Am Coll Surg* 2000;191: 381–388.
33. Poon RT, Fan ST, Lo CM, et al. Improving survival results after resection of hepatocellular carcinoma: a prospective study of 377 patients over 10 years. *Ann Surg* 2001;234:63–70.
34. Fong Y, Sun RL, Jarnagin W, Blumgart LH. An analysis of 412 cases of hepatocellular carcinoma at a Western center. *Ann Surg* 1999;229:790–799.
35. Grazi GL, Ercolani G, Pierangeli F, et al. Improved results of liver resection for hepatocellular carcinoma on cirrhosis give the procedure added value. *Ann Surg* 2001;234:71–78.
36. Fan ST, Lo CM, Liu CL, et al. Hepatectomy for hepatocellular carcinoma: toward zero hospital deaths. *Ann Surg* 1999;229:322–330.
37. Poon RT, Fan ST, Ng IO, Wong J. Significance of resection margin in hepatectomy for hepatocellular carcinoma: a critical reappraisal. *Ann Surg* 2000;231:544–551.
38. Poon RTP, Fan ST, Wong J. Risk factors, prevention, and management of postoperative recurrence after resection of hepatocellular carcinoma. *Ann Surg* 2000;232:10–24.
39. Yamaoka Y, Kumada K, Ino K, et al. Liver resection for hepatocellular carcinoma (HCC) with direct removal of tumor thrombi in the main portal vein. *World J Surg* 1992;16:1172–1176.
40. Ikai I, Yamaoka Y, Yamamoto Y, et al. Surgical intervention for patients with stage IV-A hepatocellular carcinoma without lymph node metastasis: proposal as a standard therapy. *Ann Surg* 1998;227:433–439.
41. Ohkubo T, Yamamoto J, Sugawara Y, et al. Surgical results for hepatocellular carcinoma with macroscopic portal vein tumor thrombosis. *J Am Coll Surg* 2000;191:657–660.
42. Wu CC, Hsieh SR, Chen JT, et al. An appraisal of liver and portal vein resection for hepatocellular carcinoma with tumor thrombi extending to portal bifurcation. *Arch Surg* 2000; 135:1273–1279.
43. Minagawa M, Makuuchi M, Takayama T, Ohtomo K. Selection criteria for hepatectomy in patients with hepatocellular carcinoma and portal vein tumor thrombus. *Ann Surg* 2001; 233:379–384.
44. Satoh S, Ikai I, Honda G, et al. Clinicopathologic evaluation of hepatocellular carcinoma with bile duct thrombi. *Surgery* 2000;128:779–783.
45. Shiomi M, Kamiya J, Nagino M, et al. Hepatocellular carcinoma with biliary tumor thrombi: aggressive operative approach after appropriate preoperative management. *Surgery* 2001;129:692–698.
46. Chiu JH, Wu LH, Kao HL, et al. Can determination of the proliferative capacity of the nontumor portion predict the risk of tumor recurrence in the liver remnant after resection of human hepatocellular carcinoma? *Hepatology* 1993;18:96–102.
47. Adachi E, Maeda T, Matsumata T, et al. Risk factors for intrahepatic recurrence in human small hepatocellular carcinoma. *Gastroenterology* 1995;108:768–775.
48. Shirabe K, Takenaka K, Taketomi A, et al. Postoperative hepatitis status as a significant risk factor for recurrence in cirrhotic patients with small hepatocellular carcinoma. *Cancer* 1996;77:1050–1055.
49. Ko S, Nakajima Y, Kanehiro H, et al. Significant influence of accompanying chronic hepatitis status on recurrence of hepatocellular carcinoma after hepatectomy. Result of multivariate analysis. *Ann Surg* 1996;224:591–595.
50. Bilimoria MM, Lauwers GY, Doherty DA, et al., International Cooperative Study Group on Hepatocellular Carcinoma. Underlying liver disease, not tumor factors, predicts long-term survival after resection of hepatocellular carcinoma. *Arch Surg* 2001;136:528–535.

51. Yamamoto M, Iizuka H, Matsuda M, Nagahori K, Miura K, Itakura J. The indications for tumor mass reduction surgery and subsequent multidisciplinary treatments in stage IV hepatocellular carcinoma. *Surg Today* 1993;23:675–681.
52. Shimada M, Takenaka K, Kawahara N, et al. Surgical treatment strategy for patients with stage IV hepatocellular carcinoma. *Surgery* 1996;119:517–522.
53. Yamamoto K, Takenaka K, Kawahara N, et al. Indications for palliative reduction surgery in advanced hepatocellular carcinoma. The use of a remnant tumor index. *Arch Surg* 1997;132:120–123.
54. Sato Y, Fujiwara K, Furui S, et al. Benefit of transcatheter arterial embolization for ruptured hepatocellular carcinoma complicating liver cirrhosis. *Gastroenterology* 1985;89:157–159.
55. Shuto T, Hirohashi K, Kubo S, et al. Delayed hepatic resection for ruptured hepatocellular carcinoma. *Surgery* 1998;124:33–37.
56. Sonoda T, Kanematsu T, Takenaka K, Sugimachi K. Ruptured hepatocellular carcinoma evokes risk of implanted metastases. *J Surg Oncol* 1989;41:183–186.
57. Ikeda Y, Shimada M, Hasegawa H, et al. Prognosis of hepatocellular carcinoma with diabetes mellitus after hepatic resection. *Hepatology* 1998;27:1567–1571.
58. Yamanaka J, Yamanaka N, Nakasho K, et al. Clinicopathologic analysis of stage II-III hepatocellular carcinoma showing early massive recurrence after liver resection. *J Gastroenterol Hepatol* 2000;15:1192–1198.
59. Matsumata T, Ikeda Y, Hayashi H, Kamakura T, Taketomi A, Sugimachi K. The association between transfusion and cancer-free survival after curative resection for hepatocellular carcinoma. *Cancer* 1993;72:1866–1871.
60. Yamamoto J, Kosuge T, Takayama T, et al. Perioperative blood transfusion promotes recurrence of hepatocellular carcinoma after hepatectomy. *Surgery* 1994;115:303–309.
61. Lauwers GY, Terris B, Balis UJ, et al., The International Cooperative Study Group on Hepatocellular Carcinoma. Prognostic histologic indicators of curatively resected hepatocellular carcinomas: a multi-institutional analysis of 425 patients with definition of a histologic prognostic index. *Am J Surg Pathol* 2002;26:25–34.
62. Poon RT, Ng IO, Lau C, et al. Serum vascular endothelial growth factor predicts venous invasion in hepatocellular carcinoma: a prospective study. *Ann Surg* 2001;233:227–235.
63. Chau GY, Wu CW, Lui WY, et al. Serum interleukin-10 but not interleukin-6 is related to clinical outcome in patients with resectable hepatocellular carcinoma. *Ann Surg* 2000; 231:552–558.
64. Donato MF, Arosio E, Del Ninno E, et al. High rates of hepatocellular carcinoma in cirrhotic patients with high liver cell proliferative activity. *Hepatology* 2001;34:523–528.
65. Yamanaka N, Tanaka T, Tanaka W, et al. Correlation of hepatitis virus serologic status with clinicopathologic features in patients undergoing hepatectomy for hepatocellular carcinoma. *Cancer* 1997;79:1509–1515.
66. Roayaie S, Haim MB, Emre S, et al. Comparison of surgical outcomes for hepatocellular carcinoma in patients with hepatitis B versus hepatitis C: a western experience. *Ann Surg Oncol* 2000;7:764–770.
67. Ono T, Yamanoi A, Nazmy El Assal O, Kohno H, Nagasue N. Adjuvant chemotherapy after resection of hepatocellular carcinoma causes deterioration of long-term prognosis in cirrhotic patients: metaanalysis of three randomized controlled trials. *Cancer* 2001;91:2378–2385.
68. Takayama T, Sekine T, Makuuchi M, et al. Adoptive immunotherapy to lower postsurgical recurrence rates of hepatocellular carcinoma: a randomised trial. *Lancet* 2000;356:802–807.
69. Suou T, Mitsuda A, Koda M, et al. Interferon alpha inhibits intrahepatic recurrence in hepatocellular carcinoma with chronic hepatitis C: a pilot study. *Hepatol Res* 2001;20:301–311.
70. Kubo S, Nishiguchi S, Hirohashi K, et al. Effects of long-term postoperative interferon-alpha therapy on intrahepatic recurrence after resection of hepatitis C virus-related hepatocellular carcinoma. A randomized, controlled trial. *Ann Intern Med* 2001;134:963–967.

71. Ikeda K, Arase Y, Saitoh S, et al. Interferon beta prevents recurrence of hepatocellular carcinoma after complete resection or ablation of the primary tumor-A prospective randomized study of hepatitis C virus-related liver cancer. *Hepatology* 2000;32:228–232.
72. Muto Y, Moriwaki H, Ninomiya M, et al. Prevention of second primary tumors by an acyclic retinoid, polyprenoic acid, in patients with hepatocellular carcinoma. Hepatoma Prevention Study Group. *N Engl J Med* 1996;334:1561–1567.
73. Lau WY, Leung TW, Ho SK, et al. Adjuvant intra-arterial iodine-131-labelled lipiodol for resectable hepatocellular carcinoma: a prospective randomised trial. *Lancet* 1999;353: 797–801.
74. Nakashima O, Kojiro M. Recurrence of hepatocellular carcinoma: multicentric occurrence or intrahepatic metastasis? A viewpoint in terms of pathology. *J Hepatobiliary Pancreat Surg* 2001;8:404–409.
75. Nagasue N, Yukaya H, Ogawa Y, Sasaki Y, Chang YC, Niimi K. Second hepatic resection for recurrent hepatocellular carcinoma. *Br J Surg* 1986;73:434–438.
76. Poon RT, Fan ST, Lo CM, Liu CL, Wong J. Intrahepatic recurrence after curative resection of hepatocellular carcinoma: long-term results of treatment and prognostic factors. *Ann Surg* 1999;229:216–222.
77. Arii S, Monden K, Niwano M, et al. Results of surgical treatment for recurrent hepatocellular carcinoma; comparison of outcome among patients with multicentric carcinogenesis, intrahepatic metastasis, and extrahepatic recurrence. *J Hepatobiliary Pancreat Surg* 1998;5:86–92.
78. Lam CM, Lo CM, Yuen WK, Liu CL, Fan ST. Prolonged survival in selected patients following surgical resection for pulmonary metastasis from hepatocellular carcinoma. *Br J Surg* 1998;85:1198–2000.

10 Liver Transplantation for Hepatocellular Carcinoma

C. Andrew Bonham, MD,
Martin Goodman, MD,
Sydney D. Finkelstein, MD,
Igor Dvorchik, PhD, *and J. Wallis Marsh,* MD

CONTENTS

1. INTRODUCTION

Hepatocellular carcinoma (HCC) is one of the most common cancers worldwide, with an estimated annual incidence of approx 1 million. The incidence of HCC in the United States is increasing, related for the most part to hepatitis C virus (HCV) infection *(1,2)*. Although complete surgical resection or ablation can provide cure for a small minority of patients with this disease, the vast majority of cases of HCC develops in the setting of cirrhosis, the implications of which are twofold *(3–10)*. First, the underlying liver disease is frequently the limiting factor in making treatment decisions, because patients with advanced cirrhosis or portal hypertension, or both, often cannot tolerate therapies targeted against the tumor. Second, the underlying liver disease essentially constitutes a

From: *Current Clinical Oncology: Hepatocellular Cancer: Diagnosis and Treatment*
Edited by: B. I. Carr © Humana Press Inc., Totowa, NJ

premalignant condition. Thus, standard therapies aimed at localizable tumor(s) may fail to treat synchronous lesions present in other parts of the liver; further, they do nothing to address the underlying liver disease itself. As a consequence, the diseased liver parenchyma can give rise to new lesions indefinitely.

The underlying liver disease and late presentation of HCC historically have limited the options available for treatment in most patients; the median survival from time of diagnosis to death has been reported to be 6 months in untreated patients *(11)*. Aggressive screening of patients identified at high risk for HCC has led to earlier diagnosis, making complete extirpation of the tumor(s) at such an early point feasible; however, it has become apparent that recurrence in these patients is virtually 100% if follow-up is long enough *(12–14)*. Thus, the optimal treatment of HCC should include not only removal of all tumor(s), but also correction of the underlying hepatic disease process that incites the formation of these tumors. Currently, the only treatment method that can achieve both of these goals is complete hepatectomy and orthotopic liver transplantation (OLT).

2. HISTORICAL ASPECTS OF LIVER TRANSPLANTATION FOR HCC

With the successful development of liver transplantation, there was hope that this procedure would provide a new and potentially curative treatment for patients with HCC, because OLT allows the removal of tumors deemed unresectable, while expunging the premalignant liver tissue *(15)*. However, as experience grew, the initial enthusiasm faded because early recurrences developed in most patients *(16–23)*. In the early Pittsburgh experience, Iwatsuki et al. *(17)* observed tumor recurrence in 72% of patients (13 of 18) transplanted for unresectable HCC but none of the 13 patients were found to have incidental tumors (median follow-up: 16 months). The Cincinnati Transplant Tumor Registry reported a 39% recurrence rate for nonincidental tumors, with only 9% of patients (34 of 365) surviving tumor-free for more than 2 years *(21)*. Similarly, Ringe et al. *(23)* reported a 25% tumor-free survival rate in 52 patients at a median follow-up of 19 months. A statistically significant correlation between pTNM stage and actuarial survival was demonstrated in these early series (Table 1), a trend that has been verified by a number of investigators *(23–27)*.

A review of data collected by the United Network for Organ Sharing (UNOS) for all cadaveric liver transplants performed in the United States confirmed the inferior outcomes for patients transplanted with HCC compared with those with other diagnoses (Tables 2 and 3). Such poor outcomes led to the exclusion of these patients at several transplant centers and were considered, until recently, a contraindication to OLT by the Health Care Financing Administration (now the Centers for Medicare & Medicaid Services). Without this approval, Medicare

Table 1
Early Experience With Orthotopic Liver Transplantation for Hepatocellular Carcinoma

Series	*No. patients*	*Results*		
		5-year patient survival (%)	*Recurrence, n (%)*	*Tumor-related death, n (%)*
		Median survival (mos)		
Penn *(21)*				
Incidental	31	57	4 (13)	2 (50)
Nonincidental	365	18	141(39)	128 (91)
Iwatsuki et al. *(17)*				
Incidental	13	16	0 (0)	—
Nonincidental	18	3.8	13 (72)	—
Ringe et al. *(23)*				
pTNM stage				
I	1	0.4	0	
II	6	—	56	
III	6	11.9	17	
IVA	36	8.8	14	
IVB	12	0.9	0	

and, consequently, most third-party payers denied financial reimbursement for transplantation for those with HCC, effectively eliminating any chance for prolonged survival or cure in these patients. Despite this, a number of transplant centers continued to perform transplants in these patients, obtaining excellent results in some. It eventually became apparent that accurate diagnosis and staging could identify subgroups of patients for whom OLT is curative or provides long-term tumor-free survival; this led to a change of policy by the Health Care Financing Administration in 2001 to offer reimbursement for OLT in patients with HCC under the following strict circumstances: the patient is not a liver resection candidate; the patient's tumor(s) is 5 cm or less in diameter; there is no macrovascular involvement; and there is no identifiable extrahepatic spread of tumor to surrounding lymph nodes, lungs, abdominal organs, or bone.

Although the inclusion criteria are narrow, it is an appropriate beginning.

Table 2
Patient Survival Rates at 3 Months and at 1, 3, and 5 Years After Liver Transplantation

Primary diagnosis	$N_{96–97}$[a]	*3-Month survival* %	*3-Month survival* *Standard error*	*1-Year survival* %	*1-Year survival* *Standard error*	N[b]	*3-Year survival* %	*3-Year survival* *Standard error*	*5-Year survival* %	*5-Year survival* *Standard error*
Noncholestatic cirrhosis	4083	91.2	0.5	87.1	0.6	14,638	78.0	0.4	71.8	0.5
Cholestatic liver disease or cirrhosis	993	95.9	0.6	93.1	0.8	4227	86.0	0.6	82.4	0.7
Acute hepatic necrosis	459	84.2	1.8	81.4	1.9	1713	73.1	1.2	70.4	1.3
Biliary atresia	296	91.2	1.7	86.2	2.1	1644	85.2	0.9	83.7	1.0
Metabolic disease	293	93.5	1.5	91.9	1.7	1196	83.9	1.1	81.5	1.3
malignant neoplasms	180	95.6	1.6	87.0	3.0	884	52.3	2.0	40.9	2.2
Other	242	84.0	2.5	79.0	2.8	757	77.3	1.7	75.0	1.8
Unknown	31	n.c.	n.c.	n.c.	n.c.	56	n.c.	n.c.	n.c.	n.c.
Overall	6577	91.3	0.4	87.5	0.4	25,115	78.9	0.3	73.9	0.3

Source: UNOS Scientific Registry Data.
[a]Denotes the number of transplants in 1996–1997 for which a survival time could be determined.
[b]Denotes the overall number of transplants from January 1989 through December 1997 for which a survival time could be determined.
Abbreviations:n.c., not calculated for the unknown categories; n.d., not determined because of insufficient follow-up.

TTable 3

Graft Survival Rates at 3 Months and at 1, 3, and 5 Years

Primary diagnosis	$N_{96–97}$[a]	*3-Month survival*		*1-Year survival*		N[b]	*3-Year survival*		*5-Year survival*	
		%	*Standard error*	*%*	*Standard error*		*%*	*Standard error*	*%*	*Standard error*
Noncholestatic cirrhosis	4083	85.7	0.6	79.6	0.6	14,638	68.8	0.4	62.1	0.5
Cholestatic liver disease or cirrhosis	993	91.6	0.9	86.4	1.1	4227	76.3	0.7	71.9	0.8
Acute hepatic necrosis	459	78.3	1.9	73.7	2.1	1713	60.3	1.2	57.3	1.3
Biliary atresia	296	81.6	2.3	75.1	2.6	1644	68.8	1.2	66.8	1.2
Metabolic disease	293	86.9	2.0	84.7	2.1	1196	73.7	1.3	70.5	1.4
malignant neoplasms	180	87.8	2.5	77.3	3.4	884	46.5	1.9	36.1	2.0
Other	242	75.0	2.8	66.9	3.1	757	65.7	1.8	63.0	1.9
Unknown	31	n.c.	n.c.	n.c.	n.c.	56	n.c.	n.c.	n.c.	n.c.
Overall	6577	85.4	0.4	79.6	0.5	25,115	68.9	0.3	63.4	0.3

Source: UNOS Scientific Registry Data.

[a]Denotes the number of transplants in 1996–1997 for which a survival time could be determined.

[b]Denotes the overall number of transplants from January 1989 through December 1997 for which a survival time could be determined.

Abbreviations:n.c., not calculated for the unknown categories; n.d., not determined because of insufficient follow-up.

3. DIAGNOSIS

Chronic active hepatitis B infection is one of the most common causes of HCC worldwide, particularly in the setting of cirrhosis. Likewise, hepatitis C infection increases the risk of HCC and, in the Western hemisphere, is currently the most commonly associated condition *(28)*. Other types of postnecrotic cirrhosis also have a high association with HCC (e.g., hemochromatosis, tyrosinemia, and α-1-antitrypsin deficiency), but the overall incidence of these diseases is significantly less than viral hepatitis, making the total occurrence less. Cholestatic liver diseases such as primary biliary cirrhosis, primary sclerosing cholangitis, and biliary atresia rarely give rise to HCC; the association between alcohol-induced cirrhosis and HCC is in between these extremes.

Several studies have demonstrated the benefit of screening for HCC in high-risk patient populations *(12,13)*. This typically consists of serial measurements of serum α-fetoprotein (AFP) levels and imaging of the liver by ultrasound or computed tomography (CT). However, this is not a widespread practice in the United States (as opposed to the developed Asian countries such as Japan) because of the lack of demonstrated cost-effectiveness.

Currently, all patients evaluated for liver transplantation at the University of Pittsburgh undergo a triphasic CT with noncontrast, arterial, and portal venous phases. Patients found to have lesions suspicious for tumor undergo further evaluation to exclude metastatic disease, including a chest CT and bone scan; if metastatic disease is found, these patients are deemed unsuitable for OLT.

A presumptive diagnosis of HCC often is based on characteristic CT findings such as hypodensity on noncontrast or portal venous phases, or both, with tumor enhancement in the arterial phase *(29)*. When there is doubt as to the diagnosis and this diagnosis is critical to the patient's treatment, the diagnosis is confirmed by percutaneous, laparoscopic, or open liver biopsy. If portal or hepatic vein thrombosis is present on preoperative imaging studies, percutaneous biopsy of the thrombus can be performed to differentiate bland from tumor thrombus. (This differentiation often can be made on CT because bland thrombus does not enhance on arterial imaging but tumor thrombus often does.) Patients with malignant, venous thrombosis should not be transplanted because the results are uniformly poor, resulting in rapid recurrence and death resulting from HCC, usually within the first postoperative year *(30)*.

4. STAGING OF HCC

Because the number of organs available for transplantation is grossly inadequate to meet demand, the selection criteria for potential transplant candidates must simultaneously maximize the number of viable candidates and reject the smallest number who could have benefited from this treatment. Unfortunately, the pTNM system has not proved to be predictive of tumor-free survival *(30–32)*.

In addition to the shortage of organs, the waiting time for OLT is sufficiently long that many patients experience disease progression and become unsuitable for transplant while awaiting the surgery. UNOS, which uses an alternative staging system based on the American Liver Tumor Study Group (Table 4), currently allows patients with stage I or II disease who meet the following criteria to be upgraded on the transplant candidate waiting list in an effort to shorten their waiting time.

1. The patient has known HCC and has undergone a thorough assessment to evaluate the number and size of tumors and to rule out any extrahepatic spread, macrovascular involvement (i.e., portal or hepatic veins), or both. A prelisting biopsy is not mandatory, but the lesion must meet established imaging criteria. Histological grade and the presence of encapsulation or histological classification (fibrolamellar versus nonfibrolamellar) are not considered in determining the patient's listing as status 2B because a prelisting biopsy is not required. The assessment of the patient should include ultrasound of the patient's liver, a CT or magnetic resonance imaging (MRI) scan of the abdomen and chest, and a bone scan. A reassessment of the patient must be performed every 3 months that the patient is on the UNOS waiting list.
2. The patient has stage I or stage II HCC in accordance with the modified Tumor-Node-Metastasis (TNM) classification, or the patient has an AFP level that is rising on three consecutive occasions with an absolute value of 500 ng or more although there is no evidence of a tumor based on imaging studies.
3. The patient is not a resection candidate.

A patient with HCC at stage III or higher may continue to be considered a liver transplant candidate in accordance with each center's own specific policy or philosophy, but the patient must be listed as status 3, unless the candidate meets the other criteria specified for status 2B or 2A. In addition, a patient with HCC must be reviewed by the applicable UNOS liver regional review board before being upgraded to status 2B.

Although the increase from UNOS status 3 to UNOS status 2B does shorten the time from listing to transplantation, the waiting time is still far too long given that the HCC doubling time is estimated to be 100–200 days (Table 5) *(33–35)*.

5. CURRENT EFFORTS TO DEVELOP ACCURATE STAGING SYSTEMS

Given that current staging systems do not accurately predict tumor-free survival and, therefore, have limited clinical applicability, we are engaged in ongoing efforts to develop and refine a staging system that could assign to each patient an individual prognostic risk score of recurrence (Table 6). Our initial work on this topic considered only the pathological features included in the pTNM staging system plus patient gender *(30)*. An array of statistical techniques, including

Table 4
American Liver Tumor Study Group Modified TNM Staging Classification

TX, NX, MX	Not assessed
T0, N0, M0	Not found
T1	One nodule <1.9 cm
T2	One nodule 2.0–5.0 cm; two or three nodules, all <3.0 cm
T3	One nodule >5.0 cm; two or three nodules, at least one >3.0 cm
T4a	Four or more nodules, any size
T4b	T2, T3, or T4a plus gross intrahepatic portal or hepatic vein involvement as indicated by CT, MRI, or US
N1	Regional nodes involved
M1	Metastatic disease
Stage I	T1
Stage II	T2
Stage III	T3
Stage IVA1	T4a
Stage IVA2	T4b
Stage IVB	Any N1, any M1

proportional hazard model, back-propagation artificial neural networks, and logistic regression, were used for the analysis *(30,36–39)*. Although the same tumor characteristics (vascular invasion, tumor number, tumor size, and lobar distribution) plus patient gender had similar effects on tumor-free survival regardless of statistical technique used, the techniques differed in the proportion of between-patient variance that each model could explain. The model that best explained the largest proportion of this variance was based on an artificial neural network *(30)*. Using this model, it was possible to identify the values of the joint distribution of risk factors that unambiguously prognosticated recurrence outcome for approx 70% of all patients in the study (Tables 7 and 8). However, the other 30% fell into a prognostication gray area, that is, the probability scores corresponding to the regions in the joint distribution of risk factors that lead to recurrence in some, but not all, cases. This shortfall, in conjunction with the failure of any existing system to constitute a reliable predictive tool for HCC recurrence, suggested that other factors were playing an important role in recurrence.

The recent explosion in biotechnology has led to a flood of reports of various cellular or molecular markers that may be related to HCC development and progression *(12,38,40–43)*; however, these tools have not yet been incorporated into HCC clinical outcome prediction models. In an attempt to incorporate such factors, we applied microdissection-based genotyping to the individual tumors in the explanted liver specimens in an attempt to identify surrogates of tumor suppressor gene loss based on loss of heterozygosity (LOH) in microsatellites spatially associated with known tumor suppressor genes.

Table 5
Median Waiting Time in Days for UNOS Status at Time of Listing

UNOS status at listing	*Year listed*	*No. registrations*	*Median waiting time (days)*	*95% Confidence interval*
Liver status 2A	1997–1998	373	12	(8, 16)
Liver status 2B	1997–1998	2403	179	(166, 196)
Liver status 3	1997–1998	13084	680	(651, 715)
Liver status 2A	1999–2000	756	15	(12, 18)
Liver status 2B	1999–2000	5791	288	(271, 302)
Liver status 3	1999–2000	12655	*	(., .)

Source: Organ Procurement and Transplantation Network, Liver Kaplan–Meier Median Waiting Times For Registrations Listed: 1995–2000, Based on OPTN data as of February 22, 2002.

Data subject to change based on future data submission or correction.

*An M was not computed because *N* was less than 10.

The finding of tumor suppressor gene loss was based on the determination of loss of heterozygosity for informative loci situated within or adjacent to specific genes of interest (APC, CDKN2A, DCC, MET, MYC1, OGG1, p34, p53, PTEN). DNA polymorphisms were in the form of polymorphic microsatellites with polymerase chain reaction primers based on GenBank references as follows: D1S407[L18040], MYCL[M19720], D3S1539[L16393], D3S2303 [L17972], D5S592[L16423], D5S615[L18737], MCC[M62397], D7S1530 [L30387], D8S373[L16320], D9S251[L18726], D9S254[L18050], D10S-520[L16357], D10S1173[L30341], D17S1163[30445], TP53[M13121], D17-S974[G07961], D17S1289[G09615], D18S814[L17776].

Because not all genes of interest were informative in all patients, we used the fractional allelic loss (FAL) rate, defined as the percent mutated markers in each patient divided by the total number of informative markers for that patient, as an index of the total mutational load. An FAL rate of more than 0.3 proved to be an important predictor of posttransplant HCC recurrence (Fig. 1). Of 50 patients, only one with an FAL of less than 0.3 had recurrence.

An additional benefit of the performance of mutational profiling is that in patients with multiple tumors, this method can discriminate intrahepatic metastases from synchronous, independent (i.e., *de novo*) tumor formation by comparing the mutational changes between tumors (Fig. 2A,B). Tumors that represent metastatic spread have similar genetic mutational profiles, whereas *de novo* tumors have discordant profiles indicating different sites of origin. The implications for this distinction are clear: patients previously assigned to stage IV because of the presence of bilobar tumors but who really have multiple T1 or

Table 6
Risk Factors of Tumor-Free Survival
and Prognostic Risk Score Grading for Tumor Recurrence

Variable	*Relative risk*	*95% Confidence interval*
Bilobar tumor ($p < 0.0001$)[a]	3.1	(1.7, 5.4)
Tumor size ($p < 0.0003$)[b]		
2–5 cm	4.5	(1.5, 13.0)
>5 cm	6.7	(2.2, 19.9)
Vascular invasion ($p < 0.0001$)[c]		
Microscopic	4.4	(2.1, 9.5)
Macroscopic	15.0	(6.7, 33.8)
Risk score (RS)		
Grade 1	0 < RS < 7.5	
Grade 2	7.5 < RS < 11.0	
Grade 3	11.0 < RS < 15.0	
Grade 4	RS > 15.0	
Grade 5	Positive margins, lymph nodes, or metastasis	

[a]Compared with unilobar.
[b]Compared with size ≤2 cm.
[c]Compared with none.

Table 7
Values of Risk Factor That Should Not Lead to HCC Recurrence After OLT

Vascular invasion	*Lobar distribution*	*Tumor number*	*Gender*	*Tumor size*
None	Unilobar	Single	Any	Any
None	Unilobar	Multiple	Any	≤8.0 cm
None	Unilobar	Multiple	Female	Any
None	Bilobar	Single	Male	≤4.0 cm
None	Bilobar	Single	Female	Any
None	Bilobar	Multiple	Female	Any
Micro	Unilobar	Single	Any	≤4.0 cm
Micro	Unilobar	Multiple	Any	≤2.0 cm
Micro	Unilobar	Multiple	Female	≤4.0 cm
Micro	Bilobar	Single	Female	≤4.0 cm
Micro	Bilobar	Multiple	Female	≤2.0 cm

T2 tumors can now be designated as stage I or II and offered transplantation with a high expectation of cure or an acceptable tumor-free survival (Fig. 3). It should be noted that not all patients designated as having intrahepatic metastases expe-

Table 8
Values of Risk Factors That Should Lead to HCC Recurrence After OLT

Vascular invasion	*Lobar distribution*	*Tumor number*	*Gender*	*Tumor size*
Micro	Unilobar	Single	Male	>8.0 cm
Micro	Bilobar	Single	Male	>4.0 cm
Micro	Bilobar	Single	Female	>8.0 cm
Macro	Unilobar	Single	Male	Any
Macro	Unilobar	Single	Female	>2.0 cm
Macro	Unilobar	Multiple	Male	>2.0 cm
Macro	Unilobar	Multiple	Female	>8.0 cm
Macro	Bilobar	Single	Any	>4.0 cm
Macro	Bilobar	Multiple	Male	>2.0 cm
Macro	Bilobar	Multiple	Female	>4.0 cm

rience HCC recurrence; therefore, candidacy for transplantation should not be based on genetic mutational profiling alone.

6. CURRENT RECOMMENDATION FOR TRANSPLANTATION

As stated above, for patients with HCC awaiting transplantation, UNOS currently allows upgrading to status 2B only for patients with stage I or II disease. And although this is understandable in the light of the tremendous organ shortage, problems exist, as outlined below.

1. Some patients with HCC will become ineligible for transplant because of tumor progression while on the waiting list (patients must be reassessed every 3 months).
2. Patients previously classified as stage IV but who really should be classified as stage II will never receive this curative therapy because of the inadequacies of current guidelines.

Regardless of which patients can actually receive OLT under the current guidelines, the following steps can be used to determine which patients constitute high and low risk for HCC recurrence after transplantation (given our current understanding of the biology of this disease). Obviously, these recommendations are based to a large degree on information obtained from the explanted liver, and it is conceded that full application of models such as those described herein must wait until radiological imaging improves significantly. Nonetheless, these recommendations are applicable to those patients in whom the diagnosis of HCC is made before surgery, and these outcomes models also can be used to guide the decision for adjuvant therapies in the postoperative period.

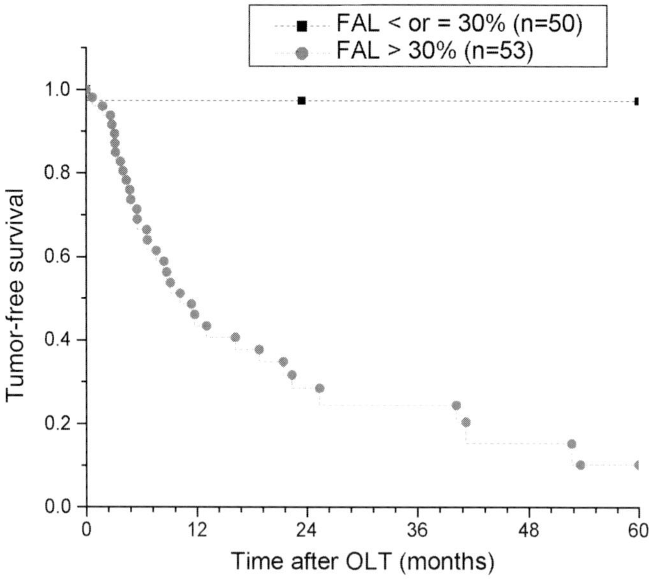

Fig. 1. Tumor-free survival stratified by FAL ($p < 0.0001$).

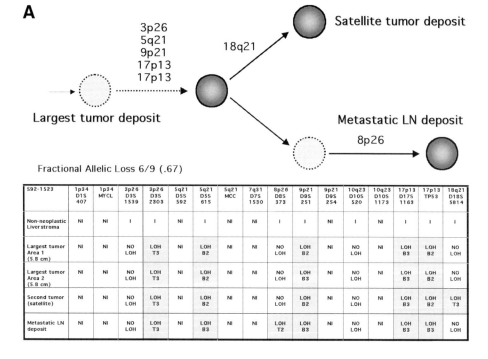

A

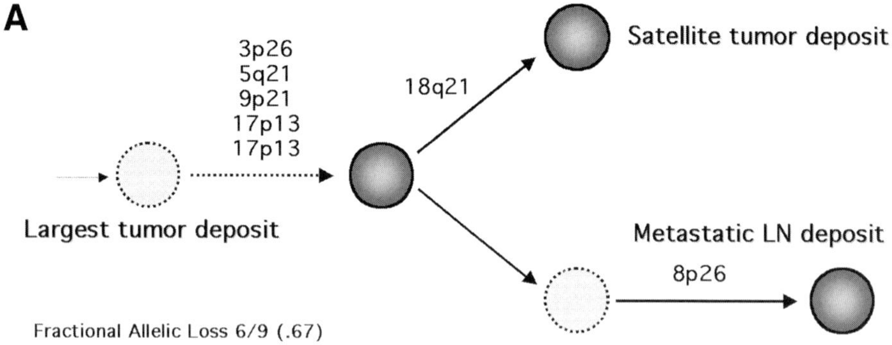

Fractional Allelic Loss 6/9 (.67)

S92-1523	1p34 D1S 407	1p34 MYCL	3p26 D3S 1539	3p26 D3S 2303	5q21 D5S 592	5q21 D5S 615	5q21 MCC	7q31 D7S 1530	8p26 D8S 373	9p21 D9S 251	9p21 D9S 254	10q23 D10S 520	10q23 D10S 1173	17p13 D17S 1163	17p13 TP53	18q21 D18S 5814
Non-neoplastic Liver stroma	NI	NI	I	I	NI	I	NI	NI	I	I	NI	I	NI	I	I	I
Largest tumor Area 1 (5.8 cm)	NI	NI	NO LOH	LOH T3	NI	LOH B2	NI	NI	NO LOH	LOH B2	NI	NO LOH	NI	LOH B3	LOH B2	NO LOH
Largest tumor Area 2 (5.8 cm)	NI	NI	NO LOH	LOH T3	NI	LOH B2	NI	NI	NO LOH	LOH B3	NI	NO LOH	NI	LOH B3	LOH B2	NO LOH
Second tumor (satellite)	NI	NI	NO LOH	LOH T3	NI	LOH B2	NI	NI	NO LOH	LOH B2	NI	NO LOH	NI	LOH B3	LOH B2	LOH T3
Metastatic LN deposit	NI	NI	NO LOH	LOH T3	NI	LOH B3	NI	NI	LOH T2	LOH B3	NI	NO LOH	NI	LOH B3	LOH B3	NO LOH

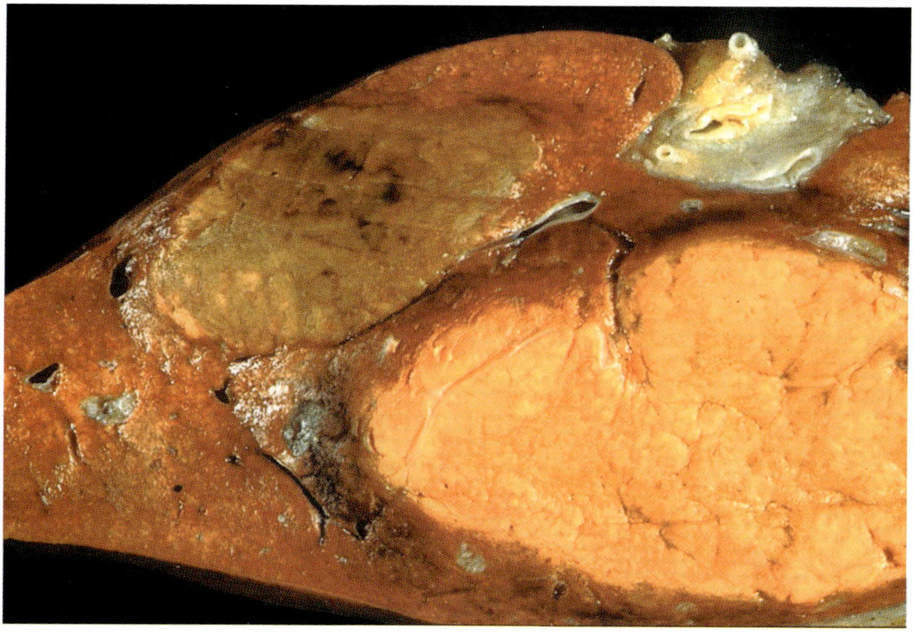

Color Plate 1, Fig. 1 (*see* discussion in Ch. 4, and full caption on p. 79). Two mass lesions arising in a noncirrhotic liver.

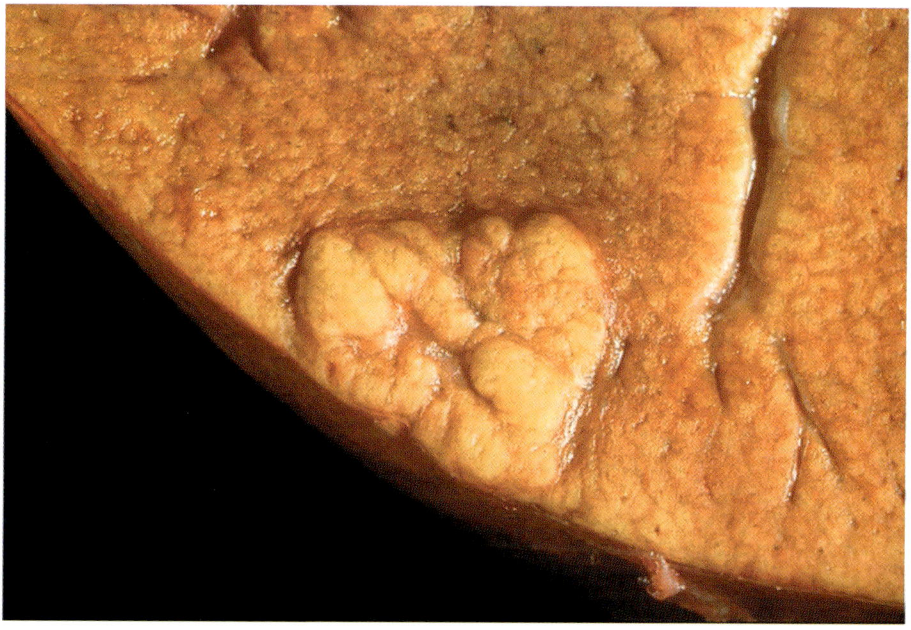

Color Plate 2, Fig. 3 (*see* discussion in Ch. 4, and full caption on p. 84). Focal nodular hyperplasia.

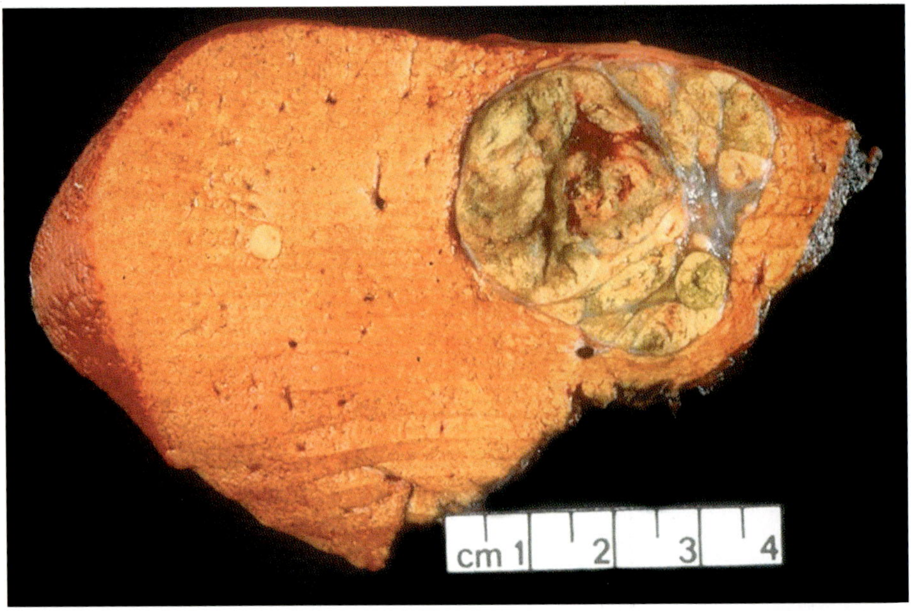

Color Plate 3, Fig. 4 (*see* discussion in Ch. 4, and full caption on p. 85). Hepatocellular carcinoma.

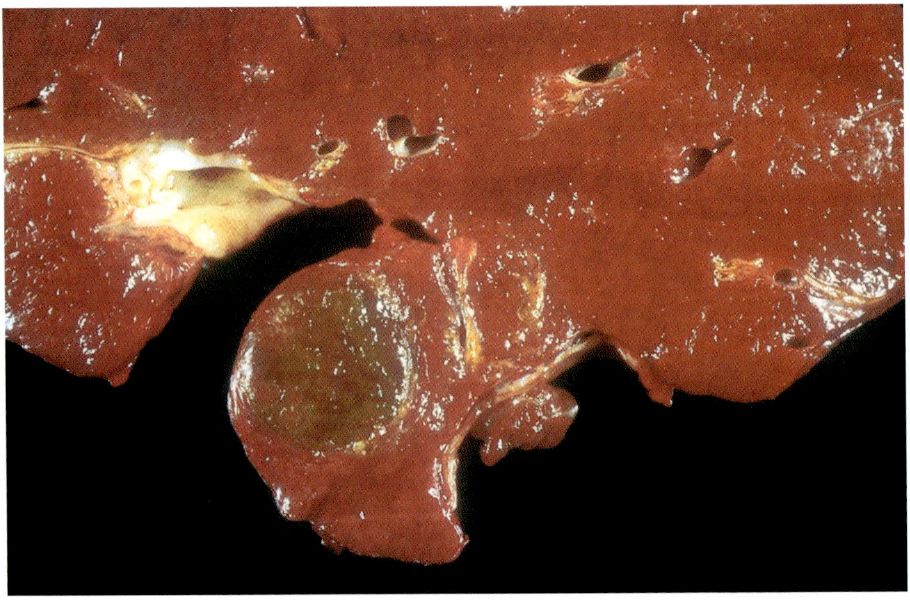

Color Plate 4, Fig. 5 (*see* discussion in Ch. 4, and full caption on p. 86). Hepatocellular carcinoma with portal vein invasion.

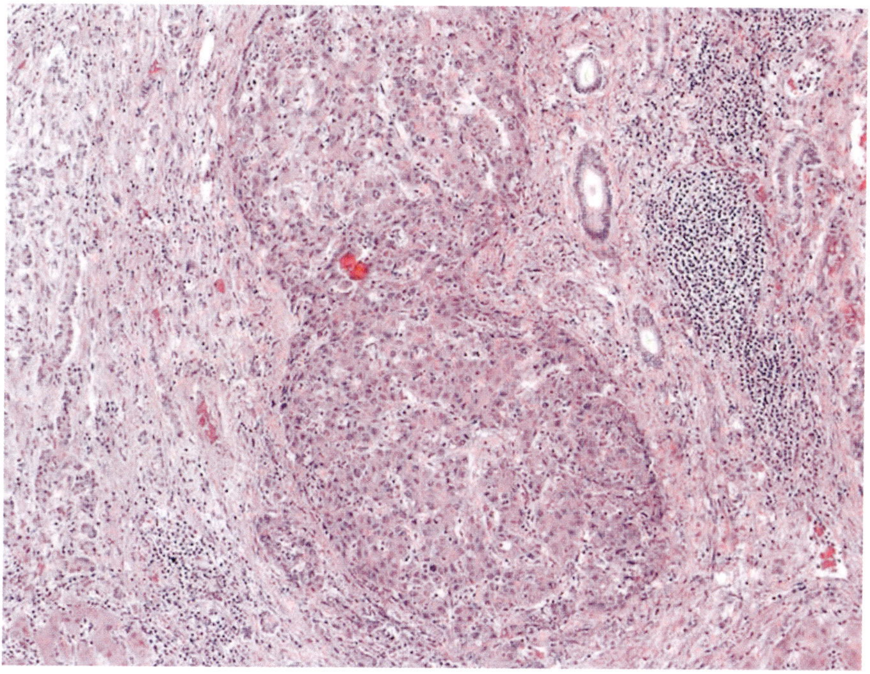

Color Plate 5, Fig. 8 (*see* discussion in Ch. 4, and full caption on p. 93). Hepatocellular carcinoma.

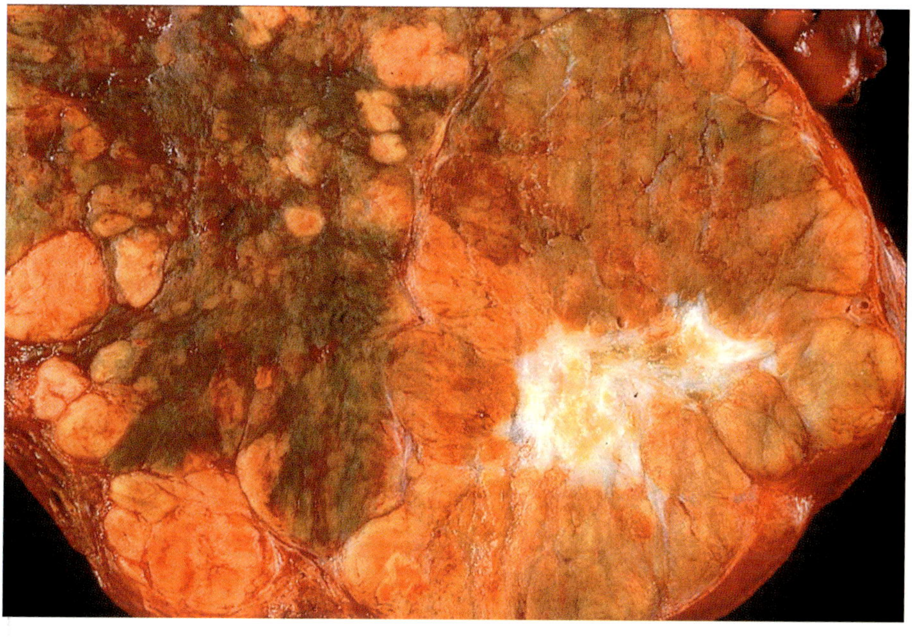

Color Plate 6, Fig. 10 (*see* discussion in Ch. 4, and full caption on p. 100). Hepatocellular carcinoma, fibrolamellar subtype.

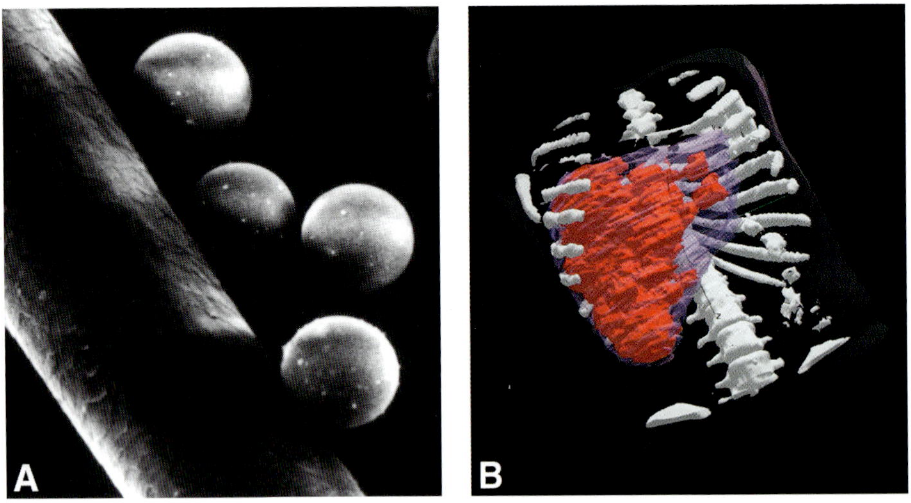

Color Plate 7, Fig. 1A,B (*see* discussion in Ch. 8, and full caption on p. 274). **(A)** An electron micrograph of glass microspheres adjacent to a human hair for perspective. **(B)** CT-based reconstruction from radiation therapy treatment planning software of a predominently right-sided tumor (red) with transparent (purple) liver volume.

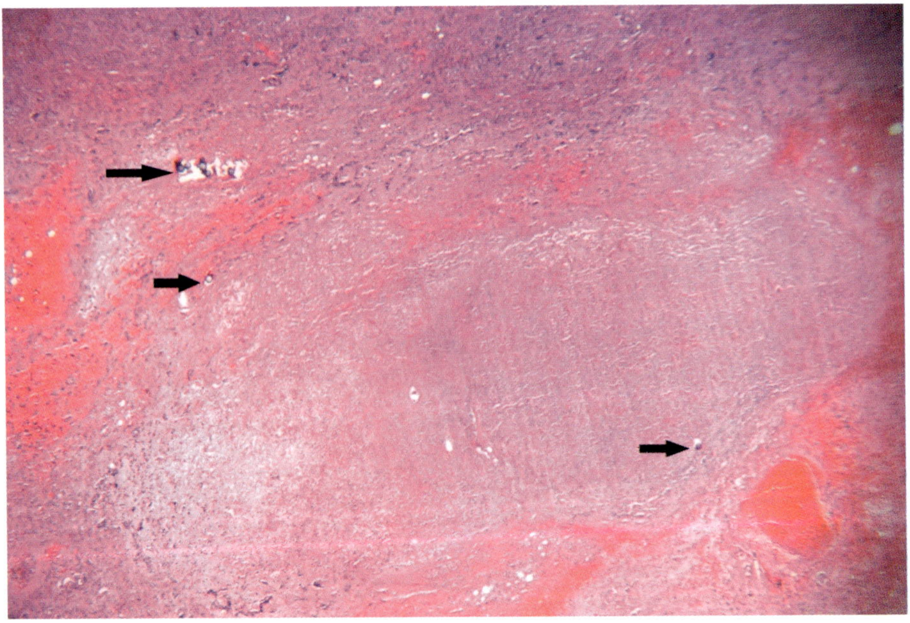

Color Plate 8, Fig. 2 (*see* discussion in Ch. 8, and full caption on p. 276). Photomicrograph of glass microspheres (arrows) in clusters within a tumor nodule of HCC.

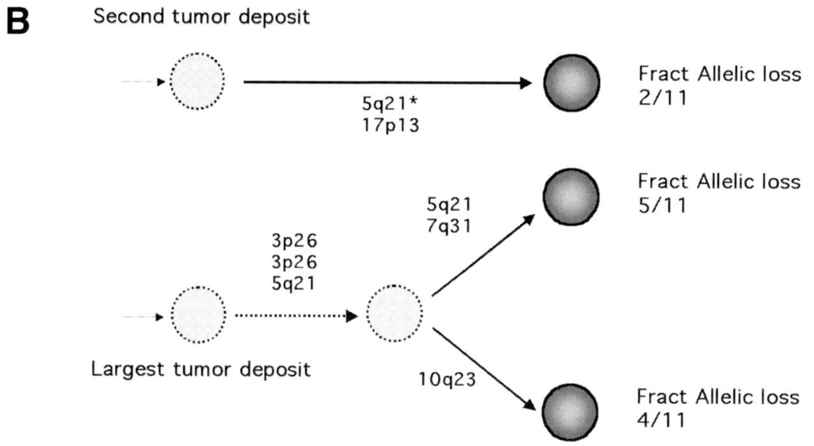

Fractional Allelic Loss 5/11 (.45)

S92-12624	1p34 D1S 407	1p34 MYCL	3p26 D3S 1539	3p26 D3S 2303	5q21 D5S 592	5q21 D5S 615	5q21 MCC	7q31 D7S 1530	8p26 D8S 373	9p21 D9S 251	9p21 D9S 254	10q23 D10S 520	10q23 D10S 1173	17p13 D17S 1163	17p13 TP53	18q21 D18S 5814
Non-neoplastic Liver stroma	I	NI	I	I	I	I	NI	I	I	NI	NI	I	I	I	NI	I
Largest tumor Area 1 (4.5 cm)	NO LOH	NI	LOH T3	LOH T3	LOH T2	LOH B2	NI	NO LOH	NO LOH	NI	NI	LOH T3	NO LOH	NO LOH	NI	NO LOH
Largest tumor Area 2 (4.5 cm)	NO LOH	NI	LOH T2	LOH T2	LOH T2	LOH B2	NI	LOH B3	NO LOH	NI	NI	NO LOH	NO LOH	NO LOH	NI	NO LOH
Second tumor	NO LOH	NI	NO LOH	NO LOH	NO LOH	LOH T2	NI	NO LOH	NO LOH	NI	NI	NO LOH	NO LOH	LOH B2	NI	NO LOH

Fig. 2. (A) (*opposite and above*) Similar genetic mutational profile indicating intrahepatic metastases. **(B)** Discordant genetic mutational profile indicating *de novo* tumors.

1. Patients with positive lymph nodes, extrahepatic metastases, and those who cannot be transplanted with negative margins should be excluded from OLT.
2. Patients not excluded by step 1 should next be evaluated by the criteria outlined in Tables 6–8.
3. Those patients not classified by steps 1 or 2 should be evaluated by mutational profiling. Patients with FAL of 0.3 or greater should be transplanted. If the FAL >0.3, the recurrence outcome is uncertain; OLT for these patients must be based on the individual institutional policies.

7. CONCLUSIONS

Although early reports of OLT for HCC described poor results secondary to high rates of recurrence and tumor-associated death, it has become clear that a

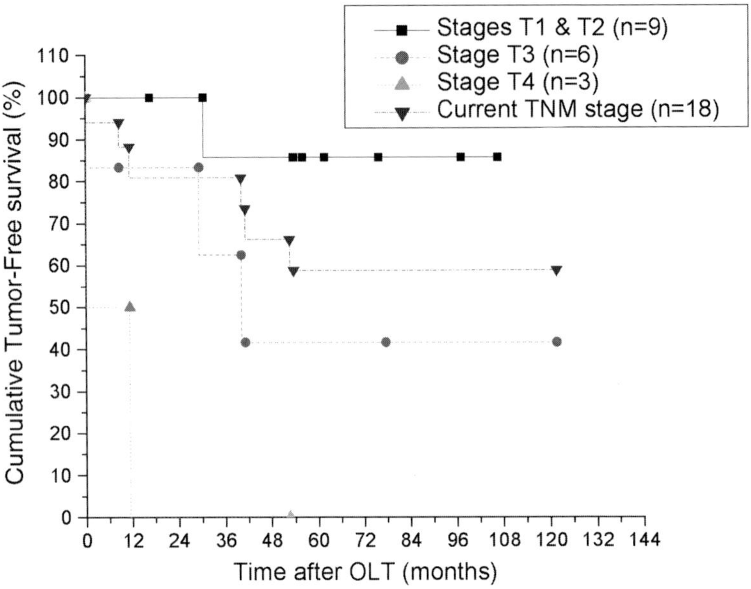

Fig. 3. Tumor-free survival for all patients calculated as T4 by current TNM stage and by recalculated stage based on mutational profile.

subpopulation clearly benefits from transplantation. Therefore, it is of paramount importance to stage patients accurately to identify those for whom OLT offers the greatest potential benefit. Unfortunately, the current shortage in suitable cadaveric organs prevents the use of transplantation as definitive therapy for all patients, and the wait for cadaveric transplantation prolongs the interval from diagnosis to treatment. Therefore, patients with well-compensated cirrhosis should be considered for resectional or ablational therapy, although tumor recurrence is high compared with that associated with transplantation *(18,39)*. For patients with more advanced cirrhosis awaiting liver transplantation, it is reasonable to provide less radical, palliative therapies such as radiofrequency ablation or transarterial chemoembolization in an effort to slow tumor growth while these patients await surgery. For those who experience tumor recurrence after resection, ablation, or chemoembolization, transplant can be considered according to the criteria outlined above.

REFERENCES

1. el-Serag HB. Epidemiology of hepatocellular carcinoma. *Clin Liver Dis* 2001;5:87–107, vi.
2. el-Serag HB, Mason AC. Risk factors for the rising rates of primary liver cancer in the United States. *Arch Intern Med* 2000;160:3227–3230.
3. Okuda K. Hepatocellular carcinoma. *J Hepatol* 2000;32(Suppl):225–237.

4. Colombo M, de Franchis R, Del Ninno E, et al. Hepatocellular carcinoma in Italian patients with cirrhosis. *N Engl J Med* 1991;325:675–680.
5. Tsukuma H, Hiyama T, Tanaka S, et al. Risk factors for hepatocellular carcinoma among patients with chronic liver disease. *N Engl J Med* 1993;328:1797–1801.
6. Johnson PJ, Williams R. Cirrhosis and the aetiology of hepatocellular carcinoma. *J Hepatol* 1987;4:140–147.
7. Poynard T, Aubert A, Lazizi Y, et al. Independent risk factors for hepatocellular carcinoma in French drinkers. *Hepatology* 1991;13:896–901.
8. Pateron D, Ganne N, Trinchet JC, et al. Prospective study of screening for hepatocellular carcinoma in Caucasian patients with cirrhosis. *J Hepatol* 1994;20:65–71.
9. Cottone M, Turri M, Caltagirone M, et al. Screening for hepatocellular carcinoma in patients with Child's A cirrhosis: an 8-year prospective study by ultrasound and alphafetoprotein. *J Hepatol* 1994;21:1029–1034.
10. Akriviadis EA, Llovet JM, Efremidis SC, et al. Hepatocellular carcinoma. *Br J Surg* 1998;85:1319–1331.
11. Olubuyide IO. The natural history of primary liver cell carcinoma: a study of 89 untreated adult Nigerians. *Cent Afr J Med* 1992;38:25–30.
12. Tong MJ, Blatt LM, Kao VW. Surveillance for hepatocellular carcinoma in patients with chronic viral hepatitis in the United States of America. *J Gastroenterol Hepatol* 2001;16: 553–559.
13. Yuen MF, Cheng CC, Lauder IJ, Lam SK, Ooi CG, Lai CL. Early detection of hepatocellular carcinoma increases the chance of treatment: Hong Kong experience. *Hepatology* 2000;31:330–335.
14. Poon RT, Ng IO, Fan ST, et al. Clinicopathologic features of long-term survivors and disease-free survivors after resection of hepatocellular carcinoma: a study of a prospective cohort. *J Clin Oncol* 2001;19:3037–3044.
15. Starzl TE. *Experience in Hepatic Transplantation*, WB Saunders, Philadelphia, 1969, pp. 4–8.
16. Bismuth H, Chiche L, Adam R, Castaing D, Diamond T, Dennison A. Liver resection versus transplantation for hepatocellular carcinoma in cirrhotic patients. *Ann Surg* 1993;218: 145–151.
17. Iwatsuki S, Gordon RD, Shaw BW Jr, Starzl TE. Role of liver transplantation in cancer therapy. *Ann Surg* 1985;202:401–407.
18. Iwatsuki S, Starzl TE, Sheahan DG, et al. Hepatic resection versus transplantation for hepatocellular carcinoma. *Ann Surg* 1991;214:221–228; discussion 8–9.
19. Jenkins RL, Pinson CW, Stone MD. Experience with transplantation in the treatment of liver cancer. *Cancer Chemother Pharmacol* 1989;23(suppl):S104–S109.
20. McPeake JR, O'Grady JG, Zaman S, et al. Liver transplantation for primary hepatocellular carcinoma: tumor size and number determine outcome. *J Hepatol* 1993;18:226–234.
21. Penn I. Hepatic transplantation for primary and metastatic cancers of the liver. *Surgery* 1991;110:726–734; discussion 734,735.
22. Ringe B, Wittekind C, Bechstein WO, Bunzendahl H, Pichlmayr R. The role of liver transplantation in hepatobiliary malignancy. A retrospective analysis of 95 patients with particular regard to tumor stage and recurrence. *Ann Surg* 1989;209:88–98.
23. Ringe B, Pichlmayr R, Wittekind C, Tusch G. Surgical treatment of hepatocellular carcinoma: experience with liver resection and transplantation in 198 patients. *World J Surg* 1991;15: 270–285.
24. Colella G, Rondinara GF, De Carlis L, et al. Liver transplantation for hepatocellular carcinoma: prognastic factors associated with long-term survival. *Transpl Int* 1996;9(Suppl 1):S109–S111.
25. Herrero JI, Sangro B, Quiroga J, , et al. Influence of tumor characteristics on the outcome of liver transplatation among patients with liver cirrhosis and hepatocellular carcinoma. *Liver Transpl* 2001;7:631–636.

26. Regalia E, Fassati LR, Valente U, et al. Pattern and management of recurrent hepatocellular carcinoma after liver transplantation. *J Hepatobiliary Pancreat Surg* 1998;5:29–34.
27. Wittekind C. Prognostic factors in liver tumors. *Verh Dtsch Ges Pathol* 1995;79:109–115.
28. El-Serag HB, Mason AC. Rising incidence of hepatocellular carcinoma in the United States. *N Engl J Med* 1999;340:745–750.
29. Peterson MS, Baron RL, Marsh JW Jr, Oliver JH 3rd, Confer SR, Hunt LE. Pretransplantation surveillance for possible hepatocellular carcinoma in patients with cirrhosis: epidemiology and CT-based tumor detection rate in 430 cases with surgical pathologic correlation. *Radiology* 2000;217:743–749.
30. Marsh JW, Dvorchik I, Subotin M, et al. The prediction of risk of recurrence and time to recurrence of hepatocellular carcinoma after orthotopic liver transplantation: a pilot study. *Hepatology* 1997;26:444–450.
31. Llovet JM, Bruix J, Fuster J, et al. Liver transplantation for small hepatocellular carcinoma: the tumor-node-metastasis classification does not have prognostic power. *Hepatology* 1998;27:1572–1577.
32. Hermanek P, Sobin LH. 1987. TNM classification of malignant tumours. In: *UICC, International Union against Cancer* (Hermanek P, Sobin LH, eds.), Springer-Verlag, Berlin, New York, 53–55.
33. Nakajima T, Moriguchi M, Mitsumoto Y, et al. Simple tumor profile chart based on cell kinetic parameters and histologic grade is useful for estimating the natural growth rate of hepatocellular carcinoma. *Hum Pathol* 2002;33:92–99.
34. Okada S, Okazaki N, Nose H, et al. Follow-up examination schedule of postoperative HCC patients based on tumor volume doubling time. *Hepatogastroenterology* 1993;40:311–315.
35. Okazaki N, Yoshino M, Yoshida T, et al. Evaluation of the prognosis for small hepatocellular carcinoma based on tumor volume doubling time. A preliminary report. *Cancer* 1989;63: 2207–2210.
36. Marsh JW, Dvorchik I, Bonham CA, Iwatsuki S. Is the pathologic TNM staging system for patients with hepatoma predictive of outcome? *Cancer* 2000;88:538–543.
37. Iwatsuki S, Dvorchik I, Marsh JW, et al. Liver transplantation for hepatocellular carcinoma: a proposal of a prognostic scoring system. *J Am Coll Surg* 2000;191:389–394.
38. Kirimlioglu H, Dvorchick I, Ruppert K, et al. Hepatocellular carcinomas in native livers from patients treated with orthotopic liver transplantation: biologic and therapeutic implications. *Hepatology* 2001;34:502–510.
39. Yamamoto J, Iwatsuki S, Kosuge T, et al. Should hepatomas be treated with hepatic resection or transplantation? *Cancer* 1999;86:1151–1158.
40. Libbrecht L, Craninx M, Nevens F, Desmet V, Roskams T. Predictive value of liver cell dysplasia for development of hepatocellular carcinoma in patients with non-cirrhotic and cirrhotic chronic viral hepatitis. *Histopathology* 2001;39:66–73.
41. Itano O, Ueda M, Kikuchi K, et al. A new predictive factor for hepatocellular carcinoma based on two-dimensional electrophoresis of genomic DNA. *Oncogene* 2000;19:1676–1683.
42. Sun CA, Wang LY, Chen CJ, et al. Genetic polymorphisms of glutathione *S*-transferases M1 and T1 associated with susceptibility to aflatoxin-related hepatocarcinogenesis among chronic hepatitis B carriers: a nested case- control study in Taiwan. *Carcinogenesis* 2001;22: 1289–1294.
43. Wong N, Lai P, Lee SW, et al. Assessment of genetic changes in hepatocellular carcinoma by comparative genomic hybridization analysis: relationship to disease stage, tumor size, and cirrhosis. *Am J Pathol* 1999;154:37–43.

11 Interventional Radiology Techniques for Intra-Arterial Chemoembolization

Nikhil B. Amesur, MD,
Albert B. Zajko, MD,
and Philip D. Orons, DO

CONTENTS

1. INTRODUCTION

Transcatheter arterial chemoembolization (TACE) of hepatic malignancies has been described in the medical literature for more than two decades *(1–3)*. This method exploits the fact that the liver has a unique dual blood supply. Although most of the blood flow to the liver is derived from the portal venous system, hepatic malignancies in general tend to derive their blood supply solely from the hepatic artery (Fig. 1). This unique property has led to the popular but controversial treatment method commonly referred to as TACE. TACE allows

From: *Current Clinical Oncology: Hepatocellular Cancer: Diagnosis and Treatment*
Edited by: B. I. Carr © Humana Press Inc., Totowa, NJ

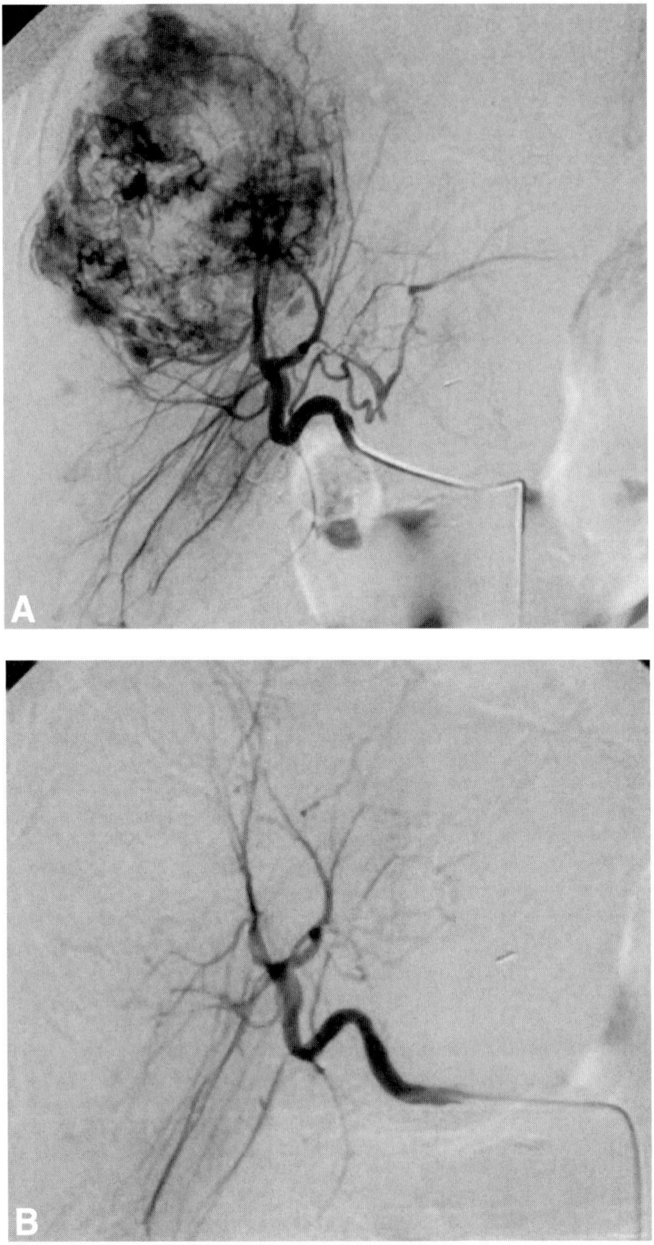

Fig. 1. (A) Right hepatic arteriogram shows the presence of a large hypervascular lesion in the right hepatic artery distribution. **(B)** Same patient as above after several cycles of chemotherapy infusion and Gelfoam embolization no longer demonstrates presence of the hypervascular lesion.

the interventionalist to catheterize branches of the hepatic artery selectively and to deliver high doses of chemotherapy and embolization agents directly to the target lesions.

Because the agent is delivered directly to the liver, systemic side effects are decreased. We have been using TACE for more than 14 years at our institution. This chapter describes TACE itself and discusses some of the complications related to the procedure. Clinical results from TACE have been published previously and are discussed in greater detail in other chapters in this book *(4,5)*.

2. PATIENT SELECTION AND PREPARATION

Initial patient selection is a complex process and is described in detail in the introductory chapters. In summary, patients who are not candidates for surgical resection or radiofrequency ablation, those with advanced bilobar disease, those who have not responded to systemic chemotherapy agents, and patients with recurrent hepatocellular carcinoma after liver transplantation are offered this procedure at our institution. If all the appropriate criteria are met, the patient is scheduled to undergo the procedure. All cross-sectional imaging studies, such as computed tomography (CT) and magnetic resonance imaging, are reviewed. Visceral arterial anatomy is evaluated. Patency of the portal vein is documented. Routine blood work obtained before the procedure includes coagulation studies, such as PT, PTT, and INR. Renal function and platelet counts are also checked. Liver enzyme levels also are obtained routinely as part of the oncology work-up to assess baseline liver function before TACE. Patients with elevated bilirubin levels (>2.5 mg/dL) are at higher risk of liver injury with intra-arterial chemotherapy. Depending on the clinical situation and after careful discussion with the patient, some of these patients with elevated bilirubin levels may still be offered the treatment. In these patients, we often infuse chemotherapeutic agents only and will not embolize the vessels, or may embolize them less aggressively, in an attempt to minimize hepatic injury.

Patients maintain a clear liquid diet from midnight the evening before the procedure and are encouraged to drink as much water as possible. The patient reports to the radiology outpatient unit early in the morning. Informed consent for the procedure and conscious sedation is obtained. Two large-bore intravenous lines usually are placed. If the patient has a venous tunneled catheter or port, these can be used. Intravenous fluid hydration is administered for 2–4 hours at a rate of 250 mL/hour if the cardiac status will allow it.

A Foley catheter or a condom catheter is placed to allow adequate monitoring of urine output during and after the procedure. Mild sedation before Foley catheter placement is helpful. Intravenous antibiotics and antiemetics are administered. If a patient is not allergic to penicillin, we usually use 1 g Cefazolin intravenously. Oral anxiolytics, such as lorazepam, are given to reduce procedure-related anxiety as needed before the patient is transported to the angiography suite.

3. HEPATIC ARTERIAL ANATOMY ESSENTIAL TO TACE

Considerable variation exists in the arterial supply to the liver, and variant hepatic arterial anatomy may be seen in up to 42% of patients *(6,7)*. A thorough understanding of visceral arterial anatomy is required before performing chemoembolization procedures to ensure adequate treatment of the patient and to avoid nontarget organ embolization.

Classically, the celiac axis gives rise to three vessels: the splenic artery, common hepatic artery (CHA), and left gastric artery (LGA; Fig. 2). The CHA gives rise to the gastroduodenal artery (GDA) and then becomes the proper hepatic artery (PHA). The PHA divides most commonly into the left hepatic artery (LHA) and right hepatic artery (RHA). A single LHA may divide into a medial segment and a lateral segment or such segments may originate independently from the PHA or in some cases from the CHA. The cystic artery most commonly arises from the RHA. The caudate lobe of the liver usually is supplied by branches from the right hepatic artery. The GDA gives rise to the superior pancreaticoduodenal artery (sPDA). The inferior pancreaticoduodenal artery (iPDA) usually is a branch of the superior mesenteric artery (SMA). Both the sPDA and iPDA have anterior and posterior divisions that join together to form the pancreaticoduodenal arcade (PDA). These collateral pathways between the celiac axis and SMA become especially important in cases of celiac artery or common hepatic artery occlusion, where alternate routes of selective hepatic artery catheterization may have to be used.

4. VARIANT ARTERIAL ANATOMY

As many as 20% of patients may have some vascular supply to the liver originating from the SMA. Variations include replaced RHA from the SMA (Fig. 3A), accessory RHA (in which case there is a main RHA originating from the celiac trunk), or replaced CHA (Fig. 4). Another 23% of patients may have the entire LHA or the left lateral segment hepatic artery originating from the left gastric artery (Fig. 5) or arising from the SMA (as part of a replaced CHA in 2.5% of patients). The CHA or RHA also rarely may originate directly from the aorta. Arterial anatomy also may be confounded when the patient has undergone an orthotopic liver transplant and is being treated for recurrent tumor in the al-

Fig. 2. (*opposite page*) **(A)** CT arteriogram demonstrating conventional hepatic artery anatomy. **(B)** Common hepatic arteriogram demonstrates similar appearance of the common hepatic artery.

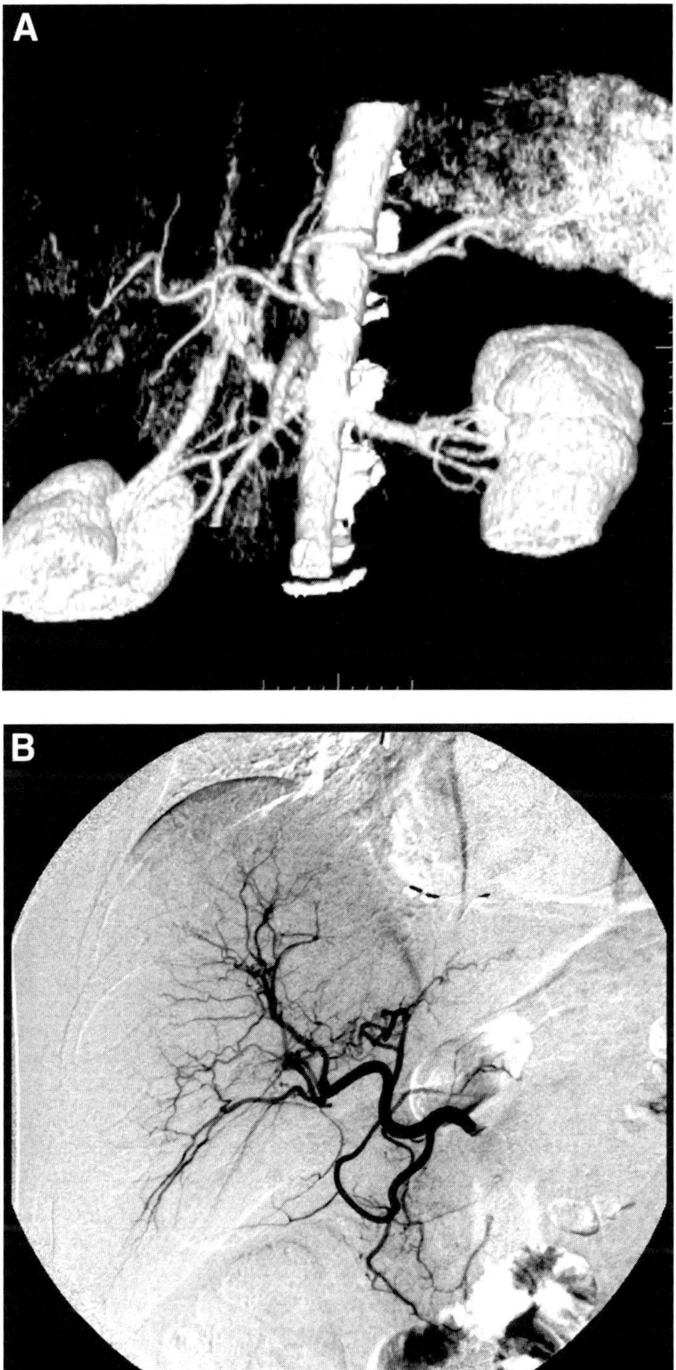
A
B

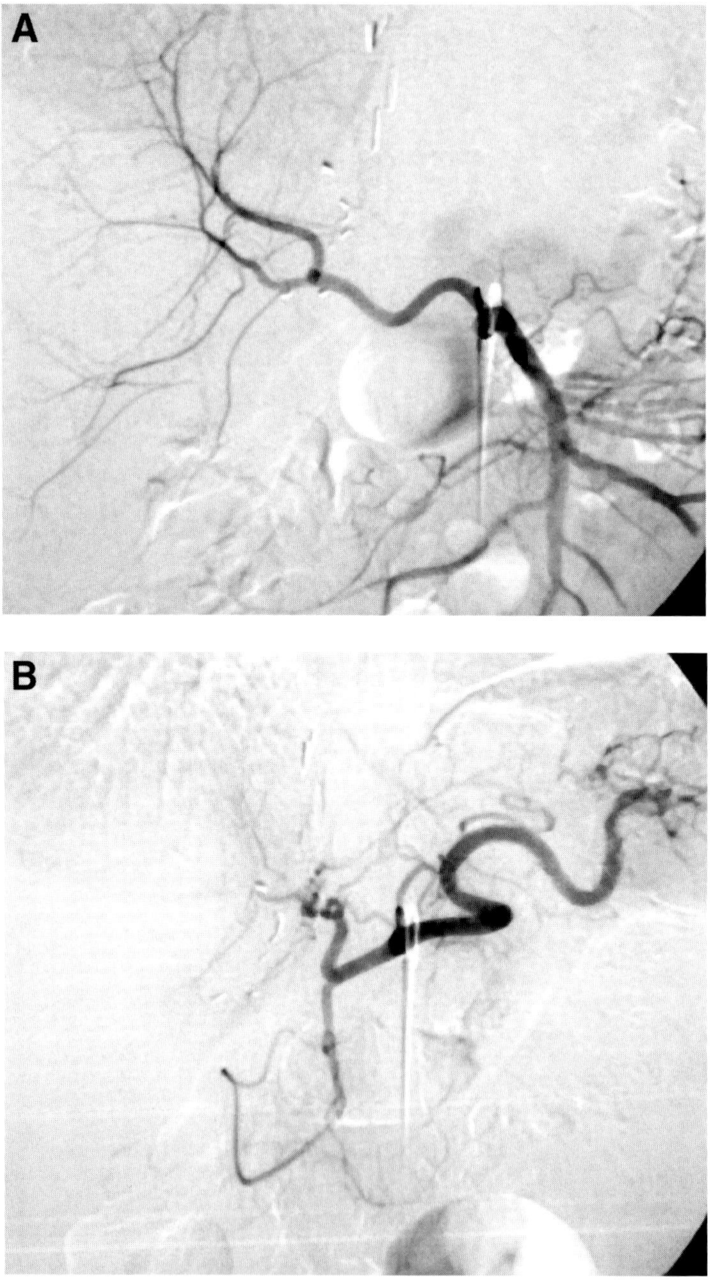

Fig. 3. (A) Replaced right hepatic artery seen originating from the SMA. **(B)** Same patient as above demonstrates only the LHA, GDA, and splenic artery from the celiac axis.

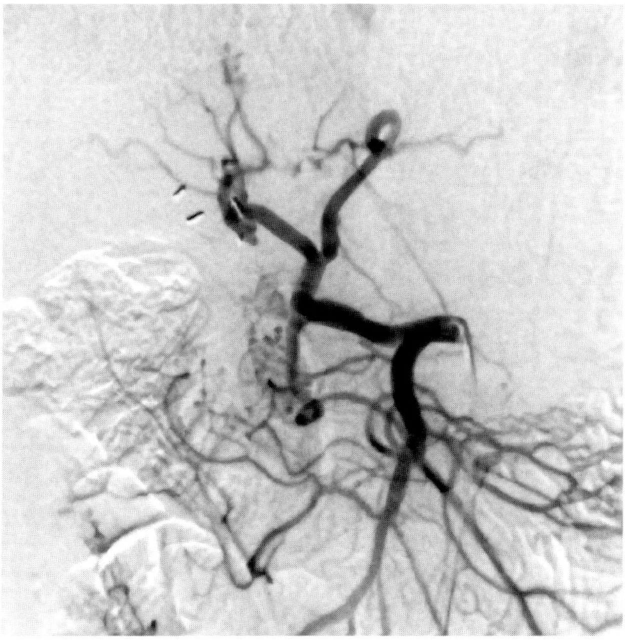

Fig. 4. Replaced common hepatic artery arising from the SMA.

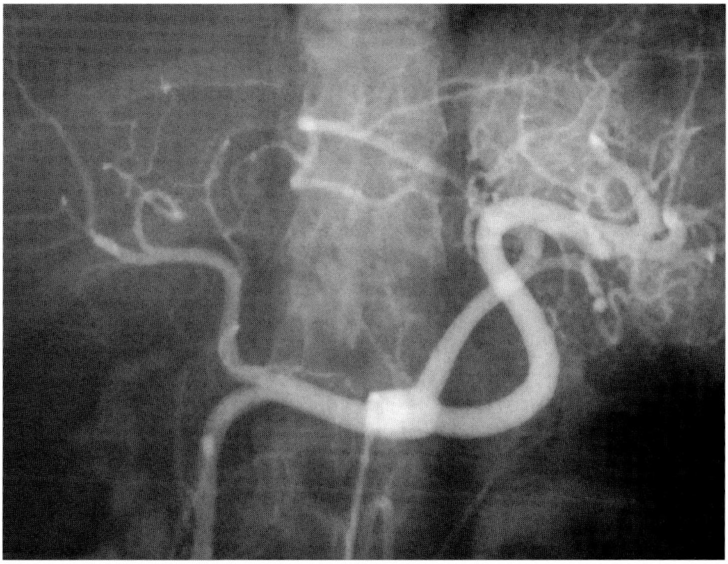

Fig. 5. Replaced left hepatic artery seen originating from the left gastric artery.

lograft. These patients often will have a graft directly arising from the infrarenal aorta. The operative note should be reviewed before TACE.

5. TACE PROCEDURE

The patient is placed on cardiac monitors and given intravenous conscious sedation, usually a combination of an anxiolytic such as midazolam hydrochloride, and pain medication such as fentanyl citrate. The femoral artery is accessed using a standard Seldinger technique or, in some cases, a micropuncture set (Cook Inc, Bloomington, IN) if there is a coagulopathy or thrombocytopenia. The advantage of the micropuncture set is that the initial puncture is made using a single-wall 21-gauge needle. A C2 catheter (Angiodynamics, Queensbury, NY) is used to catheterize the origin of the SMA. Hand injection of contrast is performed to exclude the presence of a replaced RHA or an accessory RHA originating from the SMA. This needs to be assessed, because missing such a replaced vessel can result in incomplete treatment. In many cases, this information can be determined from the arterial phase of the CT.

The celiac axis is then cannulated and a celiac arteriogram is performed to obtain a general overview of the axis and to look for a replaced LHA off the left gastric artery. In some patients, the celiac axis can have an acute angle at its origin; such vessels often need to be accessed using either a reversed curve catheter such as a Sos catheter (Angiodynamics) or by creating a Waltman loop *(8)*. Briefly, this is carried out by advancing the C2 catheter into the SMA or opposite iliac artery. Using a series of twists and advances, the catheter is advanced up into the aorta. This results in the C2 catheter bending back on itself in the aorta. As soon as this is achieved, the catheter is pulled back down into the aorta and the celiac axis is cannulated.

A complete hepatic arteriogram is performed. If conventional hepatic arterial supply is present, this can be accomplished by catheter placement in the CHA. Tumor vascularity is assessed and compared with that seen on CT scan. As soon as all these data are collected, a decision is made in conjunction with the oncologist as to which vessels need to be treated and if concomitant embolization agents are to be used. After this decision is made, the appropriate vessel is cannulated. Most often, we try to treat only one lobe of the liver in a single session. If the vessel to be treated is large enough and fairly straight, the 5-French catheter is negotiated out into it, usually with the aid of a 0.38-inch angled glide wire (Boston Scientific, Watertown MA). If the vessel is of a smaller caliber or is tortuous, microcatheters are used.

There are many microcatheter choices. They include the Cragg wire (Boston Scientific), the Turbo Tracker Infusion Catheter (Boston Scientific), and the Renegade Hi-Flo (Boston Scientific) microcatheters. The first catheter has a larger inner diameter and can accommodate guide wires up to 0.025 inches in diameter, whereas the others accept guide wires up to 0.018 inches in diameter. Numerous wire choices are available. These include the 0.018- or 0.025-inch glide wires, glide gold wire (Boston Scientific), Seeker 0.014 or Seeker 0.016 wire (Boston Scientific), and Headliner wire (Boston Scientific). Each of these different catheter and wire combinations has advantages, and the choice often depends on operator preference.

As soon as final catheter position is confirmed, we administer 5 mg of morphine sulfate and 20 mg of Decadron intra-arterially into the vessel being treated. The morphine is used to reduce the pain associated with embolization and the Decadron is used to decrease the inflammatory response created by the chemotherapy in the normal hepatocytes. Many presized embolic agents are commonly available in the United States for patients requiring embolization; these include Embogold Microspheres (Biosphere Medical, Rockland, MA) and Contour SE particles (Boston Scientific). These particles are prepackaged in different size ranges and are suspended in saline. Predictable diameters, hydrophilic surfaces, and elastic compressibility of these particles may result in a more complete embolization of the vessel. We are currently evaluating response to chemoembolization with different size particles, and they have become our main embolization vector.

Prior to availability of these newer agents, the most commonly used embolization agent at our institution was gel foam (Surgifoam, Ethicon, A Johnson & Johnson Company, Somerville, NJ), which we still use on select patients. The 2 cm × 6 cm gel foam wafer is pressed down and then cut into 1- to 2-mm longitudinal strips using a pair of scissors (Fig. 6). The strips are them cut at a 90° angle to form the 1- to 2-mm pledgets. These pledgets are placed in a glass syringe and sterilized. Alternatively, they can be cut at the time of embolization. A mixture of 50% contrast and saline is mixed with the pledgets just prior to use and allowed to soak in it. The syringe is then attached to another syringe by means of a three-way stpocock. The gel foam slurry is forced back and forth between the syringes, resulting in further breakdown of the gel foam. The stopcock can be partially turned off to decrease the size of the hole that the gel foam is forced through. This results in gel foam fragments of a smaller size. This is especially important when embolizing through microcatheters to prevent clogging the catheter. The embolization particles (Gelfoam or Microspheres) are infused into the vessel under fluoroscopy to minimally slow antegrade flow prior to chemotherapy administration. Chemotherapy infusion is then initiated at a rate that would allow us to infuse the entire volume in about 30 to 40 minutes. Frequent fluoroscopic monitoring of the catheter during the infusion is imperative to ensure that the catheter does not move from the desired location. This means that the patient must remain on the angiography table during the chemotherapy infusion. Upon completion of the chemotherapy infusion, further embolization is performed to either further

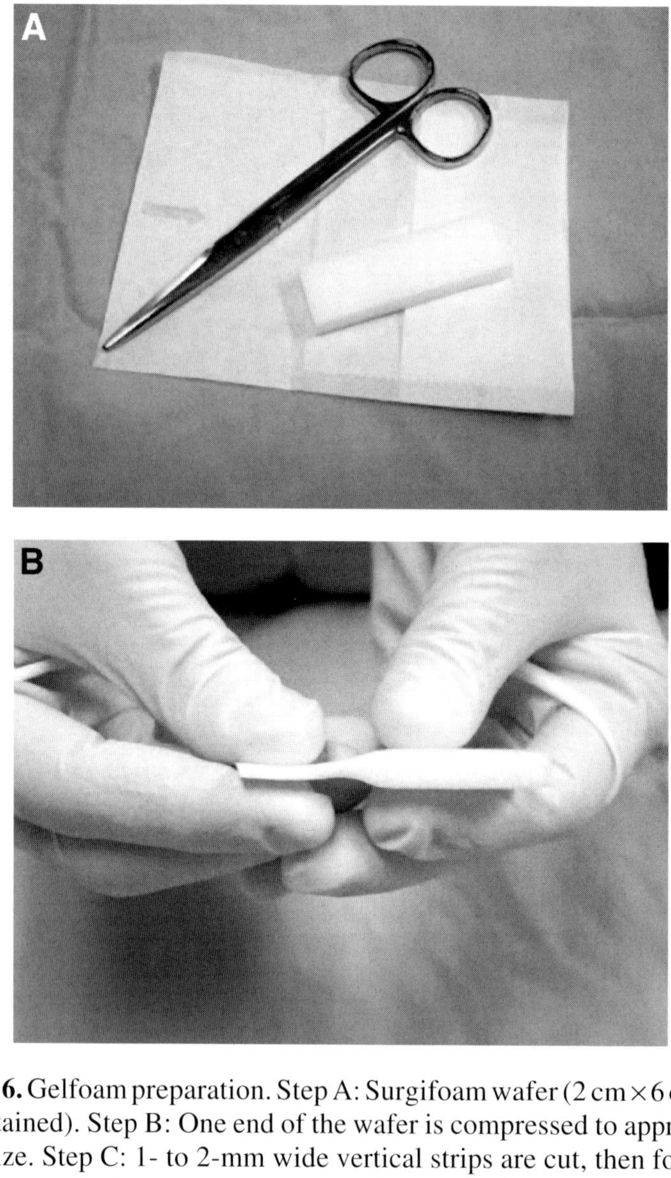

Fig. 6. Gelfoam preparation. Step A: Surgifoam wafer (2 cm × 6 cm × 7 mm size is obtained). Step B: One end of the wafer is compressed to approximately half the size. Step C: 1- to 2-mm wide vertical strips are cut, then followed by horizontal cuts of the same size. Step D: Gelfoam pledgets are collected in a sterile cup. Step E: The pledgets are then placed into a glass syringe. Step F: Just

slow antegrade flow or occlude antegrade flow. If the bilirubin level is not elevated and the portal vein is patent, we generally occlude antegrade flow. Embolization is usually only performed on one side of the liver, even if the

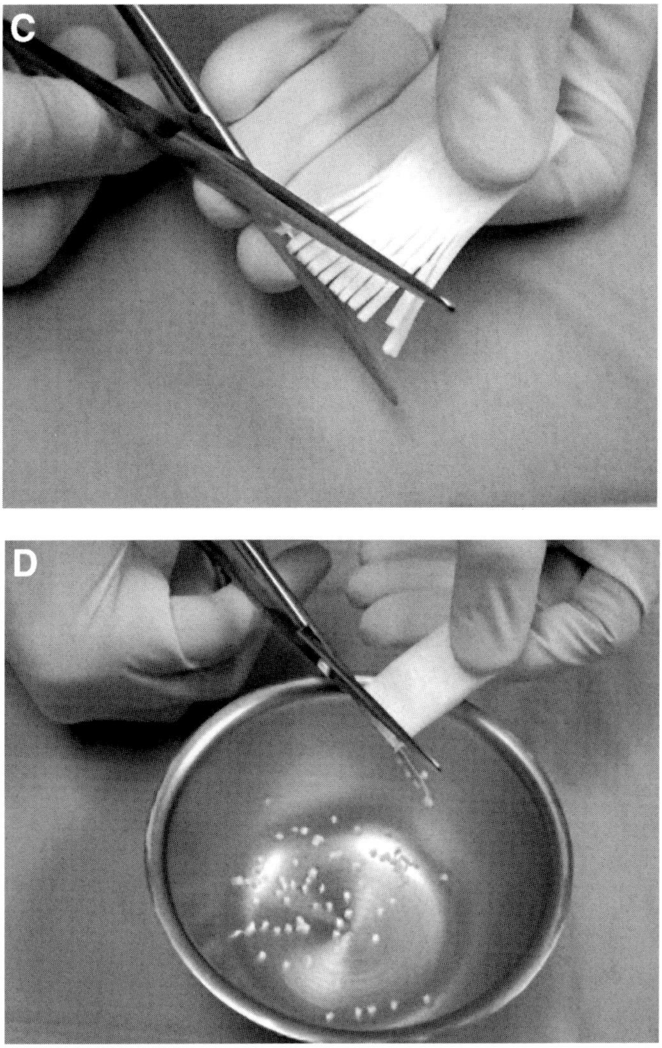

Fig. 6. (*continued*) before use, a mixture of saline and contrast is mixed into the pledgets. Step G: The contents of the glass syringe are pushed into a plastic sterile syringe. The Gelfoam is moved back and forth between the two plastic syringes to break it down further. Note that the stopcock is partially in the off position. This results in further breakdown of the Gelfoam.

chemotherapy is split into both lobes. The catheter is removed, and after hemostatis is obtained, the patient is admitted for overnight observation and continued hydration.

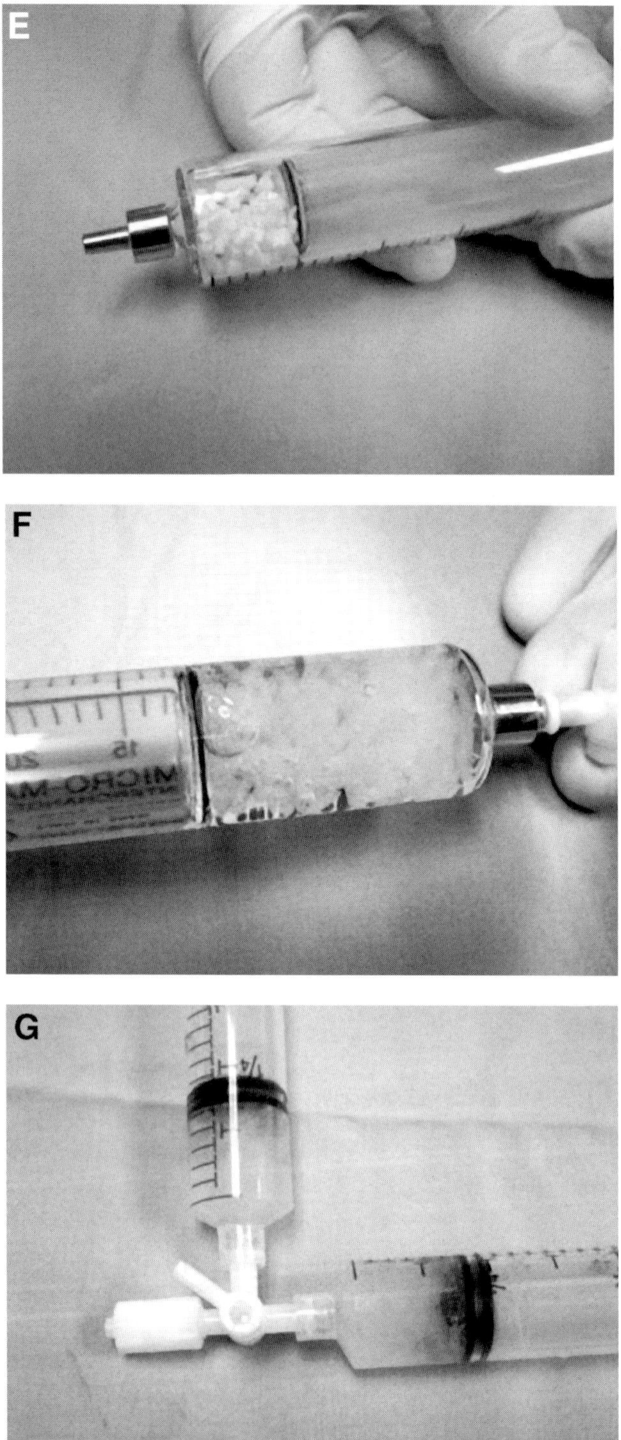
E
F
G

6. COMPLICATIONS FROM TACE

Multiple complications can arise as a consequence of TACE *(9)*. These can be broken down into direct procedural-related complications such as arterial dissection or occlusion, contrast reaction, puncture site hematomas, inadvertent chemoembolization of adjacent organs, and liver infarction. Late complications include liver failure, abscess formation *(10,11)*, and chronic arterial occlusion.

Complications related to catheterization such as hematomas, arterial dissections, and occlusions are relatively small, occurring in less than 2% of patients in the hands of experienced angiographers. In the case of hepatic arterial occlusions, an experienced angiographer can take advantage of collateral pathways to treat the tumor. Collaterals can arise from all adjacent vessels, such as the phrenic arteries, branches of the internal mammary arteries, and branches from the pancreaticoduodenal arcade, and have to be vigorously sought.

Inadvertent chemoembolization of adjacent organs theoretically can occur unless meticulous attention is paid to the patient's vascular anatomy. Patients have to be monitored closely for any clinical signs of nontarget embolization, such as bowel ischemia.

Abscess formation rates after TACE are variable, with published data indicating a range of 0.2–4.5%. Abscess formation is believed to result from the ascending biliary infection after TACE *(10,11)*. A prior surgical biliary anastomosis may lead to increased risk of abscess formation. Prophylactic antibiotics, especially to cover gastrointestinal flora before TACE, are imperative to minimize this risk.

7. ADVANCED CATHETERIZATION TECHNIQUES AND ADJUVANT THERAPY

Complex anatomy can be encountered in patients. Also, as soon as a patient has undergone multiple TACE procedures, occlusions of the vessels can result. These may be related to the toxicity of the drugs used, repeated catheterizations, or tumor encasement. As soon as this occurs, collateral vessels usually develop, and angiographic assessment often will provide information on alternate arterial access. In many cases, TACE is still possible through the use of collateral vessels *(12)*. If a celiac artery or CHA occlusion occurs, flow often will reverse in the GDA. This can be exploited by advancing a microcatheter up from the iPDA to the sPDA and up the GDA to catheterize the LHA or RHA (Fig. 7). Collaterals also may arise from the inferior phrenic artery or from the internal mammary artery. These may need to be assessed selectively and catheterized.

In some patients, stenoses of the intrahepatic arterial branches or PHA may make selective catheterization impossible. The PHA bifurcation may arise very close to, or at the level of, the GDA. In such cases, the CHA may need to be treated with TACE. Because chemotherapeutic agents are toxic to small bowel, the GDA

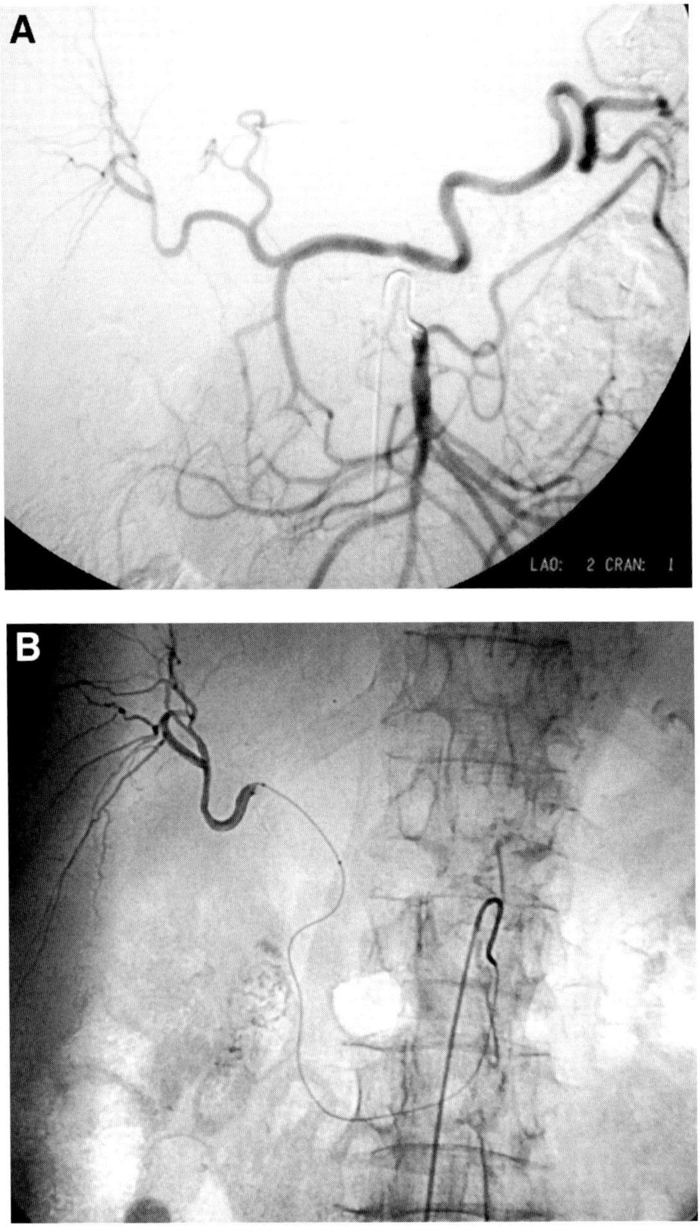

Fig. 7. (A) SMA arteriogram demonstrates complete filling of the celiac axis via the pancreaticoduodenal arcade, indicating complete occlusion of the celiac axis. **(B)** Tracker microcatheter has been advanced via the pancreaticoduodenal arcade all the way into the right hepatic artery for selective chemoembolization.

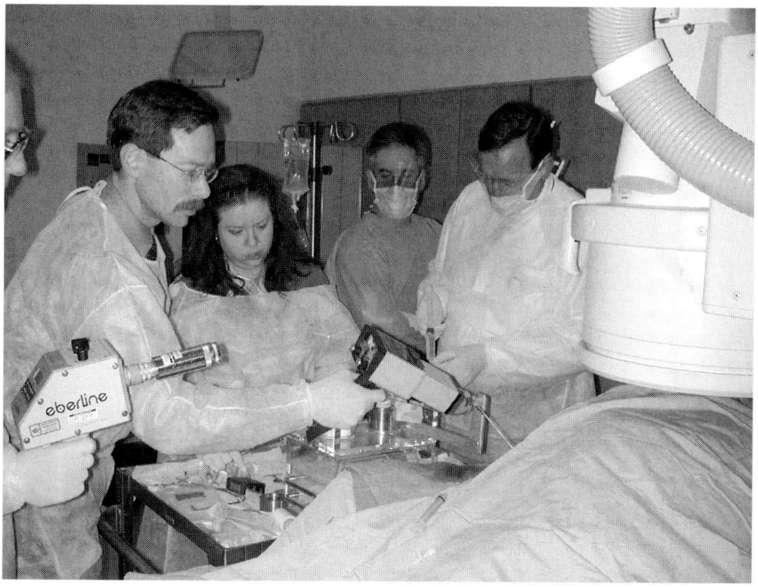

Fig. 8. Complex setup involved in treating a patient with Therasphere particles. Therasphere particles being injected into a patient by the physician while radioactivity levels are recorded.

may be embolized using coils, effectively changing the CHA to the PHA, allowing bilobar treatment with a single infusion site.

8. NEW HORIZONS IN TREATMENT OF LIVER TUMORS

Catheter-directed delivery of a local burst of radiation offers an exciting new treatment method. Yttrium 90 glass spheres, either imbedded in a resin or in glass beads (TheraSphere; MDS Nordion, Ottawa, Ontario, Canada) has been used at our institution for approx 3 years *(13)*. The use of TheraSphere and other similar β emitters may prove to be a more effective and tolerable treatment method. When such β emitters are used, care must be taken to limit its infusion only to the liver. Even infusion of a tiny fraction into the cystic artery potentially can result in decay of the gallbladder. Thus, high-magnification arteriography and careful evaluation of the cystic artery is imperative. We have been embolizing the cystic artery routinely with coils to prevent administration of Therasphere into the cystic artery (Figs. 8 and 9).

9. CONCLUSIONS

TACE offers an effective method of delivering high doses of chemotherapeutic agent directly to the area of the liver affected by the tumor as well as

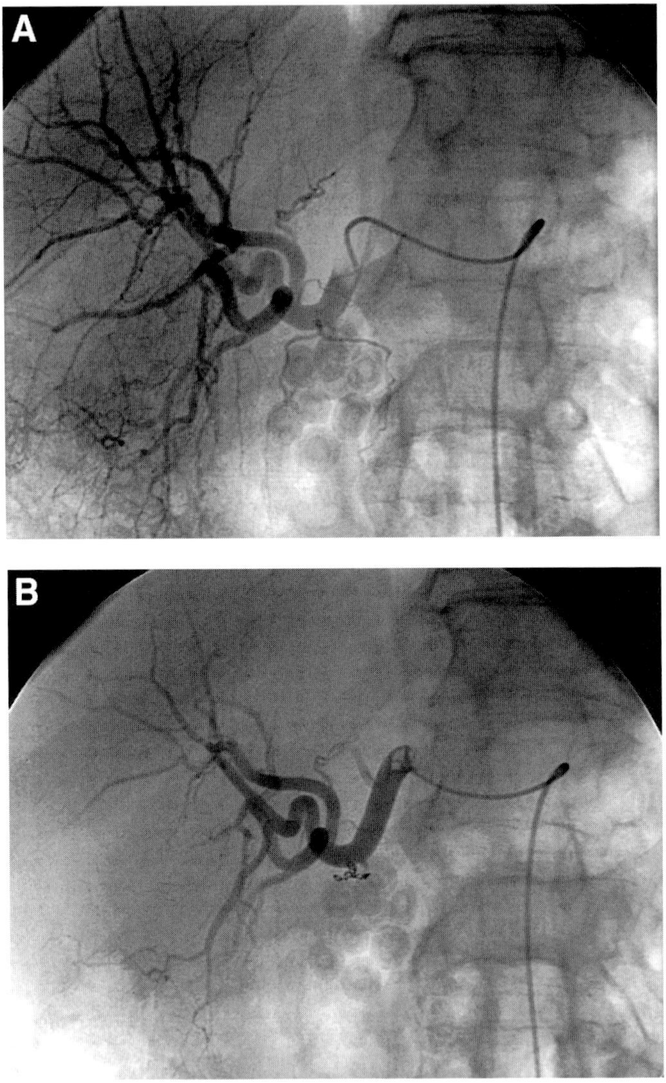

Fig. 9. (A) Selective right hepatic artery arteriogram showing filling of the cystic artery. Note the presence of gallstones in the gallbladder. **(B)** Selective right hepatic artery arteriogram after coil embolization of the cystic artery.

embolizing the vessels to decrease tumor vascularity and increase tumor necrosis. Optimal treatment requires experienced angiographers with expertise in the use of microcatheterization techniques. A close working relationship needs to exist between the interventionalist and oncologist to develop and maintain a successful intra-arterial chemoembolization practice.

REFERENCES

1. Goldstein HM, Wallace S, Anderson JH, Bree RL, Gianturco C. Transcatheter occlusion of abdominal tumors. *Radiology* 1976;120:539–545.
2. Chuang VP, Wallace S. Hepatic artery embolization in the treatment of hepatic neoplasms. *Radiology* 1981;140:51–58.
3. Yamada R, Sato M, Kawabata M, Nakatsuka H, Nakamura K, Takashima S. Hepatic artery embolization in 120 patients with unresectable hepatoma. *Radiology* 1983;148:397–401.
4. Kamada K, Nakanishi T, Kitamoto M, Aikata H, Kawakami Y, Ito K, et al. Long-term prognosis of patients undergoing transcatheter arterial chemoembolization for unresectable hepatocellular carcinoma: comparison of cisplatin lipiodol suspension and doxorubicin hydrochloride emulsion. *Vasc Interv Radiol* 2001;12:847–854.
5. Ebied OM, Federle MP, Carr BI, Pealer KM, Li W, Amesur N, et al. Evaluation of responses to chemoembolization in patients with unresectable hepatocellular carcinoma. *Cancer* 2003;97:1042–1050.
6. Kadir S. *Diagnostic Angiography*, WB Saunders, Philadelphia, 1986.
7. Kadir S, Lundell C, Saeed M. Celiac, superior and inferior mesenteric arteries. In: *Atlas of Normal and Variant Angiography Anatomy* (Kadis S, ed.), WB Saunders, Philadelphia, 1991, pp. 297–364.
8. Waltman AC, Courey WR, Athanasoulis C, Baum S. Technique for left gastric artery catheterization. *Radiology* 1973;109:732–734.
9. Gates J, Hartnell GG, Stuart KE, Clouse ME. Chemoembolization of hepatic neoplasms: safety, complications and when to worry. *Radiographics* 1999;19:399–414.
10. Song SY, Chung JW, Han JK, Lim HG, Koh YH, Park JH, et al. Liver abscess after transcatheter oily chemoembolization for hepatic tumors: incidence, predisposing factors, and clinical outcome. *JVIR* 2001;12:313–320.
11. Kim W, Clark TWI, Baum RA, Soulen MC. Risk Factors for liver abscess formation after hepatic chemoembolization. JVIR 2001;12:965–968.
12. Shibata T, Kojima N, Itoh K, Konishi J. Transcatheter arterial chemoembolization through collateral arteries for hepatocellular carcinoma after arterial occlusion. *Radiat Med* 1998;16:251–256.
13. Salem R, Thurston KG, Carr BI, Goin JE, Geschwind JFH. Yttrium-90 microspheres: radiation therapy for unresectable liver cancer. *JVIR* 2002;13:S223–S229.

12 Medical Therapy of Hepatocellular Carcinoma

Brian I. Carr, MD, FRCP, PhD

CONTENTS

1. PRINCIPLES

1.1. Clinical Presentation

The principles underlying medical management of hepatocellular carcinoma (HCC) are based on an understanding of the clinical setting, the tumor characteristics, and the underlying biology. Reviewing our patient population, we found that 81% had cirrhosis and 19% had no evidence of cirrhosis by biopsy or computed tomography (CT) scan (Table 1). The male/female ratio was 2.5:1, and 72% of our patients were caucasian. Interestingly, 24% of our patients had no symptoms at all but were diagnosed either by the finding of elevated liver function test results on routine physical examination or as an incidental finding, such as a work-up for some unrelated disease. A further 17% of patients were diagnosed because of a planned surveillance CT scan screening because of a known

From: *Current Clinical Oncology: Hepatocellular Cancer: Diagnosis and Treatment*
Edited by: B. I. Carr © Humana Press Inc., Totowa, NJ

Table 1
Clinical Presentation of HCC, University of Pittsburgh, Liver Cancer Center (n = 547), 1989–2001

Symptom	*No. patients*	*%*
No symptom	**129**	**24**
Abdominal pain	219	40
Other (work-up of anemia and various diseases)	64	12
Routine physical examination finding, elevated LFTs	129	24
Weight loss	112	20
Appetite loss	59	11
Weakness or malaise	83	15
Jaundice	30	5
Routine CT scan screening of known cirrhosis	92	17
Cirrhosis symptoms (ankle swelling, abdominal bloating, increased girth, pruritus, encephalopathy, gastrointestinal bleed)	98	18
Diarrhea	7	1
Tumor rupture	1	1
Patient characteristics		
Mean age (years)	56 ± 13	
Male/female ratio	205:1	
Ethnicity		
White	72%	
Middle Eastern	10%	
Asian	13%	
Black	5%	
Cirrhosis	**81%**	
No cirrhosis	**19%**	
Tumor characteristics		
Hepatic tumor numbers		
1	20%	
2	25%	
3 or more	65%	
Portal vein invasion	75%	
Unilobar	25%	
Bilobar	75%	

Abbreviations: LFTs, liver function test results.

history of hepatitis B or C, cirrhosis, or both. Eighteen percent of patients had the symptoms of cirrhosis, which include ankle swelling, abdominal bloating, increased girth, pruritus, encephalopathy, or a gastrointestinal (GI) bleed, and a full 40% of patients had abdominal pain at presentation. This seemed to be the

Table 2
Treatment Options for HCC

Potentially curative options
Liver resection
Liver transplantation
Other treatments
Regional therapies
Ablative therapies: cytoreductive therapies
Palliative resection
Cryosurgery
Microwave ablation
Ethanol injection
Acetic acid injection
Radiofrequency ablation
Transcatheter hepatic artery treatments
Transarterial chemotherapy
Transarterial embolization
Transarterial chemoembolization
Transarterial radiotherapy
^{90}Y microspheres
^{131}I lipiodol
Gene therapies
External beam conformal radiation
Systemic therapies
Chemotherapy
Immunotherapy
Hormonal therapy
Growth factor or antibody control of cell cycle
Supportive palliative care

most common presenting symptom in our patient population. We also found a significant proportion of our patients had experienced weight loss, general malaise or weakness, and loss of appetite. We recently found (unpublished data) that more than 80% of patients report loss of sexual function or desire within the proceeding 12 months of the diagnosis. This seems to be a sensitive but nonspecific correlate of our cancer patients and was found on analysis of our systematic study of quality-of-life questionnaires. The tumor characteristics tend to display interesting patterns. In our experience, HCC is typically a multifocal and bilobar cancer (Table 1, tumor characteristics), and is thus typically not a surgeon's disease. In addition, portal vein invasion of either the main portal or main branch portal vein, as judged by occlusion of flow or expansion of the vein on CT scan, occurred in 75% of our patients (Table 2).

1.2. Underlying Liver Disease

Metastatic cancer that spreads to the liver from organs such as the breast, colon, or lung, spread to a normal liver. By contrast, most patients with HCC typically have a diseased underlying liver as well as the cancer. Although this varies from country to country, between 60 and 90% of patients with HCC have underlying cirrhosis *(1)*. The cause of this may vary, but the most common factors are hepatitis B virus (HBV), hepatitis C virus (HCV), chronic alcohol consumption, and probably chronic exposure to mycotoxins, such as aflatoxin B_1 in Africa and Asia. This has major implications for therapy, because the cirrhosis limits the ability of the surgeon to resect a liver mass safely without risk of liver failure in the remaining liver and limits the ability of the chemotherapist to deliver cytotoxic drugs without risk of liver failure because of the additional damage to a liver that is already damaged as a result of chronic disease.

1.3. HCC Is a Multifocal Disease

Because HCC typically arises in the setting of cirrhosis, and there are millions of cirrhotic nodules in an individual liver, HCC is often multifocal and bilobar (Table 1, tumor characteristics). Although countries with screening programs are able to diagnose earlier and smaller HCCs, its natural history includes the development of multiple satellite lesions in both lobes of the liver over time. The cause of this is twofold. First, studies with HBV integration sites show that multiple distinct primary tumors can arise in different parts of the liver either synchronously or metachronously. Second, a clonal HCC can spread throughout the liver via portal vein invasion or arteriovenous connections. In addition, the evidence from liver transplantation indicates that HCC is commonly a whole-organ disease.

1.4. HCC Is a Vascular Tumor

A characteristic of HCC that distinguishes it from most metastases to the liver is the fact that it is a highly vascular tumor. The vascularity typically is found on the arterial phase of triple phase helicalcomputed atial tomography (CAT) scans (Fig. 1) or on hepatic angiography (Fig. 2). This is in contrast to metastases resulting from colon cancer, which are typically hypovascular. This vascularity provides an opportunity for selective delivery of drugs to the tumor, because the vascular supply to HCC typically arises from hepatic arteries, whereas the delivery of 90% of the oxygenated blood to the underlying nontumorous liver is mainly from the portal vein. This provides a partial basis for intrahepatic chemoembolization or intrahepatic chemotherapy, which permits a relatively selective delivery of chemotherapy to the tumors in the liver via the tumor neovasculature that typically grows in response to the presence of an HCC.

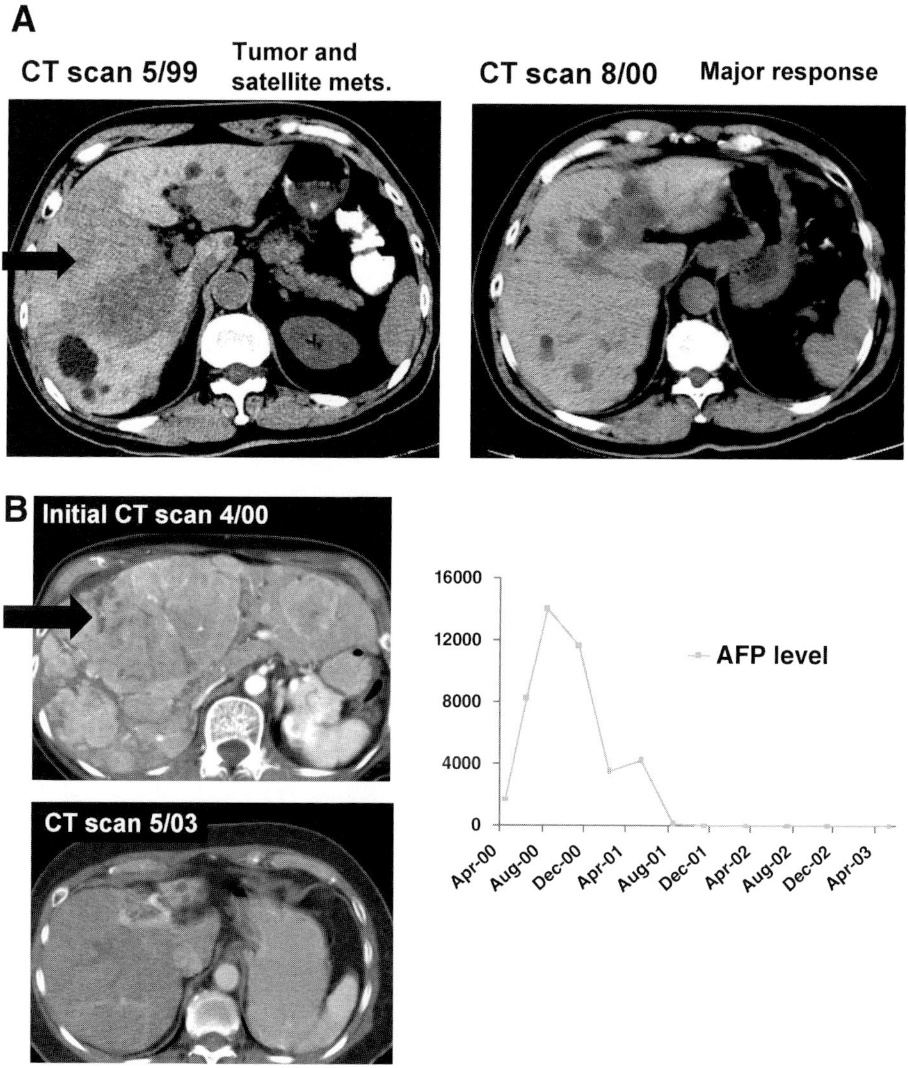

Fig. 1. CATY scan of two patients (**A** and **B**) who experience major shrinkage of their HCCs after TACE therapy.

1.5. Portal Vein Invasion: A Key Prognostic Characteristic of HCC

The tendency of HCC to invade the portal vein is a characteristic of HCC and distinguishes it from most metastases to the liver. It is manifested clinically as thrombosis of a major portal vein or a major portal vein branch (Fig. 1), seen as

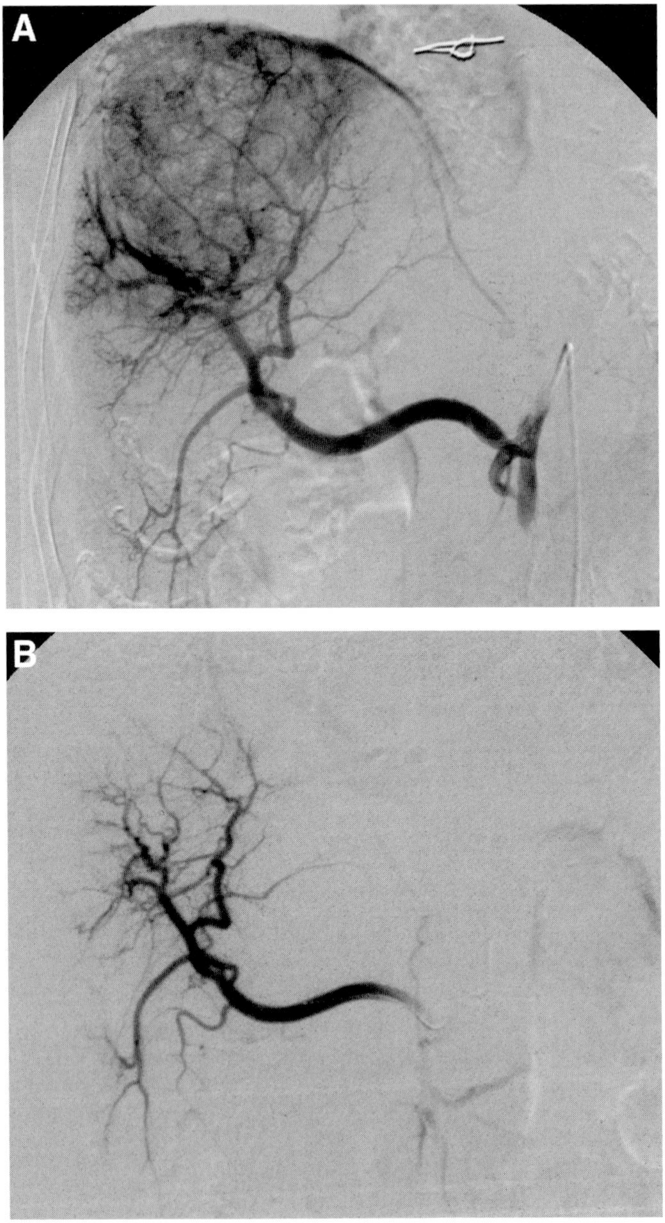

Fig. 2. Hepatic angiograms showing tumor vascularity associated with an HCC of a patient before **(A)** and after **(B)** responding to TACE.

occlusion or expansion of the portal vein on CAT scan, or both, or microscopically, it is seen as presence of HCC in the walls or lumens of normal hepatic vessels. It is also probably the most important negative prognostic factor in the evaluation of the patient with HCC for any form of surgery, but particularly for liver transplantation. Because the portal vein is thrombosed, it can be biopsied safely by a percutaneous needle, and this provides proof of the malignant nature of portal vein thrombosis in the presence of HCC *(2,3)*. Portal vein invasion (thrombosis) is currently deemed to be a major contraindication for liver transplantation. Portal vein thrombosis previously was thought to be a contraindication for hepatic artery chemotherapy, because if the portal vein is blocked by tumor and the hepatic artery is embolized for therapeutic purposes, then that lobe of the liver is thought to undergo necrosis, with resultant liver failure. However, as shown here, most of our patients with advanced HCC have portal vein thrombosis, at least of a major branch, and most of these are unresectable. Despite this, most of the cases of thrombosis have been treated with intrahepatic chemo-occlusion with little deleterious effect on the underlying liver, provided certain precautions are observed, as discussed here. These include treating only one lobe of the liver at any single chemotherapy session, as well as using subocclusion but never complete embolization of the treated hepatic artery.

1.6. HCC Is Relatively Resistant to the Toxic Effects of Most Chemotherapeutic Agents

It has been known for more than 70 years, since the experiments of Haddow *(4)*, that the liver that has been damaged by carcinogenic or other toxic chemicals and then recovers becomes remarkably resistant to a subsequent challenge by a variety of toxic agents *(5)*. Most other cancers such as breast cancer adapt to chemotherapy by developing acquired resistance to the toxic effects of the chemotherapy. It is thought that most HCC arises *ab initio* as a drug-resistant tumor. This was most clearly demonstrated in the drug resistance–growth inhibition model of rodent carcinogenesis first described by Solt and Farber *(6)*, but many other studies have shown the carcinogen-altered liver to be remarkably resistant to toxicity by various poisons or cancer chemotherapy agents *(7)*. The clinical consequence of this is that most clinical trials of phase 2 and phase 3 chemotherapy drugs have shown responses to single drugs in less than 20% of the patients and have no beneficial effect on survival (Table 3 *[13–35]*). However, when given by the hepatic artery route, the same drugs have been found to result in tumor shrinkage and partial responses (PRs) in 30–70% of the patients, usually in association with some form of hepatic artery occluding agent (Tables 4 *[36–68]* and 7). Hepatic artery occlusion alone does not seem to impact the tumor, which the results of hepatic artery ligation showed long ago. Several recent randomized trials have shown the benefits of transarterial catheter embolization (TACE) in causing tumor shrinkage (PRs), as seen in Table 5 *(69–81)*, but only recently did two recent randomized clinical trials comparing TACE with no therapy as a control arm convincingly show a survival advantage for TACE therapy (Table 6 *[82–90]*).

Table 3
Selected Recent Studies of Chemotherapy

Investigation	*Drug*	*Partial response rate (%)*
Systemic chemotherapy		
Sciarrino et al., 1985 *(23)*	Doxorubicin	0
Chlebowski et al., 1987 *(13)*	Doxorubicin	11
Ihde et al., 1977 *(14)*	Doxorubicin	15
Falkson et al, 1984 *(15)*	Doxorubicin, 5-fluorouracil, methyl-CCNU	19
Falkson et al., 1984 *(16)*	Neocarzinostatin	8
Ravry et al., 1984 *(17)*	Doxorubicin, bleomycin	16
Cavalli et al., 1981 *(18)*	VP-16	13
Melia et al., 1983 *(19)*	VP-16	18
Melia et al., 1981 *(20)*	Cisplatin	1
Ravry et al., 1986 *(21)*	Cisplatin	0
Falkson et al., 1987 *(22)*	Cisplatin	17
Falkson et al., 1987 *(22)*	Mitoxantrone	8
Colleoni et al., 1993 *(24)*	Mitoxantrone	23
Chao et al., 1998 *(25)*	Paclitaxel	0
Patt et al., 2003 *(26)*	5-FU + IFN	18
Patt et al., 1999 *(27)*	5-FU + IFN + Cisplatin + Doxorubicin	20
Okada et al., 1999 *(29)*	Cisplatin, Mitoxantrone + 5-FU	33
Reviews *(30–35)*		

Abbreviations: 5-FU, 5-fluorouracil; IFN, interferon.

2. SPECIAL CONSIDERATIONS FOR THE ONCOLOGIST

HCC arises on the basis of a diseased liver, which is more sensitive to toxic damage by chemotherapeutic agents than normal liver. In addition, cirrhosis causes portal hypertension, which poses additional hazards for the chemotherapist.

2.1. Myelosuppression

Portal hypertension is associated with splenomegaly and associated leukopenia and thrombocytopenia. Unlike the myelosuppression that results from systemic chemotherapy and can be attributed to chemotherapy-mediated damage to the cells of the bone marrow, the leukopenia and thrombocytopenia consequent to splenomegaly is thought to be the result of sequestration of blood cells in the spleen, in the presence of a normal marrow. Although the starting values of white blood cells (WBCs) and platelets in the patient with cirrhosis typically are lower

Table 4
Intrahepatic Artery Chemotherapy for Hepatocellular Carcinoma

Investigation	*Agents*	*Response rate (%)*
Sasaki et al., 1987 *(36)*	Platinum, gelatin sponge	65
Kasugai et al., 1989 *(37)*	Platinum, ethiodized oil	38
Ohnishi et al., 1984 *(38)*	MMC, microcapsules	32
Lin et al., 1988 *(39)*	5-FU, Ivalon	32
Fujimoto et al., 1985 *(40)*	5-FU/MMC, starch	68
Audisio et al., 1990 *(41)*	MMC + microcapsules	43
Kobayashi et al., 1986 *(42)*	Doxorubicin + ethiodized oil	42
Kanematsu et al., 1989 *(43)*	Doxorubicin + ethiodized oil	47
Shibata et al., 1989 *(44)*	Platinum + ethiodized oil	47
Konna et al., 1983 *(45)*	SMANCS + ethiodized oil	90
Pelletier et al., 1990 *(46)*	Doxorubicin + gelatin sponge	17
Carr et al., 1991 *(47)*	Doxorubicin/Cisplatin	50
Venook et al., 1990 *(48)*	Doxorubicin/Cisplatin/MMC + gelatin sponge	24
Ohnishi et al., 1987 *(49)*	MMC + microcapsules	28
Ohnishi et al., 1987 *(49)*	MMC + gelatin sponge + microcapsules	57
Beppu et al., 1991 *(51)*	Cisplatin + ethiodized oil + aclarubicin microspheres	50
Trinchet et al., 1995 *(52)*	Cisplatin + ethiodized oil vs. 0 0	16
Chang et al., 1994 *(53)*	Cisplatin + Gelfoam + ethiodized oil vs. Gelfoam + ethiodized oil	68[a] 67[a]
Stuart et al., 1993 *(54)*	Doxorubicin, ethiodized oil + Gelfoam	43
Bruiz et al., 1994 *(55)*	Gelfoam, no chemotherapy	81
Carr et al., 1996 *(56)*	Doxorubicin, cisplatin + Spherex	63
Carr et al., 1993 *(57)*	Doxorubicin, cisplatin + ethiodized oil vs. doxorubicin + cisplatin	57 47

(continued)

Table 4 (Continued)
Intrahepatic Artery Chemotherapy for Hepatocellular Carcinoma

Investigation	*Agents*	*Response rate (%)*
Carr et al., 2002 *(58)*	Cisplatin	58
Ngan et al., 1993 *(59)*	Cisplatin, ethiodized oil, Gelfoam	41
Yamamoto et al., 1993 *(60)*	IL-2	
Kawai et al., 1994 *(61)*	Epirubicin + Gelfoam vs. doxorubicin + Gelfoam	[a]
Yoshimi et al., 1992 *(62)*	Resection vs TAE	[a]
Epstein et al., 1991 *(63)*	Cisplatin + hepatic radiation	48
Rougier et al., 1993 *(64)*	Doxorubicin + Gelfoam	41
Onohara et al., 1988 *(65)*	Cisplatin	55
Kajanti et al., 1986 *(66)*	Cisplatin	40
Ando et al., 1987 *(67)*	Epirubicin	15
Carr et al., 1996 *(68)*	Cisplatin dose escalation	50

Abbreviations: 5-FU, 5-fluorouracil; MMC, mitomycin C; SMANCS, styrene maleic acid conjugates of neocarzinostatin and mitomycin C; IFN, interferon; IL-2, interleukin 2; TAE, transarterial embolization.

[a]Similar survival.

Table 5
Some Randomized Clinical Trials Involving Transhepatic Artery Chemoembolization vs Other Chemotherapy for HCC

Author/year	*Agents 1*	*Agents 2*	*Effects on survival*
Kawai et al., 1992 *(69)*	Doxorubicin + Embo	Embo	None
Kawai et al.,1997 *(70)*	Epirubicin + Embo	Doxorubicin + Embo	None
Watanabe et al., 1994 *(71)*	Epirubicin + Embo	Doxorubicin + Embo	None
Chang et al., 1994 *(72)*	Cisplatin + Embo	Embo	None
Hatanaka et al., 1995 *(73)*	Cisplatin, Doxorubicin + Embo	Same + Lipiodol	None
Uchino et al., 1993 *(74)*	Cisplatin, Doxorubicin + oral FU	Same + Tamoxifen	None
Madden et al., 1993 *(75)*	Cisplatin + ADMOS	5-epi-doxorubicin	None
Chang et al., 2000 *(76)*	Cisplatin + 1FN	Cisplatin	None
Lin et al., 1988 *(77)*	Embo	Embo + Intravenous FU	None
Yoshikawa et al., 1994 *(78)*	Epirubicin + Lipiodol	Epirubicin	None
Kajanti et al., 1992 *(79)*	Epirubicin + FU	Intravenous Epirubicin + FU	None
Tzoracoleftherakis et al., 1999 *(80)*	Doxorubicin	Intravenous Doxorubicin	None
Bhattachariya et al., 1995 *(81)*	Epirubicin + Lipiodol	^{131}I, Lipiodol	None

Abbreviations: FU, ; fluorouracil; IFN, interferon; Embo, embolization.

Table 6
Randomized Clinical Trials Involving Transhepatic Arterial Chemoembolization (TACE) Chemotherapy vs No Treatment Controls

Author/year	*Agents*	*Effects on survival*
Pelletier et al., 1990 *(82)*	Doxorubicin + Gelfoam	None
Trinchet et al., 1995 *(83)*	Cisplatin + Gelfoam	None
Bruix et al., 1998 *(84)*	Coils and Gelfoam	None
Pelletier et al., 1998 *(85)*	Cisplatin + Lipiodol	None
Lo et al., 2002 *(86)*	Cisplatin + Lipiodol	Yes
Llovet et al., 2002 *(87)*	Doxorubicin + Lipiodol	Yes
Reviews *(88–90)*		

Table 7
University of Pittsburgh Experience: Effects of Hepatic Arterial Cisplatin Dose Intensity *(9,10)*

Patients treated: 57
Cisplatin alone, n = 26
Cisplatin + Gelfoam = 31

A. Responses (PR)

Cisplatin alone, 11 of 26 (42%)
Cisplatin + Gelfoam, 18 of 31 (58%)

B. Effects of response on median survival (months) ± SE

	Cisplatin alone	Cisplatin + Gelfoam
Responders	29.0 ± 3.5	25.5 ± 1.7
Nonresponders	11.1 ± 1.5	15.6 ± 3.1
	p <0.0001	p <0.003

C. Effect of treatment type on median survival (months) ± SE

Cisplatin Alone	Cisplatin + Gelfoam
19.53 ± 6.3	30.73 ± 0

p <0.137

D. Effect of dose density on median survival (months) ± SE

	Cisplatin alone + Gelfoam	Cisplatin
Dose = 125 mg/m^2/mo	9.9 ± 1.66	16.4 ± 2.8
Dose = ≥ 125 mg/m^2/mo	19.5 ± 7.2	30.7 ± 0
	p <0.07	p <0.69

than are permitted in most cancer clinical chemotherapy trials, it is our experience that patients rarely come to any harm from chemotherapy with an initial WBC count ofmore than 3,000/mL or platelet count more than 40,000/mL. The recent introduction of granulocyte colony-stimulating factors into clinical practice means that the WBC count can be restored to safe levels by the oncologist at will.

2.2. GI Bleeding

Portal hypertension is associated with esophageal and gastric variceal bleeding in addition to colonic bleeding. This is a hazard for the cancer chemotherapist to consider, because the consequence of the chemotherapy is often a decrease in platelet counts. Our experience is that preventive banding or sclerosing of varices does not seem to make any difference compared with treating the varices only after there is a bleed.

2.3. Decreased Xenobiotic Metabolizing Capacity

The decreased metabolic capacity, and particularly the ability to detoxify xenobiotics, results in the increased half-life of many of the common chemotherapeutic agents. This can result in life-threatening prolongation in the myelosuppression. Careful dose adjustment to the individual tolerance of the patient needs to be taken into account by the experienced oncologist. Whereas most patients tolerate cisplatin, doxorubicin, or fluorouracil deoxyribuse (FUDR), prolonged and frightening thrombocytopenia can result from use of mitomycin C.

2.4. Decreased Liver Synthetic Activity Associated With Portal Hypertension

An increased prothrombin time from decreased synthetic capacity of the liver poses hazards for the vascular interventional radiologist. We typically treat patients with fresh frozen plasma or platelet transfusions for a platelet count less than 50,000/mL before femoral artery puncture, but, in our experience, any chemotherapy delivered with a baseline international normalization ratio (INR) higher than 1.5 risks hepatocellular failure because of the failure of the diseased liver. Also , in our experience, a low serum albumin level, especially when associated with more than minimal ascites, is a poor prognostic sign.

3. HEPATIC ARTERY CHEMOTHERAPY AND CHEMOEMBOLIZATION

3.1. Hepatic Artery Drug Delivery as a Semiselective Means for Delivering High Concentrations of Drugs to the Tumor

The hepatic artery delivery of drugs such as chemotherapeutic agents is carried out with two aims. First, because the HCC is supplied mainly by hepatic arterial blood in contrast to the portal delivery of blood to the underlying liver, this offers a semiselective means for delivering drug to the tumor rather than to the underlying liver. In clinical practice, the resulting transient elevation of several of the liver function test results suggests that the underlying liver is not really spared. Second, delivery of many drugs into the liver via the hepatic artery seems to result in much higher hepatic extraction of drug compared with systemic delivery (Table 8). As a consequence, because most HCCs are vascular, quite high concentrations of drugs can be delivered to individual HCC tumor masses.

3.2. Commonly Used Drugs

Chemotherapeutic agents that have been used in many centers include cisplatin or cisplatinum (Platinol), Doxorubicin (Adriamycin), 5-fluorouracil (5-FU) or 5-FUdR, and mitomycin C, in addition to the much lower experience with neocarzinostatin (SMANCS), vincristine, gemcitabine, and, recently, oxaliplatinum (Table 4). They have been used as single agents and in combinations, with (usually) or without some form of embolizing agent to produce chemo-embolization or chemo-occlusion. The most commonly used agent in addition to chemotherapy is Lipiodol (Ethiodol), which is an oily radio-opaque material that produces an emulsion with the injected drugs. This emulsion is believed to keep the drugs in longer contact with the tumor.

3.3. Hepatic Arterial Occlusion

Various agents have been introduced into the hepatic artery (Table 7) together with chemotherapy to cause vascular slowing (occlusion) or embolization (TACE). These include Gelfoam (a degradable gelatin sponge and our preferred agent, Pharmacia and Upjohn), Ivalon (polyvinyl alcohol, which is irreversible and, in our experience, more dangerous), blood clots, degradable starch microspheres (Spherex, a relatively safe and attractive product, Pharmacia), and steel coils. Recently, particles of defined size ranges have been introduced, such as Embogold (trisacrylpolymer, Biosphere Medical) compressible microspheres (Biosphere) with particle sizes of 40–120 μm, 100–300 μm, and 300–500 μm. A similar product is contour SE polyvinyl alcohol particles (Boston Scientific). Our main experience has been with Gelfoam, Spherex starch spheres, and Biospheres, because they are all degradable and seem to be the least hepatotoxic and to cause only transient vascular occlusion, allowing further chemotherapy sessions after several weeks. Lipiodol (Ethiodol) has been widely used, particularly in Europe and Japan. We have not noted any particular added effect of Lipiodol to chemotherapy in terms of tumor response *(28)*. In addition, it often obscures the subsequent interpretation of CAT scans. Therefore, we have abandoned its use. The hepatic artery approach is based on two considerations. First, because the hepatic artery supplies more than 90% of oxygenated blood to the HCC and

Table 8
University of Pittsburgh Experience: Cisplatin Hepatic Artery Chemoembolization, Prognostic Factors for Survival (n = 155)

	Patient characteristics (%), patient survival		
	>24 months (n = 49)	*4–24 months (n = 80)*	*<4 months (n = 26)*
Liver disease			
Cirrhosis	73	84	88
HBV	28	29	31
HCV	0	36	35
Alcohol	12	15	19
Laboratory results			
Bilirubin <1.6 mg/dL	96	71	42
Albumin >3.4 g/dL	76	47	35
No ascites	92	90	38
INR <1.2	80	60	31
Platelets $>150 \times 10^9$/L	71	55	27
Portal hypertension (CT)	35	45	85

the portal vein acts similarly for the underlying liver, this permits a selective drug delivery. Second, as the hepatic arterial flow rate is reduced by use of an embolizing agent, enhanced hepatic uptake has been shown *(8)* for many cancer chemotherapy drugs (Table 8).

3.4. University of Pittsburgh Protocol for Chemo-Occlusion Therapy of HCC

Our largest experience has been with cisplatin, because it has moderate tumor-shrinking ability and has minimal myelosuppressive activity compared with most other agents. This is a useful property in the setting of portal hypertension. It is also relatively well tolerated by the cirrhotic liver. It is usually given at a starting dose of 125 mg/m^2 of body surface area. This dose is essentially tolerated by everyone with a bilirubin of less than 1.5 mg/dL, a normal INR, and without gross ascites. Patients who tolerate this well, without change in their blood count or increase in their liver functions, typically have the dose increased after two or three cycles to 150 mg/m^2 and then to 175 mg/m^2. The cisplatin is given in 100 mL of normal saline and infused into the hepatic artery over 30 minutes, together with 20 mg of dexamethasone (to limit hepatic inflammation), 5 mg of morphine sulfate (for pain), as well as intravenous antibiotics (Ancef or Vancomycin) given before TACE. A pressure pump is used to deliver the drug. Simultaneously, 250 mL of 3% saline is administered intravenously. In addition, intravenous hydration is administered to the patients aggressively. This is carried out using D5 normal saline or just normal saline with 20 mEg KCl/L at 250 mL/hour for a minimum of 3 hours. As soon as the patient is in the vascular procedure room, the fluid rate is increased to 2 L over 2 hours immediately before the cisplatin infusion, together with immediate intravenous infusion of the diuretics (12.5 g of Mannitol and 40 mg of Furosemide) during the cisplatin infusion. This diuretic regimen is designed to prevent cisplatin from being retained in the kidney and causing nephrotoxicity. Aggressive triple antiemetics consisting of a combination of Reglan, Benadryl (or Kytril), or Anzemet and Dexamethasone are all given repetitively for the next 24 hours. Before cisplatin, we give a single intravenous dose of 1 mg of Kytril (Granisetron) or 32 mg of Zofran (Ondansetron), together with 4 mg of dexamethasone (Decadron) . After cisplatin, we give 2 mg/kg of intravenous Reglan (Metoclopramide), 25 mg of Benadryl, and 4 mg of Decadron every 3 hours for the next 12 hours. Zofran, Anzemet, or Kytril is continued at 10 mg intravenously every 8 hours. In addition, we give an intravenous bolus of 9 g/m^2 of sodium thiosulfate immediately before the chemotherapy and a 6-hour intravenous infusion of 1.5 g/m^2 per hour afterward. This has resulted in essential disappearance of cisplatin-mediated ototoxicity and neurotoxicity. Intravenous hydration at 150 mL/hour is continued after chemotherapy until the patient is discharged from hospital. Patients are typically hospitalized overnight and are discharged the following morning. However, whether they need to be kept as an inpatient overnight is not clear. Most patients require some form of bolus intravenous morphine sulfate, typically 2- or 5-mg injections, every 3–4 hours for two or three administrations after the vascular occlusion. The pain of postembolization syndrome is likely caused in part by arterial spasm. Lab work is rechecked the morning after treatment for electrolyte imbalances or potassium or magnesium losses that need to be replaced, as needed.

Gelfoam sponge particles (not powder), which are made by cutting up Gelfoam sponge sheets with scissors and then autoclaving, typically are injected hepatic-arterially at the beginning of the administration of chemotherapy, halfway through and again at the end of the cisplatin administration. The idea is to cause vascular slowing but never complete occlusion. Thus, we do not actually perform complete embolization. This has resulted in a much larger safety margin for our protocol. The arterial flow is monitored during the chemotherapy by regular bolus injections of angiographic dye to monitor the vascular flow. Gelfoam powder is thought to be too toxic and is not used in our institution. Similarly, Ivalon is not given because of its hepatotoxicity and irreversibility, limiting the ability to give future doses of chemotherapy.

The chemotherapy (TACE) is typically repeated every 8–12 weeks, depending on the hepatic tolerance, the tumor response, and recovery of the WBCs, platelets, liver transaminases, or bilirubin and on the time required for clinical patient recovery. The main toxicity seems to be tiredness and loss of appetite for

7–10 days after treatment. With this regimen of intravenous triple antibiotic and intra-arterial morphine sulfate, we have found that nausea and vomiting are minimal and hepatic pain is also limited. The patients thus do not typically fear repeated treatments.

4. SAFETY CONSIDERATIONS OF HEPATIC ARTERY CHEMO-OCCLUSION

4.1. Unilobar Treatments

It is possible to administer chemotherapy safely to the whole liver through the proper hepatic artery to an entirely normal liver with metastatic cancer. It is also possible to do this with multifocal bilobar HCCs with completely normal liver function and no ascites and in the complete absence of portal vein thrombosis, hepatitis, or cirrhosis. However, our experience is that chemo-occlusion is much safer when only one lobe of the liver is given TACE treatment at any one treatment session. This is now our standard operating procedure. The lobe of the liver with the maximum amount of tumor is normally selected for initial treatment, and several treatments are given to this lobe until tumor control is achieved. Then, the other liver lobe is treated on subsequent treatment sessions.

4.2. Vascular Slowing Is Performed Without Complete Occlusion

Chemotherapy is given with regular pulses of embolizing materials to achieve vascular slowing, but complete occlusion of the arterial blood flow is avoided to minimize subsequent hepatotoxicity.

4.3. Drug Doses Are Tailored to Each Individual

Almost all patients with a bilirubin level of less than 1.5 mg/dL tolerate 125 mg/m^2 of cisplatin. Doses on subsequent treatments can be escalated (Table 7) from 150 mg/m^2 to 175 mg/m^2 to 200 mg/m^2, although few patients can tolerate 200 mg/m^2. A completely normal blood count and no change in liver function tests is used as the basis for increasing the dose of cisplatin by one dose level on a subsequent treatment. By contrast, prolongation of a prothrombin time or elevation of the bilirubin to levels greater than normal generally is used to decrease the cisplatin to 100 mg/m^2 on a subsequent treatment, or down one dose level if a higher dose than the starting dose level has been used. A nadir WBC count of more than 2,000/mL or nadir platelet count of more of than 40,000/mL rarely requires a decrease in the dose of cisplatin on subsequent treatments. The timing of repeated treatments is somewhat arbitrary. A newly diagnosed patient typically is put on a schedule of repeat treatments every 6 or 8 weeks for the first two or three treatments until some form of tumor response can be seen. After this point, the time between treatments is increased rapidly up to a maximum of 12 weeks. We think that extending the intertreatment intervals beyond 12 weeks is associated with increasing likelihood of tumor growth. However, it is our experience that tumors that decrease by more than 50% of their size can stabilize without repeat treatments for many months without regrowth.

5. RESULTS OF HEPATIC ARTERY CHEMOTHERAPY AND CHEMOEMBOLIZATION

We recently evaluated the results of treating a large number of patients with cisplatin-based chemoembolization (TACE) and have evaluated them based on prolonged survival (longer than 24 months), poor survival (less than 4 months), or intermediate survival somewhere between these two (Tables 8, 9, and 10). We found that cirrhosis alone was not a good predictor of poor survival, because many patients with cirrhosis also were in the best survival category. However, poor liver function, as judged by an elevated bilirubin, low albumin, or prolonged prothrombin time (INR) all were strongly associated with the poor survival category (Table 8). The main tumor characteristics that seemed to be important in survival of patients with HCC after TACE were portal vein invasion and very high α-fetoprotein (AFP) levels (Table 9). Tumor size or numbers of tumors did not seem to be important in our series. By contrast, any form of partial response to chemotherapy, as judged by tumor shrinkage or decreased tumor vascularity on a triple-phase helical CT scan, was strongly associated with the prolonged survival group (Table 9). Examples of this are shown in the CT scans in Fig. 1A,B and the angiograms in Fig. 2A,B. It seems that there are two types of HCC response to chemotherapy. These are formal tumor shrinkage as noted with other types of cancer, as well as a decrease in tumor vascularity *(11,12)*. Because response to chemotherapy seemed to play such an important part in enhanced survival in our large TACE patient experience, we retrospectively examined those patient or tumor characteristics that correlated with response to chemotherapy (Table 10). We found that the presence of cirrhosis was much higher in those patients who did not respond to any chemotherapy (79%), although many patients (64%) who did respond to chemotherapy also had some degree of cirrhosis. An important consideration was tumor vasculature, because only 5% of patients with tumors that were hypovascular on CT scan responded to treatment, whereas 85% of patients whose tumors were hypervascular on CT scan showed response, as judged by tumor shrinkage (Table 10). Portal vein thrombosis also was important, because 86% of the patients whose tumors progressed on TACE had main portal vein thrombus, compared with only 48% in the response category. As in survival, tumor numbers or maximum tumor size seemed to have no correlation with response or failure to respond to TACE (Table 10).

Table 9
University of Pittsburgh Experience: Cisplatin Hepatic Artery Chemoembolization, Prognostic Factors for Survival (n = 155)

	Tumor characteristics (% patient), patient survival		
	>24 months (n = 49)	*6–24 months (n = 80)*	*<6 months (n = 26)*
Tumors			
Unilobar	29	15	8
Bilobar	71	85	92
>3 Tumors	78	83	85
PV invasion	41	56	73
Vascular tumors	90	80	42
Any tumor >5 cm	76	83	85
Metastases (except LNs)	6	17	15
AFP >100 K ng/mL	12	30	46
Response to chemotherapy			
Chemo responses (PR)	84	69	8
Tumor stability	16	25	4

Abbreviations: AFP, α-fetoprotein; LN, lymph node; PR, partial response.

Table 10

University of Pittsburgh Experience: Cisplatin Hepatic Artery Embolization for HCC, Factors Associated With Tumor Responses (n = 155)

	PR (n = 98; 63%)	*Stable (n = 29; 19%)*	*Progress (n = 28; 18%)*
Survival (months)			
<6	2 (2.0%)	1 (3%)	23 (82%)
6–24	55 (56%)	20 (69%)	5 (18%)
>24	41 (42%)	8 (28%)	0
Cirrhosis			
No	34 (35%)	10 (34%)	6 (21%)
Yes	64 (65%)	19 (66%)	22 (79%)
Tumor vasculature			
–	5 (5%)	1 (3%)	14 (50%)
+/–	10 (10%)	5 (17%)	2 (7%)
++	83 (85%)	23 (79%)	12 (43%)
PV thrombus			
–	51 (52%)	17 (58%)	4 (14%)
+	47 (48%)	12 (41%)	24 (86%)
Number	No correlation		
Maximum size	No correlation		

Abbreviations: PV,portal vein; PR, partial response (of tumor seen on CAT scan) .

6. SYSTEMIC CHEMOTHERAPY

A huge number of randomized and nonrandomized studies have been performed with various single agents and some combinations of chemotherapeutic agents (Table 3). Table 3 also cites several reviews. The bottom line is that there seems to be no response rate of more than 20% of patients nor is there a survivor benefit for any single agent tested thus far. Similarly, claims of enhanced responses up to 20% for some combinations, such as platinum, interferon, adriamycin, and FU (PIAF) *(120–122)*, are associated with enhanced toxicity, but it is not clear whether there is a survival benefit there either. For this reason, much of the recent literature has focused on regional chemotherapy to try and enhance tumor exposure to the cytocidal effects of higher doses of chemotherapy.

7. OTHER SYSTEMIC THERAPIES

A variety of hormonal therapies have been assessed for their usefulness in shrinking HCCs or enhancing of the survival in patients with HCC. This has been based on the known gender bias, in which HCC has been found to be a predominantly male disease and in which antigen receptors have been found in many HCC tumors. As a consequence, both Tamoxifen and kytenizing hormone-releasing hormone (LHRH) antagonists as well as Megesterol (Megace) have been evaluated for their tumor-shrinking abilities (Table 11; refs. *91–94,96–119*). Despite initial reports of responses to Tamoxifen, subsequent controlled randomized trials have essentially shown no survival benefit for Tamoxifen, LHRH antagonists such as Leuprolide or Flutamide, or Megestrol. A similarly large number of studies have investigated the effects of interferons, both because they have an antiangiogenic action as well as antihepatitis activity. Although there are conflicting reports of benefit or no benefit to tumor shrinkage or survival, the consensus is that there is no survival benefit for the use of interferon at any dose level, including huge doses of interferon that would not normally be tolerated by Western patients. Vitamin K or its analogs are a very attractive therapy, because a biochemical hallmark of HCC is a defect in vitamin K metabolism, resulting in elevated levels of immature prothrombin or des-γ-carboxy prothrombin, which is one of the more useful HCC serum tumor markers *(8,50,95)*. Although vitamins K1 and K2 seem to be almost nontoxic in adult humans, they have very weak antitumor activity, as judged by tumor responses, even given at huge supratherapeutic doses. However, the concept is a good one, and it may be only a matter of time before more potent K vitamin analogs are introduced into clinical testing for the treatment of HCC.

Table 11
Recent Medical Treatments Evaluated for Unresectable HCC

Systemic
Tamoxifen *(91–94)*
LHRH agonists *(96)*
Interferon *(97–100)*
Sandostatin *(101,102)*
Megestrol *(103,104)*
Vitamin K *(105–108)*
Thalidomide *(109)*
EGFR antibody
Arsenic trioxide
IL-2 *(110)*
Anti-angiogenesis strategies
Hepatic arterial
^{131}I – Lipiodol *(111–113)*
^{131}I – Ferritin *(114)*
^{90}Yttrium microspheres *(115–119)*

8. NEW HORIZONS AND FUTURE DIRECTIONS

The current generation of anticancer agents is based on the idea of cell cytotoxicity. Because these agents are essentially nonselective in their action, they are effective at killing both normal cells and tumor cells. This results in what are called *side effects.* A new paradigm is needed for drugs that are developed with a quite different method and intent of action, based not on killing cells but on the manipulation of cell growth and cell differentiation. Several new agents are beginning to appear on the horizon. These include antibodies against the epidermal growth factor (EGF) receptor, because many hepatoma cells have EGF receptors and are stimulated either by EGF or transforming growth factor-α. Phase I and II clinical studies with antibodies against the EGF receptor produced by several companies are currently in progress. A second approach is to restore the function of tumor suppressor genes that are known to be rendered dysfunctional or mutated in the carcinogenic process and to include the tumor suppressor genes *pRB* and *p53*. Gene therapy trials currently are underway using gene therapy with constructs for the wild-type *p53*. The anti-HCC activity currently is not yet known. A third approach involves the use of agents directed against the angio-

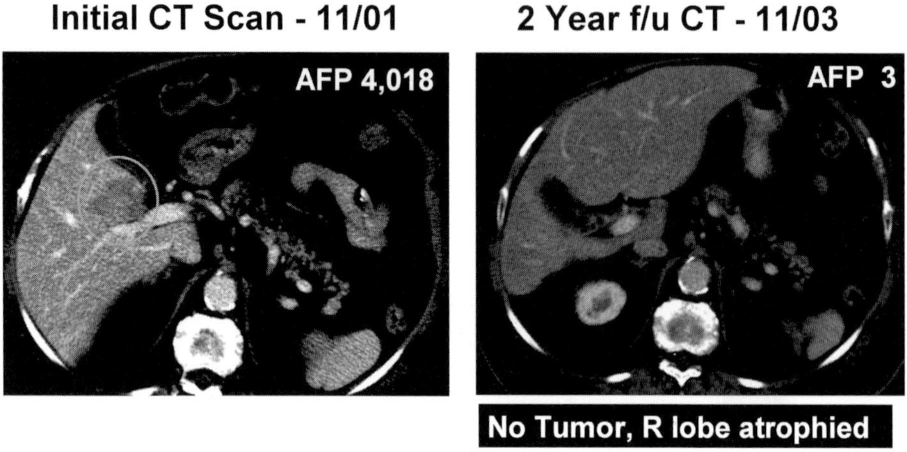

Fig. 3. CAT scan showing a complete tumor response after a single dose of Therasphere.

genesis that is a hallmark of many cancers, but particularly HCC. In our patients whose tumors respond to chemotherapy, the angiograms clearly change, and thus the tumor neovasculature is plastic. Several systemic agents currently are in clinical trials with action against neovasculature and, therefore, against the tumors that depend on the new vasculature. These agents include Thalidomide and antibodies against the growth factors that are specifically thought to be involved in angiogenesis such as vascular EGFs (VEGF). Other agents are in the process of development (Table 11).

Although HCC in general is thought to be radioresistant tumor, there is some evidence of antitumor activity with radioactively administered agents delivered into the hepatic artery, including ^{131}I-Lipiodol. These agents have only mild activity so far. A new agent that seems promising uses ^{90}Yttrium glass spheres, either imbedded in a resin or in glass beads (Therasphere). The University of Pittsburgh is currently in the middle of a phase II clinical trial using hepatic arterial Therasphere, and 85 patients have been treated so far. The main attraction of the pure β-emitting agent with a 1-cm maximum path length and 62-hour half-life is that very high doses of radiation can be given to vascular tumors with minimal hepatotoxicities so far *(118)*. In addition, only very small numbers of treatment applications are required, the tolerance is high, and the side effects are low. Thus, patients seem to have promising quality of life during such treatment. Figures 3A,B and 4A,B show CT scan and angiogram results 6 months after only

Fig. 4. (*opposite page*) Hepatic arteriogram showing a vascular response to Therashpere therapy. **(A)** Pretherapy. **(B)** Posttherapy.

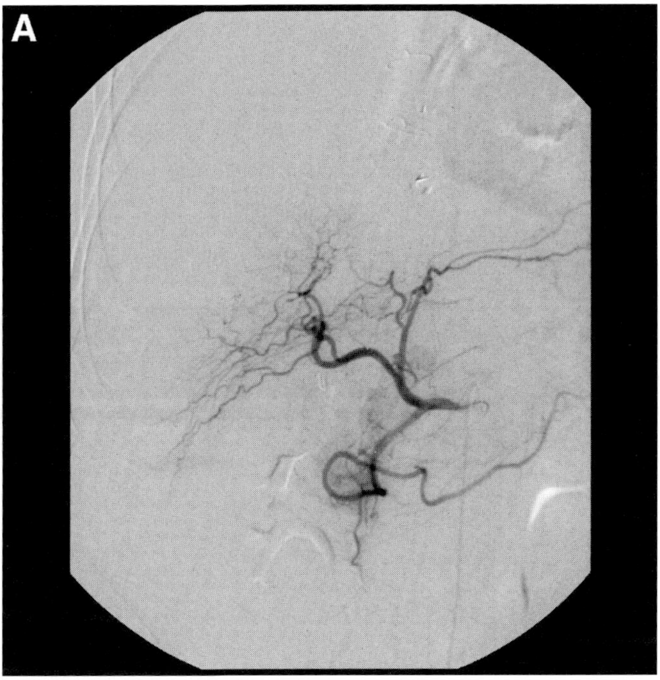
A

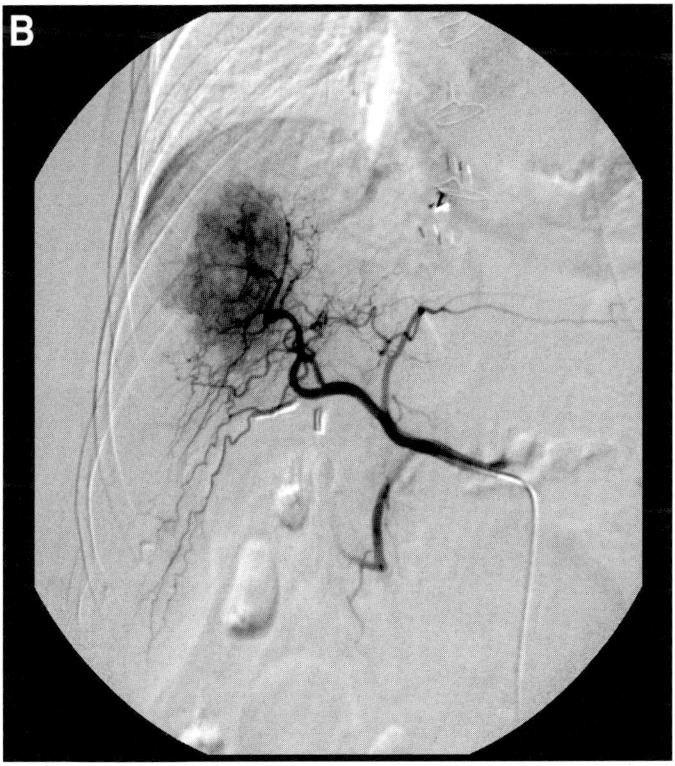
B

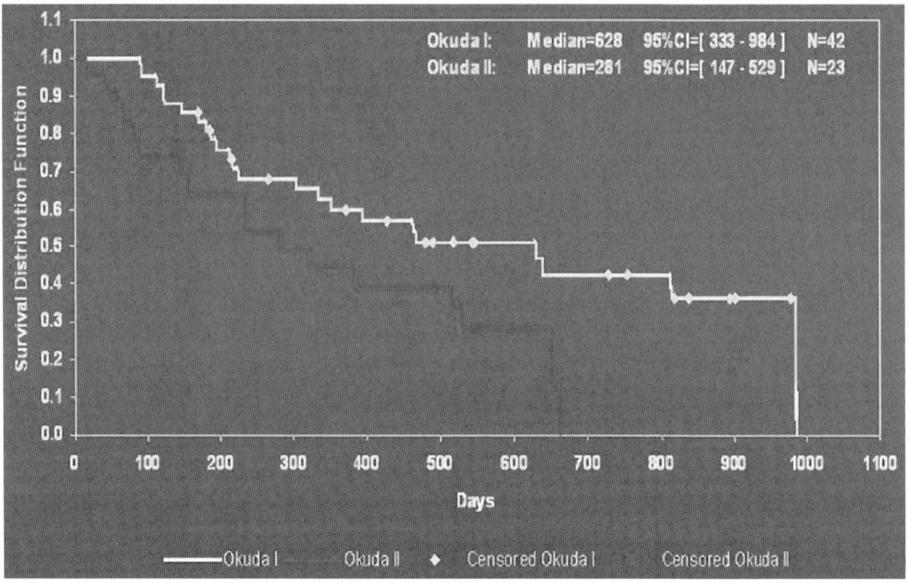

Fig. 5. Kaplan–Meier plots of survival for unresectable HCC after Therasphere therapy.

a single treatment with hepatic atery microshperes (Therashpere) and Fig. 5 shows current survival data for recent patients treated this way. A randomized comparison of Therasphere with intrahepatic chemotherapy will be needed to determine whether one treatment or the other is associated with prolonged survival and increased quality of life.

9. WHAT IS NEEDED NEXT?

9.1. Improvements in Therapy of Unresectable HCC

The greatest need is the development of newer, more active drugs that have minimal hepatotoxicity. The antiangiogenics and the cell-cycle regulatory drugs currently starting clinical testing all seem to be effective candidates.

9.2. Earlier Diagnosis

Given that survival by surgery is significantly enhanced for lower-stage HCC compared with advanced-stage HCC, screening programs resulting in earlier diagnosis with lower-stage disease would be predicted to result in enhanced survival after treatment. Any screening program is predicated on knowledge of the etiological or predisposing factors for HCC development, as well as a long interval between the action of such factors and the development of the tumor (as used in screening for carcinoma of the cervix uteri). Both of these criteria are satisfied for HCCs that develop on the basis of chronic HCV, chronic HBV, or cirrhosis from any cause, because one to two decades typically pass between infection and tumor development. Annual screening of patients by ultrasound and tumor marker (AFP and des-γ-carbotyprothrombin [DCP]) should be expected to result in the diagnosis of tumors at an earlier stage of disease in those known to have predisposing risk factors than most of the tumors currently presenting at our center.

9.3. Liver Transplantation Is Still Needed

Even if chemotherapy is completely successful in eradicating or inhibiting the growth of HCCs after diagnosis, more than 80% of the patients still have another chronic disease, namely cirrhosis. Because this probably plays a large part in the limited survival of patients with advanced-stage HCC, some form of liver replacement therapy is still needed for the treatment of HCC that is based on cirrhosis. Whether this is based on cadaveric donor liver transplantation, living-related donor liver transplantation, partial liver transplantation, hepatocyte transplantation, stem cell transplantation, or the ability to biologically reverse the fibrosis in a cirrhotic liver, these are all possibilities for the future total care of patients with HCC.

9.4. Primary Prevention of HCC

The ideal long-term advance in HCC management would be cancer prevention entirely. This is feasible, given that we know the etiological cause in such a high percentage of these patients. Two obvious strategies are immediately available and include vaccination and prevention of hepatitis or the treatment of chronic carriers of hepatitis, as well as refrigeration of stored food grains and peanuts (substrates for carcinogenic fungal growth) in the Third World. In those Third World countries where HCC is most common, most of the population is agrarian and most food staples such as rice are stored in unrefrigerated village silos. After the monsoons, the high humidity encourages the growth of carcinogenic fungi, of which *Aspergillus flavus*-producing Aflatoxins are the best studied. The provision of refrigerated granaries for stored grains is expected to go a long way to reducing the conditions under which such carcinogen-producing organisms can flourish, and thus decreasing the exposure and the risk of the population to hepatocarcinogens.

9.5. Causes of Death in Patients With HCC

Why do patients with unresectable HCC die? It may seem obvious that they die because their growing tumors physically destroy the underlying liver. But most of these patients also have cirrhosis, which is a cause of death as a result of liver failure even without presence of a tumor. Also, TACE is hepatotoxic, and several clinical trials have reported decreased survival in some patients after

TACE therapy. In a recent analysis of deaths in our patients with HCC, we gave ourselves the rule that if the CAT scan did not worsen or the AFP did not increase in the 6 months before death, then the patient probably did not die only of cancer. On that basis, 42% of our patient deaths were not attributable to cancer growth.

The field of primary prevention (HBV vaccination), early detection (surveillance screening of people at risk for cirrhosis), and the newer therapies (^{90}Yttrium, growth modulators) have brought renewed excitement to the field of HCC management, in which multiple ongoing clinical trials of newer therapies (including gene therapy) are already in progress.

REFERENCES

1. Bartlett D, Marsh W, Carr BI. Hepatocellular Carcinoma. In: *Principles and Practice of Oncology*, 7th ed. (DeVita VT, et al., eds.), Philadelphia, Lippincott Williams & Wilkins, 2004.
2. Dodd GD, Carr BI. Percutaneous biopsy of portal vein thrombus: a new staging technique for hepatocellular carcinoma. *Am J Radiology* 1993;161:229–233.
3. Duesenbery D, Dodd III GD, Carr BI. Percutaneous fine-needle aspiration of portal vein thrombi as a staging technique for hepatocellular carcinoma. *Cancer* 1995;75:2057–2062.
4. Haddow A. Cellular inhibition and origin of cancer. *Acta Unio Int Contra Cancrum* 1938;3:342–352.
5. MacNider WDB. A study of the acquired resistance of fixed tissue cells morphologically altered through process of repair. II. The resistance of liver epithelium altered morphologically as a result of an injury from uranium, followed by repair to the hepatotoxic action of chloroform. *J Pharm Exp Ther* 1936;56:373–382.
6. Solt D, Farber E. New principle for the analysis of chemical carcinogenesis. *Nature* 1976;263:701–703.
7. Carr BI, Laishes BA. Carcinogen-induced drug resistance in rat hepatocytes. *Cancer Res* 1981;41:1715–1719.
8. Liebman HA, Furie BC, Tong MJ, et al. DES-g-carboxy (abnormal) prothrombin as a serum marker of primary hepatocellular carcinoma. *N Engl J Med* 1984;310:1427–1431.
9. Carr BI, Dvorchik I. Effects of cisplatin dose-intensity on response and survival for patients with unresectable and untransplantable HCC. *Jap J Cancer Chemother* 2001;27:432–435.
10. Carr BI. Escalating cisplatin doses by intrahepatic infusion for advanced stage hepatocellular carcinoma. *Proc ASCO* 1996;15:23.
11. Katyal S, Oliver JH, Peterson MS, Chang PJ, Baron LR, Carr BI. Prognostic significance of arterial phase CT for prediction of response to transcatheter arterial chemoembolization in unresectable HCC. *Am J Roentgenol* 2000;175:1665–1672.
12. Ebied OM, Federle MP, Carr BI, et al. Evaluation of responses to chemoembolization in patients with unresectable hepatocellular carcinoma. *Cancer* 2003;97:1042–1050.
13. Chlebowski RT, Brzechwa-Adjukiewa A, Cowden A, et al. Doxorubicin (75 mg/m^2) for hepatocellular carcinoma: clinical and pharmacokinetic results. *Cancer Treat Rep* 1984;68:487–491.
14. Ihde DC, Kane RC, Cohen MH, et al. Adriamycin therapy in American patients with hepatocellular carcinoma. *Cancer Treat Rep* 1977;61:1385–1387.
15. Falkson G, MacIntyre JM, Moertel CG, et al. Primary liver cancer: an Eastern Cooperative Oncology Group trial. *Cancer* 1984:54:970–977.
16. Falkson G, MacIntyre J, Schutt A, et al. Neocarzinostatin versus m-AMSA or doxorubicin in hepatocellular carcinoma. *J Clin Oncol* 1984;2:581–584.

17. Ravry JR, Omura GA, Bartolucci AA. Phase II evaluation of doxorubicin plus bleomycin in hepatocellular carcinoma. *Eur J Cancer Clin Oncol* 1981;7:275.
18. Cavalli F, Rosencweig M, Goldhirsch A, Hansen HH. Phase II study of oral VP-16-213 in hepatocellular carcinoma. *Eur J Cancer Clin Oncol* 1981;17:1079–1082.
19. Melia WM, Johnson PG, Williams R. Induction of remission in hepatocellular carcinoma. *Cancer* 1983;51:206–210.
20. Melia WM, Westaby D, Williams R. Diamminodichloride platinum (cisplatinum) in the treatment of hepatocellular carcinoma. *Clin Oncol* 1981;7:275–280.
21. Ravry JR, Onura GA, Bartolucci AA, et al. Phase II evaluation of cisplatinum in advanced hepatocellular carcinoma and cholangiocarcinoma: a Southeastern Cancer Study Group trial. *Cancer Treat Rep* 1986;70:311,312.
22. Falkson G, Ryan LM, Johnson LA, et al. A randomized phase II study of mitoxantrone and cisplatin in patients with hepatocellular carcinoma: an ECOG study. *Cancer* 1987;60:2141–2145.
23. Sciarrino E, Simonetti R, LeMoli S, et al. Adriamycin treatment for hepatocellular carcinoma: experience with 109 patients. *Cancer* 1985;56:2751–2755.
24. Colleoni M, Buzzoni R, Bajetta E, et al. A phase II study of mitoxantrone combined with beta-interferon in unresectable hepatocellular carcinoma. *Cancer* 1993;72:3196–3201.
25. Chao Y, Chan WK, Berkhofer MJ, et al. Phase II and pharmacokinetic study of paclitaxel therapy for unresectable hepatocellular carcinoma patients. *Br J Cancer* 1998;78:34–39.
26. Patt YZ, Hassan MM, Lozano RD, et al. Phase II trial of systemic continuous fluorouracil and subcutaneous recombinant interferon alpha-IIb for treatment of hepatocellular carcinoma. *J Clin Oncol* 2003;21:421–427.
27. Patt YZ, Hassan MM, Lozano RD, et al. Durable clinical response of refractory hepatocellular carcinoma to orally administered thalidomide. *Am J Clin Oncol* 2000;23:319–321.
28. Carr BI, Selby R, Madariaga J, et al. A controlled, prospective randomized trial comparing intra-arterial cisplatin and doxorubicin with or without Lipiodol for hepatocellular carcinoma. *Hepatology* 1992;16:60.
29. Okada S, Okusaka T, Ueno H, et al. Phase II trial of cisplatin, mitroxantrone and continuous infusion 5-fluorouracil for hepatocellular carcinoma. *Proc ASCO* 1999;18:248A.
30. Martin RCG, Jarnagin WR. Randomized clinical trials in hepatocellular carcinoma and biliary cancer in prospective randomized trials in oncology. *Surg Oncol Clin N Am* 2002;11:193–205.
31. Llovet JM, Bruix J. Systemic review of randomized trials for unresectable hepatocellular carcinoma. *Hepatology* 2003;37:429–442.
32. Koda M, Murawaki Y, Mitsuda A, et al. Combination therapy with TACE and PEI compared with PEI alone for patients with small HCC. *Cancer* 2001;92:1516–1524.
33. Simonetti RG, Liberati A, Angiolini C, et al. Treatment of hepatocellular carcinoma: a systematic review of randomized control trials. *Ann Oncol* 1997;8:117–136.
34. Mathurin PE, Rixe O, Carbonell N, et al. Review article: overview of medical treatments in unresectable hepatocellular carcinoma. *Allement Pharmacol Ther* 1998;12:111–126.
35. Leung TWT, Johnson PJ. Systemic therapy for hepatocellular carcinoma. *Semin Oncol* 2001;28:514–520.
36. Sasaki Y, Imacka S, Kasugai H, et al. A new approach to chemoembolization therapy for hepatoma using iethiodized oil, cisplatin, gelatin sponge. *Cancer* 1987;60:1194–1203.
37. Kasugai H, Kojima J, Tatsuta M, et al. Treatment of hepatocellular carcinoma by transcatheter arterial embolization combined with intra-arterial infusion of a mixture of cisplatin and ethiodized oil. *Gastroenterology* 1989;97:965–971.
38. Ohnishi K, Tsuchiya S, Nakayma T, et al. Arterial chemoembolization of hepatocellular carcinoma with mitomycin C microcapsules. *Radiology* 1984;152:51–55.

39. Lin D, Liaw Y, Lee T, et al. Hepatic arterial embolization in patients with unresectable hepatocellular carcinoma: a randomized controlled trial. *Gastroenterology* 1988;94:453–456.
40. Fujimoto S, Miyazaki M, Endoh F, et al. Biodegradable mitomycin C microspheres given intra-arterially for inoperable hepatic cancer. *Cancer* 1985;56:2404–2410.
41. Audisio RA, Doci R, Mazzafero V, et al. Hepatic arterial embolization in patients with unresectable hepatocellular carcinoma: a randomized controlled trial. *Gastroenterology* 1988;94:453.
42. Kobayashi J, Hidaka H, Kajiya Y, et al. Treatment of hepatocellular carcinoma by transarterial injection of anticancer agents in iodized oil suspension or of radioactive iodized oil solution. *Acta Radiol Diagn* 1986;27:139–147.
43. Kanematsu T, Furuta T, Takenaka K, et al. A 5-year experience of lipiodolization: selective regional chemotherapy for 200 patients with hepatocellular carcinoma. *Hepatology* 1989;10:98–102.
44. Shibata J, Fujiyama S, Sata T, et al. Hepatic arterial injection chemotherapy with cisplatin suspended in an oily lymphographic agent for hepatocellular carcinoma. *Cancer* 1989;64:1586–1594.
45. Konno T, Maeda H, Iwai K, et al. Hepatic arterial injection chemotherapy with cisplatin suspended in an oily lymphographic agent for hepatocellular carcinoma. *Cancer* 1989;64:1586.
46. Pelletier G, Roche A, Ink O. A randomized trial of hepatic arterial chemoembolization in patients with unresectable hepatocellular carcinoma. *J Hepatology* 1990;11:181–184.
47. Carr BI, Starzl TE, Iwatsuki S, et al. Aggressive treatment for advanced hepatocellular carcinoma (HCC): high response rates and prolonged survival. *Hepatology* 1991;14:243.
48. Venook AP, Stagg RJ, Lewis BJ, et al. Chemoembolization for hepatocellular carcinoma. *J Clin Oncol* 1990;8:1108–1114.
49. Ohnishi K, Sugita S, Nomura F, et al. Arterial chemoembolization with mitomycin C microcapsules followed by transcatheter hepatic artery embolization for hepatocellular carcinoma. *Am J Gastroenterol* 1987;82:876–879.
50. Nakao A, Virji MA, Iwaki Y, Carr BI, Iwatsuki S, Starzl TE. Abnormal prothrombin (Des-gamma-carboxy-prothrombin) in hepatocellular carcinoma. *Hepatogastroenterology* 1991;38:450–453.
51. Beppu T, Ohara C, Yamaguchi Y. A new approach to chemoembolization for unresectable hepatocellular carcinoma using aclarubicin microspheres in combination with cisplatin suspended in iodized oil. *Cancer* 1991;68:2555–2560.
52. Trinchet J-C, Rashed A, Beaugrand M, et al. A comparison of Lipiodol chemoembolization and conservative treatment for unresectable hepatocellular carcinoma. *N Engl J Med* 1995;332:1256–1261.
53. Llovet JM, Bru C, Bruix J. Prognosis of hepatocellular carcinoma: the BCLC staging classification. *Semin Liver Dis* 1999;19:329–338.
54. Stuart K, Stokes K, Jenkins R, Trey C, Clouse M. Treatment of hepatocellular carcinoma using doxorubicin/ethiodized oil/gelatin powder chemoembolization. *Cancer* 1993;72: 3202–3209.
55. Bruix J, Castells A, Montanya X, et al. Phase II study of transarterial embolization in European patients with hepatocellular carcinoma: a need for controlled trials. *Hepatology* 1994;20:643–650.
56. Carr BI, Zajko A, Bron K, et al. Phase II study of degradable starch microspheres given into the hepatic artery in conjunction with doxorubicin and cisplatin in the treatment of advanced-stage hepatocellular carcinoma. *Semin Oncol* 1997;24:97–99.
57. Carr BI, Zajko A, Bron K, et al. Prospective randomized study of intrahepatic artery chemotherapy with cisplatin and doxorubin, with or without Lipiodol in the treatment of advanced-stage hepatocellular carcinoma. *Proc Am Soc Clin Oncol* 1993;12:668.

58. Carr BI. Hepatic artery chemoembolization for advanced-stage HCC: experience of 650 patients. *Hepatogastroastroenterology* 2002;49:79–86.
59. Ngan H, Lai CL, Fan ST, Lai EC, Yuen WK, Tso WK. Treatment of inoperable hepatocellular carcinoma by transcatheter arterial chemoembolization using an emulsion of cisplatin in iodized oil and Gelfoam. *Clin Radiol* 1993;47:315–320.
60. Kawai S, Tani M, Okamura J, et al. Prospective and randomized clinical trial for the treatment of hepatocellular carcinoma: a comparison between L-TAE with farmorubicin and L-TAE with Adriamycin: preliminary results (second cooperative study). *Cancer Chemo Pharm* 1994;33:S97–S102.
61. Yamamoto M, Iizuka H, Fujii H, Matsuda M, Miura K. Hepatic arterial infusion of interleukin-2 in advanced hepatocellular carcinoma. *Acta Oncol* 1993;32:43–51.
62. Yoshimi F, Nagao T, Inoue S, et al. Comparison of hepatectomy and transcatheter arterial chemoembolization for the treatment of hepatocellular carcinoma: necessity for prospective randomized trial. *Hepatology* 1992;16:702–706.
63. Vauthey JN, Lauwers GY, Esnaola NF, et al. Simplified staging for hepatocellular carcinoma. *J Clin Oncol* 2002;20:1527–1536.
64. Rougier P, Roche A, Pelletier G, Ducreux M, Pignon JP, Etienne JP. Efficacy of chemoembolization for hepatocellular carcinomas: experience from the Gustave Roussy Institute and the Bicetre Hospital. *J Surg Oncol* 1993;3:94–96.
65. Onohara S, Kobayashi J, Itho Y, et al. Intra-arterial cisplatinum infusion with sodium thiosulfate protection and angiotensin II induced hypertension for treatment of hepatocellular carcinoma. *Acta Radiol* 1988;29:197–202.
66. Kajanti M, Rissanen P, Virkkunen P, et al. Regional intra-arterial infusion of cisplatin in primary hepatocellular carcinoma. *Cancer* 1986;58:2386–2388.
67. Ando K, Hirai K, Kubo Y. Intra-arterial administration of epirubicin in the treatment of nonresectable hepatocellular carcinoma. *Cancer Chemother Pharmacol* 1987;19:183–188.
68. Carr BI. Escalating cisplatin doses by hepatic artery infusion (HAI) for advanced-stage hepatocellular carcinoma (HCC). Carr BI. Sixth International Congress on anti-cancer treatment 1996;367.
69. Kwai S, Okamura J, Ogawa M, et al. Prospective and randomized clinical trial for the treatment of hepatocellular carcinoma: a comparison of Lipiodol-transcatheter arterial embolization with and without Adriamycin. *Cancer Chemother Pharmacol* 1992;31:S1–S6.
70. Kwai S, Tani M, Okamura J, et al. Prospective and randomized trial of Lipiodol-transcatheter arterial chemoembolization for treatment of hepatocellular carcinoma: a comparison of epirubicin and doxorubicin. *Semin Oncol* 1997;24:S6-38–S6-45.
71. Watanabe S, Nishioka M, Ohta Y, et al. Prospective and randomized controlled study of chemoembolization therapy in patients with advanced hepatocellular carcinoma. *Cancer Chemother Pharmacol* 1994;33:S93–S96.
72. Chang JM, Tzeng WS, Pan HB, et al. Transcatheter arterial embolization with or without cisplatin treatment of hepatocellular carcinoma: a randomized controlled study. *Cancer* 1994;74:2449–2453.
73. Hatanaka Y, Yamashita Y, Takahashi M, et al. Unresectable hepatocellular carcinoma: an analysis of prognostic factors in transcatheter management. *Radiology* 1995;195:747–752.
74. Uchino J, Une Y, Sato Y, et al. Chemo-hormonal therapy of unresectable hepatocellular carcinoma. *Am J Oncol* 1993:16:206–209.
75. Madden MV, Krige JE, Bailey S, et al. Randomized trial of targeted chemotherapy with Lipiodol and 5-epidoxorubicin compared with symptomatic treatment for hepatocellular carcinoma. *Gut* 1993;35:1598–1600.
76. Chang YH, Song IH, Song BC, et al. Combined therapy consisting of intra-arterial cisplatin infusion and systemic interferon-alpha for hepatocellular carcinoma patients with major portal vein thrombosis or distant metastases. *Cancer* 2000;88:1986–1991.

77. Lin DY, Liaw YF, Lee TY. Hepatic arterial embolization in patients with unresectable hepatocellular carcinoma: a randomized controlled trial. *Gastroenterology* 1988;94: 453–456.
78. Yoshikawa M, Saisho H, Ebara M, et al. A randomized trial of intrahepatic arterial infusion of 4-epidoxorubicin with Lipiodol versus 4-epidoxorubicin alone in the treatment of hepatocellular carcinoma. *Cancer Chemother Pharmacol* 1994;33:S149–S152.
79. Kajanti M, Pyrhonen S, Mantila M, Rissanen P. Intra-arterial and intravenous use of 4-epidoxorubicin combined with 5-fluorouracil in primary hepatocellular carcinoma: a randomized comparison. *Am J Clin Oncol* 1992;15:37–40.
80. Tzoracoleftherakis EE, Spiliotis JD, Kyriakopoulou T, et al. Intra-arterial versus systemic chemotherapy for non-operable hepatocellular carcinoma. *Hepatogastroenterology* 1999;46:1122–1125.
81. Bhattacharya S, Novell JR, Dusheiko GM. Epirubicin-lipiodol chemotherapy versus 131iodine-lipiodol radiotherapy in the treatment of unresectable hepatocellular carcinoma. *Cancer* 1995;76:2202–2210.
82. Pelletier G, Roche A, Ink O, et. al. A randomized trial of hepatic artery chemo-embolization in patients with unresectable hepatocellular carcinoma. *J Hepatol* 1990;11:181–184.
83. Trinchet J-C, Rashed A, Beaugrand M, et al. A comparison of Lipiodol chemoembolization and conservative treatment for unresectable hepatocellular carcinoma. *N Engl J Med* 1995;332:1256–1261.
84. Bruix J, Llovet JM, Castells A, et al. Transarterial embolization versus symptomatic treatment in patients with advanced hepatocellular carcinoma: results of randomized control trials. *Hepatology* 1998;27:1578–1580.
85. Pelletier G, Ducreux M, Gay F, et al. Treatment of unresectable hepatocellular carcinoma with Lipiodol chemoembolization: a multicenter randomized trial. *J Hepatol* 1998;29: 129–134.
86. Lo C-M, Ngan H, Tso W-K, et al. Randomized controlled trial of transarterial Lipiodol chemoembolization for unresectable hepatocellular carcinoma. *Hepatology* 2002;35:1164–1171.
87. Llovet JM, Real MI, Montana X, et al. Arterial embolization or chemoembolization versus symptomatic treatment in patients with unresectable hepatocellular carcinoma: a randomized controlled trial. *Lancet* 2002;359:1734–1739.
88. Camma C, Schepis F, Orlando A, et al. Transarterial chemoembolization for hepatocellular carcinoma: meta-analysis of randomized controlled trials. *Radiology* 2002;224:47–54.
89. Martin RCG, Jarnagin WR. Randomized clinical trials in hepatocellular carcinoma and biliary cancer in prospective randomized trials in oncology. *Surg Oncol Clin N Am* 2002;11:193–205.
90. Llovet JM, Bruix J. Systemic review of randomized trials for unresectable hepatocellular carcinoma. *Hepatology* 2003;37:429–442.
91. Farinati F, Demaria N, Fornasiero A, et al. Prospective controlled trial with antiestrogen drug tamoxifen in patients with unresectable hepatocellular carcinoma. *Dig Dis Sci* 1992;37: 659–662.
92. Martinez Cerezo FJ, Tomas A, Donoso L, et al. Controlled trial of tamoxifen in patients with advanced hepatocellular carcinoma. *J Hepatol* 1994;20:702–706.
93. Liu CL, Fan ST, Ng IO, et al. Treatment of advanced hepatocellular carcinoma with tamoxifen and the correlation with expression of hormone receptors. A prospective randomized study. *Am J Gastroenterol* 2000;95:218–222.
94. CLIP Group. Tamoxifen in treatment of hepatocellular carcinoma: a randomized control trial. *Lancet* 1998;352:17–20.
95. Carr BI, Wang Z, Kar S. K vitamins, PTP antagonism and cell growth arrest. *J Cell Physiol* 2002;193:263–274.

96. Grimaldi C, Bleiberg H, Gay F, et al. Evaluation of anti-androgen therapy in unresectable hepatocellular carcinoma: results of an EORTC multi-center double-blind trial. *J Clin Oncol* 1998;16:411–417.
97. Lai CL, Wu PC, Lok AS, et al. Recombinant alpha II interferon is superior to doxorubicin for inoperable hepatocellular carcinoma: a prospective randomized trial. *Br J Cancer* 1989;60:928–933.
98. Llovet JM, Sala M, Castells L, et al. Randomized controlled trial of interferon treatment for advanced hepatocellular carcinoma. *Hepatology* 2000;31:54–58.
99. Lai CL, Lau JW, Wu PC, et al. Recombinant interferon alpha in inoperable hepatocellular carcinoma: a randomized controlled trial. *Hepatology* 1993;17:389–394.
100. Falkson G, Lipsitz S, Borden E, et al. Hepatocellular carcinoma. ECOG randomized phase II study of beta interferon and menogaril. *Am J Clin Oncol* 1995;18:287–292.
101. Rabe C, Pilz T, Allgaier HP, et al. Clinical outcome of a cohort of 63 patients with hepatocellular carcinoma treated with octreotide. *Z Gastroenterol* 2002;40:395–400.
102. Dimitroulopoulos D, Xinopoulos D, Tsamakidis K, et al. The role of Sandostatin in treating patients with advanced hepatocellular carcinoma. *Hepatogastroenterology* 2002;49: 1245–1250.
103. Villa E, Ferretti I, Grottola A, et al. Hormonal therapy with megestrol in inoperable hepatocellular carcinoma characterized by variant estrogen receptors. *Br J Cancer* 2001; 84:881–885.
104. Chao Y, Chan WK, Wang SS, et al. Phase II study of megestrol acetated treatment of hepatocellular carcinoma. *J Gastroenterol Hepatol* 1997;12:277–281.
105. Carr BI. A phase I/phase II study of high-dose vitamin K in patients with advanced, inoperable hepatocellular carcinoma. Proc AASLD. *Hepatology* 1994;20:727.
106. Zamibone A, Biasi L, Graffeo M, et al. Phase II study of high-dose vitamin K1 in hepatocellular carcinoma. *Proc ASCO* 1998;17:307A.
107. Carr BI, Wang Z, Kar S. K vitamins, PTP antagonism and cell growth arrest. *J Cell Physiol* 2002;193:263–274.
108. Carr BI. Complete suppression of DCP/PIVKA 2 levels by vitamin K_1 administration to patients with hepatocellular carcinoma (HCC). *Hepatology* 1993;18:500.
109. Patt YZ, Hassan MM, Lozano RD, et al. Durable clinical response of refractory hepatocellular carcinoma to orally administered thalidomide. *Am J Clin Oncol* 2000;23:319–321.
110. Yamamoto M, Iizuka H, Fujii H, Matsuda M, Miura K. Hepatic arterial infusion of interleukin-2 in advanced hepatocellular carcinoma. *Acta Oncol* 1993;32:43–51.
111. Lau WY, Leung TWT, Ho SKW, et al. Adjuvant intra-arterial iodine-131-labeled Lipiodol for resectable HCC: a prospective randomized trial. *Lancet* 1999;353:797–801.
112. Brans B, Laere KV, Gemmel F, et al. Combining iodine-131 lipiodol therapy with low-dose cisplatin as a radiosensitizer. Preliminary results in hepatocellular carcinoma. *Eur J Nucl Med* 2002;29:928–932.
113. Leung WT, Lau WY, Ho S, et al. Selective internal radiation therapy with intra-arterial iodine-131-lipiodol in inoperable hepatocellular carcinoma. *J Nucl Med* 1994;35: 1313–1318.
114. Order S, Pajak T, Leibel S, et al. A randomized prospective trial comparing full-dose chemotherapy to 131-I-antiferritin: an RTOG study. *Int J Radiat Oncol Biol* 1991;20:953–960.
115. Carr BI, Amesur N, Zajko A, et al. Safety and efficacy of hepatic artery ^{90}Y microspheres in unresectable hepatocellular carcinoma (HCC). *Proc ASCO* 2003;22:1046.
116. Lau W, Ho S, Leung T, et al. Selective internal radiation therapy for non-resectable HCC with intra-arterial infusion of 90-Yttrium microspheres. *J Radiat Oncol Biol* 1998;40:583–592.
117. Dancey J, Sheppard F, Paul K, et al. Treatment of non-resectable HCC with intrahepatic 90-Y microspheres. *J Nucl Med* 2000;41:1673–1681.

118. Carr BI. Hepatic arterial 90-Yttrium glass microspheres (Therasphere) for unresectable hepatocellular carcinoma: interim safety and survival data on 65 patients. *Liver Transplantation* 2004;10:S107–S110.
119. Salem R, Thurston KG, Carr BI, Goin JE, Geschwind JFH. Yttrium-90 microspheres: radiation therapy for unresectable liver cancer. *J Vasc Intervent Radiol* 2002;13:S223–S229.
120. Leung TWT, Tang AMY, Zee B, et al. Factors predicting response and survival in 149 patients with unresectable hepatocellular carcinoma treated by combination cisplatin, interferon-alpha, doxorubicin and 5-fluorouracil chemotherapy. *Cancer* 2002;94:421–427.
121. Leung TW, Patt YZ, Lau WY, et al. Complete pathological remission is possible with systemic combination chemotherapy for inoperable hepatocellular carcinoma. *Clin Cancer Res* 1995;5:1676–1681.
122. Patt YZ, Hoque A, Roh M, et al. Durable clinical and pathologic response of hepatocellular carcinoma to systemic and hepatic arterial administration of platinol, recombinant interferon alpha 2B, doxorubicin, and 5-fluorouracil: a communication. *Am J Clin Oncol* 1999;22: 209–213.

13 Radiation Therapy for Hepatocellular Carcinoma

Andrew S. Kennedy, MD

CONTENTS

1. INTRODUCTION

There are many factors that over time have contributed to the limited use of ionizing radiation in treating hepatocellular carcinoma (HCC). This is primarily because delivery of tumoricidal doses of radiation to a tumor will exceed tolerance of the normal surrounding liver. X-rays produce nondiscriminatory cell killing in the already diseased liver of patients with HCC. In the past, radiation beams could be delivered only in the simplest of geometric arrangements, which could not avoid enough normal liver tissue from X-rays to deliver doses of radiation to control solid tumors. Only in the past 15 years have technological advancements in radiation oncology and diagnostic radiology allowed for innovative approaches in both external beam therapy and brachytherapy for treatment of liver malignancies. Concurrent with hardware upgrades, such as megavoltage linear accelerators, have been powerful software programs that enable conversion of computed tomography (CT) or magnetic resonance imaging (MRI) data sets into three-dimensional (3D) virtual patients. With accurate 3D models of the patient to work from and estimates in real time of radiation dose deposition within the patient, radiation oncologists can attempt to deliver the higher doses of radiation that have a chance to control tumors while sparing the nonmalignant

From: *Current Clinical Oncology: Hepatocellular Cancer: Diagnosis and Treatment*
Edited by: B. I. Carr © Humana Press Inc., Totowa, NJ

hepatocytes. Most solid malignancies are successfully treated with combination therapy, and for years, it has been the desire to apply these approaches to HCC. The technology described is now widely available in all cancer centers and explains, in part, why the interest, within multidisciplinary hepatic oncology groups and ongoing clinical trials, in treating HCC is increasing. Radiobiological protectants are now in clinical trials, which may allow in the future for selective sparing of the normal liver cells found within the radiation beam. This chapter summarizes the main techniques historically and currently available in delivering ionizing radiation to HCC and describes interesting new approaches. Clinical experience over the past century suggests radiation dose parameters, above which serious and possibly fatal liver dysfunction occurs. Moreover, this occurs when the entire liver (i.e., all functional units of the organ) receives external beam radiation in excess of 30 Gy. State-of-the art radiotherapy techniques can treat small portions of the liver to cumulative doses of 90 Gy or more, as will be discussed later, but the number of patients suitable for this approach is few. Placing radiation directly in the tumor (brachytherapy) holds the promise of success because it can deliver very large doses of radiation selectively to the tumor (80–300 Gy) but spares surrounding normal liver parenchyma, which is reviewed in the microsphere section.

2. PHYSICS OF RADIATION THERAPY

2.1. External Beam Radiation Therapy

Radiation that is of sufficient energy to cause ionization of cellular contents is used therapeutically and is either an electromagnetic or particulate energy form. Electromagnetic energy, or photons, can be produced naturally by decay of radioactive isotopes (γ-rays) or by an electrical device accelerating electrons, which abruptly stop in a target, releasing energy (X-rays). Particulate energy most commonly is electrons (charge: –1; mass: 0.511 MeV), but others in limited use for cancer therapy include protons (charge: +1; mass: 2000 × electrons), α-particles (helium ions), and neutrons (same mass as proton, no charge).

External beam radiotherapy is the most commonly used method for nearly all cancers, using X-rays. Photons, which are discrete packets of electromagnetic energy, cause cell damage or cell death via apoptosis, via collision with a cell, transferring some energy to the cell. This interaction exchanges some energy to the cell, and the photon is deflected itself with a reduction in its energy. The energy absorbed by the possibly creates damage to the DNA, leading to cell death. Photons are linear in direction, and their course cannot be altered in the liver except by collision with tissue; therein lies the key disadvantage in treating hepatic tumors, because the normal tissues above and below a tumor are in the path of the photon beam and receive similar radiation dose. The rate of energy loss as a function of depth in tissue is well-known for every level of photon energy, with higher energy beams penetrating deeper into the body while giving up less energy in the first few centimeters of soft tissue.

In the 1960s through early 1980s, external beam radiation was, in fact, the delivery of photons from radioactive decay of ^{60}Cobalt. Although it yielded photon energies with sufficient penetrating power for most tumors, it could not be used for deep abdominal or pelvic tumors without delivering a much higher dose more superficially in normal tissues. In addition, the physical radiation beam itself had a relatively wide beam edge or penumbra, which made precise targeting impossible even at shallow depths of tissue.

Over the past 20 years, linear accelerators have replaced ^{60}Cobalt machines virtually everywhere and generate photons by accelerating electrons near to the speed of light before they strike a target, converting kinetic energy and mass into electromagnetic energy-photons. They generate photons of much higher energy than ^{60}Cobalt and thus are able to reach any deep tumor in the body of most patients, without excessive hot spots or doses higher than that of the tumor along the photon path in the body. In absolute numbers, ^{60}Cobalt can deliver γ-rays (photons) of two energies, 1.17 MeV (million electron volts) and 1.33 MeV; although some accelerators are capable of maximum photon energies of between 4 and 25 MeV, most centers use 6–18 MeV, which can easily safely reach the deepest parts of the liver in nearly any patient. Linear accelerators also can produce electron beams, which differ from photon beams in that electrons are particles with mass and charge, and thus have a finite range of tissue penetrance, allowing for treatment of more superficial tumors, while significantly sparing deeper normal tissues. Electron beam therapy may be appropriate in treating a mass in the liver, which is only 1–2 cm deep to the surface. The dose 4 cm below the tumor could be nearly 0 if the appropriate energy was chosen, compared with a dose of 80% of the tumor dose at that depth if photons were used. Protons can be used similarly to electrons, but with a much deeper penetration if required (*see* Section 5.).

2.2. Radiation Dose

The dose of ionizing radiation absorbed by the liver, solid tumor, or other tissues is a cornerstone of clinical trial design. Older reports used the term *roentgen* (*R*), which described ionization in air, that is, exposure, of γ-rays. Newer nomenclature uses the SI unit for absorbed dose in tissue (1 J/kg = 1 gray [Gy] = 100 rads = 100 cGy [centigray]), as the basic unit of measurement. Conversion of older literature values listed as *R* is approx *R* = 0.01 Gy for γ. Less well-known is how to convert β-radiation doses (which are low-dose, constant release radiotherapy) into equivalent external beam doses because of the differences in biologic response resulting from dose rate, fractionation, and activity *(1)*. Thus, brachytherapy doses are recorded as Gy, but these doses are not likely to be equivalent to the same dose Gy given as daily-fractionated external beam doses of X-rays. This is an area of active investigation.

2.3. 3D Conformal Radiation Treatment (3DCRT)

Advances in software allow radiation oncologists to recreate volumetric models of patients using the latest and most detailed diagnostic images from CT or MRI. Typically, CT data sets are used, and many cancer centers have dedicated spiral CT scanners in the radiation oncology department, hardwired to the treatment planning computer system. Before the mid-1990s, two-dimensional treatment planning had been the only method of planning how to arrange radiation beams targeting the tumor. This approach was limited to simple beam arrangements such as opposed beams, or those at 90° from each other (coplanar), and were designed from the standpoint of treating extra normal tissue so as to minimize the frequency of geometric miss of the target by the beam. With precise targeting and tumor delineation as seen on CT volume sets, complex and innovative beam arrangements can be used with significant reduction in the need to include extra normal tissue as a margin. These noncoplanar beams can be at virtually any angle, although the linear accelerator and patient position will make some angles unusable. This approach also benefits from powerful new radiation dose calculations, which speed up the process of comparing alternate treatment plans by displaying nearly real-time dose maps. Enhancements also include the ability to calculate more accurately dose from beams that pass through less-dense tissues (inhomogeneity corrections), such as lung, in targeting the right lobe of liver *(2)*.

2.4. Brachytherapy

It was not long after Wilhelm Conrad Roentgen discovered X-rays in 1895 that the *Lancet* reported its use in January 1896 for medical use *(3)*. Shortly after the turn of the century, it was suggested by Alexander Graham Bell that radioactive isotopes be applied directly to tissues, and thus brachytherapy was born, the term originating from the Greek *brachy,* meaning "short range." The French coined the term *endocurietherapy*, from the Greek *endo*, meaning "within." Radioactive isotopes such as iridium (^{192}Ir), cesium (^{137}Cs), and iodine (^{125}I and ^{131}I) have been used extensively since the early 1900s as primary therapy and in addition to external beam radiation as a boost to the tumor. Brachytherapy attempts to spare normal regional tissues by delivering a high dose locally in the tumor, and although γ-radiation photons are used mostly, there is relatively low dose at a distance from the tumor of several centimeters. The dose rate of radiation delivery via a brachytherapy isotope (50 cGy/hour) is much lower than photons delivered by an accelerator (100 Gy/minute). Radioactive decay from an isotope that produces electrons (charge: –1) is termed β*-decay*. These particles are used in such products as radiolabeled antibodies used in hematological malignancies or in higher energies, for bone metastases and thyroid malignancies. Currently, there is significant clinical use of pure β-emitting isotopes (no γ-photons emitted) yttrium and strontium (^{90}Y and ^{90}Sr) in brachytherapy in liver lesions (*see* Subheading 5.2.2.) and in coronary artery brachytherapy. An advantage and potential disadvantage of β-sources is that most of the effective radiation is delivered within 2–4 mm of the source, with virtually no radiation dose effect <1 cm away. Because there are no γ-rays, nuclear medicine detectors cannot readily image pure β-sources, making localization of implanted sources problematic. Brachytherapy sources can be implanted via blood infusion or needle applicator, can be applied directly and sutured into place as a permanent implant, or can be placed temporarily (minutes to hours) within a catheter that is removed from the body.

3. RADIOBIOLOGY

An understanding of radiation effects in living tissues began at the turn of the century with observations of skin reaction, primarily erythema and breakdown *(3)*. Since then, clinical experience has produced observations regarding normal and malignant tissue response and repair to ionizing radiation. The target of efficient cell killing is the DNA, with most cell death by irradiation resulting from unrepaired or misrepaired genomic injury and loss of reproductive ability. It has been estimated that in the presence of sufficient oxygen tension (>10 mmHg) *(3,4)*, any form of radiation (X-rays, γ-rays, charged or uncharged particles) will be absorbed and potentially interact directly or indirectly with the DNA. Approximately 75% of the damage to the DNA is indirect, with a photon striking a water molecule (water composes 80% of the cell) within 4 nm of the DNA strand. Kinetic energy from the incident photon is transferred to an orbital electron of the water molecule, ejecting it;the electron is then renamed a secondary electron. It can interact with a water molecule forming a free radical, which is highly reactive and breaks bonds in one of the DNA strands nearby. There also can be interaction of the secondary electron directly on the DNA strand, causing damage referred to as direct action *(3)*.

3.1. Modifiers of Radiation Response

The presence of oxygen is the single most important biologic modifier at the cellular and molecular levels *(1,5)*. Oxygen "fixes," or makes permanent, DNA damage caused by free radicals, but in low oxygen tensions, this damage can be repaired more readily. The term *oxygen enhancement ratio* (OER) is used to describe the ratio of radiation doses without and with oxygen to produce the same biological effect. For X-rays, it is estimated to be between two and three, that is, a given X-ray will be two to three times as damaging in the presence of oxygen in that tissue than if hypoxia exists *(3)*. This has significant implications clinically, because many patients with HCC are considered for embolization procedures, which can produce a relative hypoxic environment within the tumor, making them less susceptible to radiation therapy. Other factors can affect tumor sensitivity to radiation, including repair of radiation damage, reassortment of cells into more or less sensitive portions of the cell cycle (*S*-phase most radioresistant, G2–M most sensitive), and repopulation during a course of radiation, which is seen in rapidly dividing tumor populations. Repopulation also can become an issue after surgical resection, chemoembolization, cryotherapy, or radiofrequency ablation, where hepatic hypertrophy in the regional normal cells is stimulated. These normal clonogens are more susceptible to radiotherapy damage in this phase, limiting the use of radiation, which may allow for residual malignant cells to repopulate *(6)*. Repair of radiation damage, or sublethal damage repair, is enhanced in low-oxygen environments and with fractionation of radiation doses. The break between fractions in external beam radiotherapy provides an opportunity to repair DNA strand breaks in normal and malignant cells. Brachytherapy differs in this regard with continuous radiation, without a discrete fraction of radiation, but it delivers continuous lower dose rates of radiation.

4. RADIATION EFFECTS IN THE LIVER

Acute and late effects of ionizing radiation to the liver have been described in the literature since the early 1960s *(7,8)*. During radiotherapy, acute or transient effects often are reported as elevation of liver enzymes, and depending on the treated volume, hematologic effects such as neutropenia and coagulopathy can occur. However, permanent effects can be produced, occurring weeks or months after radiation (late effects), such as fibrosis, persistent enzyme elevation, ascites, jaundice, and, rarely, radiation-induced liver disease (RILD) and fatal veno-occlusive disease (VOD) *(6,9–11)*. RILD is often what is called *radiation hepatitis* and classically was described as occurring within 3 months of initiation of radiation, with rapid weight gain, increase in abdominal girth, liver enlargement, and, occasionally, ascites or jaundice, with elevation in serum alkaline phosphatase. The clinical picture resembled Budd–Chiari syndrome, but most patients survived, although some died of this condition without proven tumor progression. It was described that the whole liver could not be treated with radiation more than 30–35 Gy in conventional fractionation (1.8–2 Gy/day, 5 days per week) or else RILD or VOD was likely to occur. Interestingly, VOD also can occur without radiotherapy in patients receiving high-dose chemotherapy in hematological malignancies, alkaloids, toxic exposure to urethane, arsphenamine, and long-term oral contraceptives *(12)*, as well as patients receiving radiation combined with chemotherapy or radiation alone. The clinical presentation can differ between RILD and chemotherapy plus radiation liver disease, but the common pathological lesion associated with RILD is VOD. The pathological changes in VOD can affect a fraction of a lobe or the entire liver. It is best observed on low-power microscopy, which demonstrates severe congestion of the sinusoids in the central portion of the lobules with atrophy of the inner portion of the liver plates (zone 3) *(6,12)*. Foci of yellow necrosis may appear in the center of affected areas. If the affected area is large, it can produce shrinkage and a wrinkled, granular capsule. The sublobular veins show significant obstruction by fine collagen fibers, which do not form in larger vein (vena cava); this is a distinction between RILD and Budd–Chiari syndrome *(6,12)*. Most livers heal and display chronic changes after 6 months with little congestion but distorted lobular architecture with variable distances between central veins and portal areas. These chronic liver changes are typically asymptomatic but are reproducibly seen on liver biopsies as late as 6 years after presentation. Further investigation of the pathogenesis of VOD is difficult because most animals do not have VOD in response to radiation *(12)*.

5. CLINICAL STUDIES

5.1. External Beam Radiation Therapy

Because of the tolerance issues of normal liver to radiation as discussed earlier, there has been little activity regarding radiation alone for HCC. However, with improvements in targeting with 3DCRT there is renewed interest in combining radiation with chemotherapy and other methods. Most radiation oncologists use external beam radiation in the liver for palliation of symptoms, such as pain secondary to capsular stretching from tumor expansion or intratumor hemorrhage. Definitive therapy attempts in unresectable HCC using radiation only recently have been published with the appearance of toxicity data from carefully conducted clinical studies using CT-based 3DCRT. Seminal work by Lawrence and colleagues at the University of Michigan over the past decade has significantly increased our understanding of liver tolerance to radiotherapy and combined chemoradiotherapy *(6,10,11,13–22)*. With extensive clinical experience using 3DCRT in daily and twice-daily radiation fractions and combined with hepatic artery infusion of different chemotherapy agents, a clearer understanding now exists as to the limits of this approach, and predictive models of RILD are being created to design the next generation of clinical trials *(10,23–25)*.

Predictive models, or normal tissue complication probability (NTCP), use clinical outcomes from partial liver radiotherapy and chemoradiotherapy experiences, based on quantified volumes of the liver that received a specific dose of radiation, which lead to RILD or other toxicity. They incorporate the entire treatment plan and can describe dose-volume relationships of the liver between inhomogeneous dose distributions *(10)*. Dose escalation trials reported by Dawson have shown safety and tumor regression in HCC and other hepatobiliary cancers, with doses between 28.6 Gy and 90 Gy in combination with concurrent hepatic artery infusion of fluorodeoxyuridine *(19)*. A response rate of 68% was achieved, with only one case of RILD, grade 3 (which was reversible) and no treatment-related deaths. The team saw, not surprisingly, a dose-response advantage in progression-free survival for the 70- to 90-Gy cohorts. No maximum tolerated dose (MTD) has been reached, and radiation dose escalation is ongoing *(19)*.

Multicenter cooperative group trials have been attempted only by the Radiotherapy Oncology Group (RTOG), and these predated 3DCRT and NTCP modeling, which now enable partial liver doses >90 Gy. The first, RTOG 83-19, tested the addition of ^{131}I antiferritin monoclonal antibodies to doxorubicin plus 5-fluorouracil to patients who had first had entire liver radiotherapy to 21 Gy in large daily fractions of 3 Gy *(26)*. This study is very different in design from current liver radiotherapy practice, which uses smaller fractions once or twice, partial liver volumes, and hepatic artery infusion chemotherapy, with or without transarterial chemoembolization (TACE). Single-fraction doses of more than 2 Gy per day are known to increase late effects in the end organ, such as fibrosis, whereas small fractions given twice daily are believed to spare the organ from late injury, that is, RILD *(3)*. The outcome of the RTOG experience was negative with ^{131}I antiferritin, and the successor trial (RTOG 88-23) was also negative, with the same radiotherapy components; however, a chemotherapy change using cisplatin suggested some activity to the combination *(27)*.

External beam radiation has been delivered with 3DCRT for unresectable HCC in daily radiation fractions to more than 35 Gy with TACE and for salvage of TACE failures *(28–30)*. Seong et al. *(28)* reported the use of 3DCRT (mean tumor dose: 44 ± 9.3 Gy) in combination with chemoembolization with doxorubicin and lipiodol in 30 patients with unresectable HCC. In this small group, a 63.3% objective response was noted, along with median survival of 17 months without a treatment-related death. In a subsequent report, Seong et al. *(29)* delivered external beam radiation (mean tumor dose: 51.8 ± 7.9 Gy) to 24 patients with unresectable HCC who had progressed after TACE with lipiodol-Adriamycin (doxorubicin [generic]) mixture. They noted an encouraging response rate of 66.7%, a 3-year survival rate of 21.4%, and no treatment-related deaths. In an update on both previously reported groups with additional patients treated to a total of 158 (107 patients concurrent with TACE, 51 as salvage), Seong et al. *(30)* analyzed prognostic factors for response rate and overall survival. On univariate analysis, tumor size, portal vein thrombosis, and radiation dose were significant, but only radiation dose was significant on multivariate analysis. The mean radiation dose to the tumor for the entire cohort was 48.2 ± 7.9 Gy at 1.8 Gy/day. Park et al. *(31)* studied the same patient cohort as Seong et al. *(30)* and determined that a dose–response relationship existed, with dose groupings of <40 Gy, 40–50 Gy, and >50 Gy. An autopsy study of seven patients after radiotherapy for HCC suggested viable tumor remained despite doses of 50–70 Gy *(32)*. Using two-dimensional treatment planning to deliver external beam X-rays with TACE,

Guo et al. *(33)* reported the result in 107 patients with unresectable HCC. This retrospective study also found increasing radiation dose to be a prominent factor in objective tumor response, as well as the number of tumors. The radiation dose range was 22–55 Gy in 1.6- to 2.0-Gy/day fractionation using a moving strip technique to treat the entire liver in 78 patients.

Proton radiation therapy has been used, primarily in Japan, for HCC. A fundamental difference between X-rays of traditional external beam radiotherapy and protons is that because of charge and mass, protons can be delivered into deep tissues with lower dose deposition above and below the target than X-rays, releasing nearly all of their energy within the tumor. Because of the enormous cost of constructing these accelerators, which require a cyclotron onsite, they currently are available only at two centers in the United States and several other centers worldwide. Clinical use is mostly for central nervous system, spinal cord, ocular, cranial base, and prostate tumors. Protons have similar efficacy to X-rays in destroying tumor cells, but more normal tissue can be spared because of its physical dose deposition characteristics *(34)*. Between 1983 and 2000, the Proton Medical Research Center at the University of Tsukuba treated more than 236 patients with HCC. The dose per fraction was 4.5 Gy daily to a total dose of 72 cobalt gray equivalent (CGE) in 3.2 weeks. Dose is quoted in CGE to denote the dose in Gy multiplied by the radiation biological effectiveness unit, 1.10 (X-rays are 1.0). For small HCC tumors, Tokuuye et al. *(35)* reported a 3-year actuarial local control rate of 93%. Matsuzaki et al. *(36)* reported the use of protons for 24 patients failing TACE for HCC and found tumor response in more than 90% of these lesions. Proton beam therapy may become more common as new facilities planned worldwide become operational. Another highly conformal approach, stereotactic single-dose radiotherapy, has been studied in a phase I/II trial of mixed neoplasia in the liver, which included one HCC patient. Herfarth et al. *(37)* demonstrated feasibility of the technique to deliver 14–26 Gy in a single fraction to the liver (with the 80% isodose surrounding the planning target volume) to 60 tumors in 37 patients.

5.2. Brachytherapy

5.2.1. ^{131}I-Lipiodol

Most commonly, brachytherapy for HCC has been accomplished by hepatic artery infusion of ^{90}Y-embedded microspheres, or ^{131}I-lipiodol. The rationale for hepatic artery infusion is anatomic observation that tumors receive more than 80% of their blood supply from the hepatic artery, as opposed to normal hepatic triads, which receive the converse 80% supply of nutrients from the portal system. With the tumor/normal tissue ratio thus favorable from the hepatic artery, lipiodol, used for years in nonradiation embolic therapy in the liver (containing 38% iodine by weight), was a logical choice to add a radioisotope. In animal studies, ^{131}I-lipiodol had a significantly longer half-life in tumor as opposed to normal liver parenchyma. ^{131}I is a pure β-emitter with limited range penetration of electrons, thereby sparing normal liver adjacent to the tumor from significant dose. In an excellent review of clinical studies using ^{131}I-lipiodol by Ho et al. *(38)*, there were 14 studies between 1985 and 1997, with more than 400 patients having received this therapy *(39)*. Most patients with unresectable HCC were treated for amelioration of symptoms; response rates were 25–70% in uncontrolled studies. Raoul et al. *(39)* reported a multicenter randomized study of patients with portal vein thrombosis from HCC who received 10–100 Gy in one to five injections and had better survival than the control (untreated) group. In a separate prospective trial of 142 patients with unresectable HCC, randomization was to ^{131}I-lipiodol vs chemoembolization with cisplatin (70 mg). There was no difference in survival or tumor response between the two therapies; however, toxicity was less with ^{131}I-lipiodol *(40)*.

In the adjuvant setting, postoperative ^{131}I-lipiodol has been tested in a prospective randomized trial by Lau et al. *(41)* that was stopped early. Randomized patients after resection in the experimental arm received ^{131}I-lipiodol (1850 MBq in a single dose) or no further therapy (control group). Interim analysis of 21 treated and 22 control patients showed a statistically significant decrease in recurrence (28.5 vs 59%) and improved median disease-free survival (57.2 vs 13.6 months) for the treated patients.

5.2.2. Microspheres

The rationale for microsphere treatment is infusion of a sphere charged with ^{90}Y that will undergo β-decay with energetic electrons penetrating only 2–8 mm over a half-life of 64 hours. Microspheres range in diameter from 20 to 40 μm such that they will become embedded within the tumor vasculature; however, because the end arterioles are fewer than 10 μm in diameter, they will not pass into the venous circulation. The lungs are the next arteriole bed that would capture the spheres (Figs. 1 and 2). Pulmonary tolerance to radiation is roughly half (<20 Gy) that of the liver, and unintentional deposition of microspheres with ^{90}Y has led to deaths in past trials *(42,43)*. Arteriovenous shunts in the liver that

Fig. 1. (*opposite page*) **(A)** An electron micrograph of glass microspheres adjacent to a human hair for perspective. ^{90}Yttrium, a pure b-emitter, is permanently embedded within the ceramic matrix, becoming an active radioisotope after bombardment in a neutron flux of a nuclear reactor. A standard dose will include 4–7 million microspheres, with a decay half-life of 64.5 hours, delivering 150–350 Gy to a tumor over the entire life of the isotope (original magnification, ¥200) *(53,72,78)*. **(B)** CT-based reconstruction from radiation therapy treatment planning software of a predominately right-sided tumor (red) with transparent (purple) liver volume. The patient received two separate infusions of glass microspheres, resulting in a substantial reduction in tumor volume and tumor markers.

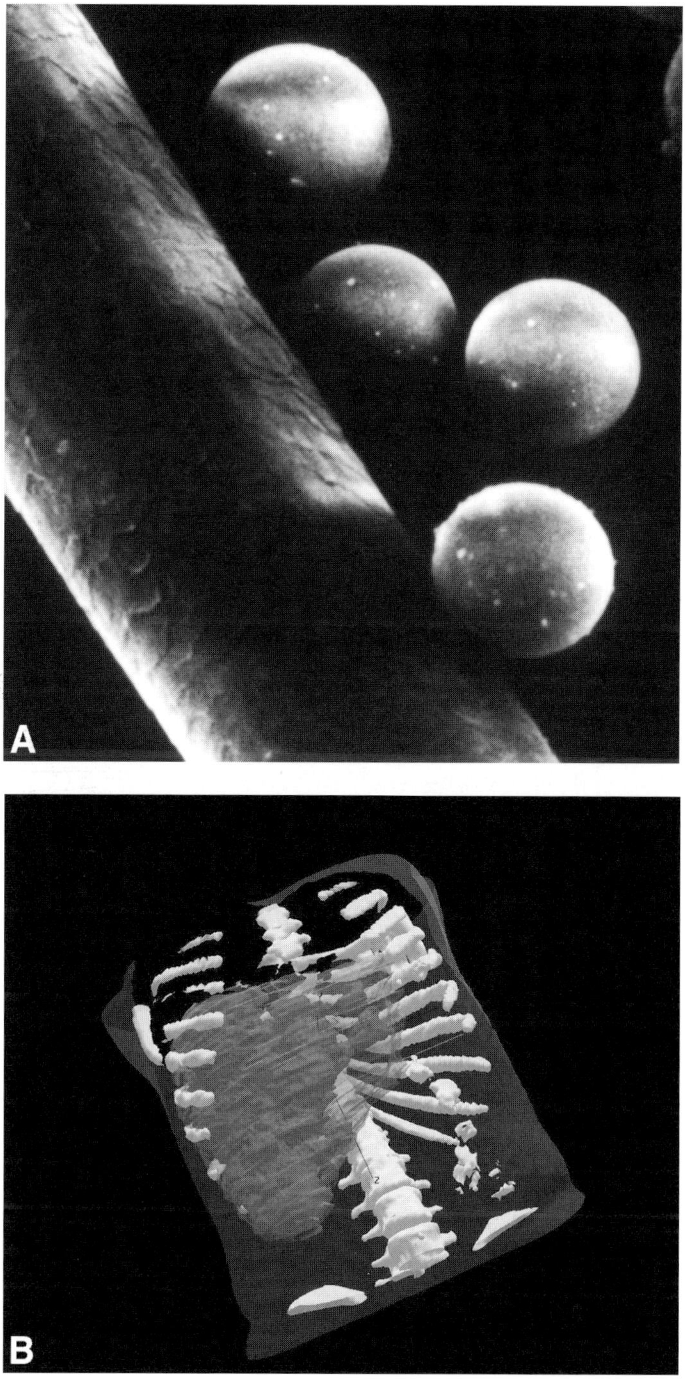
A
B

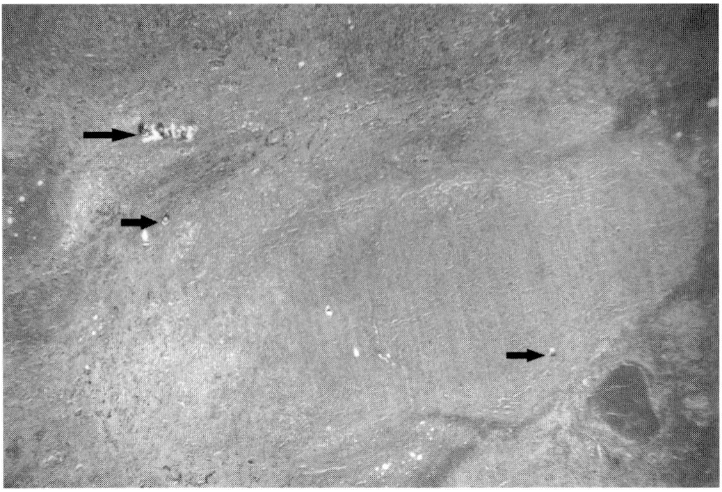

Fig. 2. Photomicrograph of glass microspheres (arrows) in clusters within a tumor nodule of HCC. Significant necrosis was seen in the region, without viable tumor cells, after a single infusion into the right lobe 4 weeks before liver transplantation (original magnification, ×100; photo courtesy of Drs. Charles Nutting and Cinthia Drachenberg).

would allow free passage of microspheres into the venous system and then to the lungs are not readily apparent on angiogram. Therefore, patient screening involves detailed hepatic angiographic mapping coupled with nuclear imaging using albumin tagged with a γ-emitter, technecium-99 (^{99m}Tc-MAA), injected into the hepatic artery. It is then possible to calculate the percentage of shunting of ^{99m}Tc in the lung compared with the known amount infused into the liver. Typically, if more than 10–15% of the dose appears in the lungs, a dose reduction of microspheres is attempted or the procedure is aborted *(44–46)*. Infusion of the entire liver can be accomplished in a single infusion; however, this will increase toxicity versus a sequential lobar approach with a 4-week interval between infusions *(44)*.

Ariel *(47)*, Ariel and Pack *(48)*, and Simon et al. *(49)* were the first investigators to perform microsphere clinical trials in humans. Most patients had metastatic carcinoid or colorectal cancers in the early 1960s–. Their pioneering work was with composite spheres and ^{90}Y, but their treatment procedures for screening, infusion, and posttreatment imaging are largely intact in modern clinical practice *(44,50–59)*. There are two microsphere devices available in the United States: the glass microsphere (TheraSphere) and the resin-based sphere (SIR-Spheres), which are similar in size and isotope (^{90}Y) but have some important differences in delivery and physical characteristics (Table 1) *(60)*. Both began in clinical trials in the late 1980s and have been used in hundreds of patients since,

Table 1
Comparison of Radioactive Microsphere Agents

Parameter	*Glass*[a]	*Resin*[b]
Size (median)	25 mm	32 mm
Isotope	^{90}Y	^{90}Y
Number of spheres in standard dose	4 million (range: 2–8 million)	40 million (range: 30–80 million)
Total activity infused in typical treatment	5 GBq (range: 3–20 GBq)	2.5 GBq (range: 0.8–3.0 GBq)
Activity per microsphere for typical treatment	2500 Bq	50 Bq
Indication(s)	HCC (United States)	Colon (USA)
Indications approved by FDA	HCC and colon (Canada)	All tumor types (Asia)
Regulatory status (FDA)	Humanitarian device exemption (HDE) for HCC only	Premarket approval (PMA) colorectal cancer liver for metastases
Limitations on treatment	High radiation dose in cirrhotic patients	High risk of embolic complications resulting from large number of microspheres

Abbreviations: FDA, Food and Drug Administration.
[a]MDS Nordian, Ottawa, Canada.
[b]Sirtex Medical, Sydney, Australia.

mostly with colorectal metastases; however, sufficient numbers of HCC patients have been treated to make some observations *(42,45,51,54,55,61–67)*. Dancey et al. *(42)* reported a phase II trial of glass microspheres for unresectable HCC in 22 patients. Whole-liver treatment in a single infusion was delivered, with a target dose of 100 Gy (median: 104 Gy; range: 46–145 Gy). There was one death related to pulmonary complications in a patient with a known high shunt fraction, but other toxicities were judged to be acceptable. The response rate was 20%, the median duration of response was 127 weeks, and the median survival was 54 weeks.

Carr et al. *(64)* and Carr *(67)* presented a report of a phase II trial of glass microspheres via lobar approach, with a nominal target dose of 135 Gy and a quality-of-life companion study *(65,68)*. They also statistically compared survival of published untreated Okuda I and II patients *(69–71)* with their study cohort (Fig. 3) *(65,67)*. Tumor reductions were documented in 42 patients (64.6%) via decreased vascularity, with 25 patients (38.4%) having a partial response by CT. Median survival for Okuda stage 1 (42 patients) was 649 days

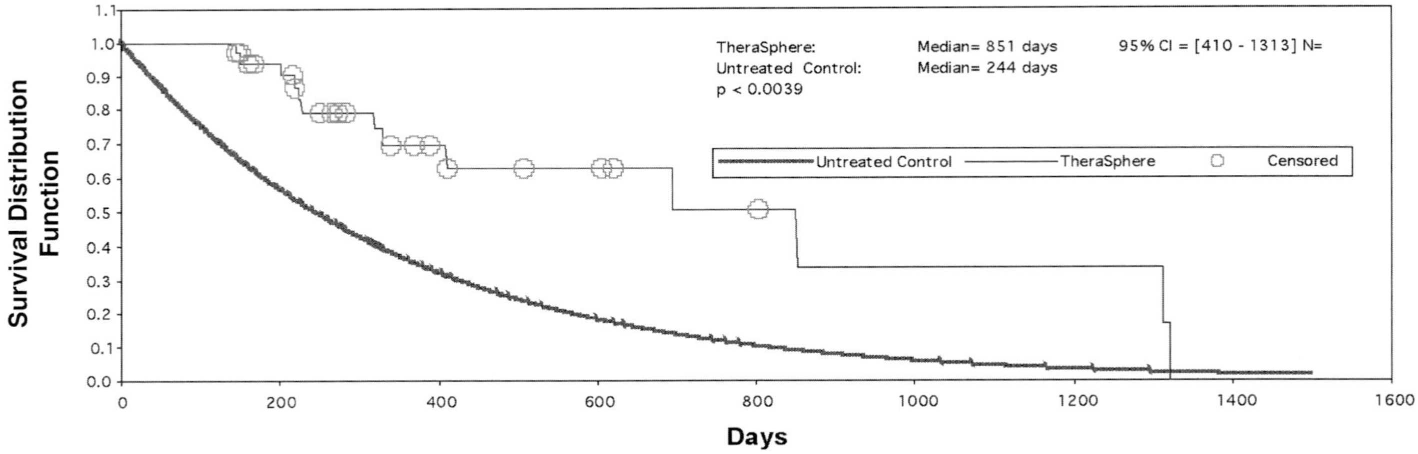

Fig. 3. Kaplan–Meier survival plots comparing results of TheraSphere-treated patients with historical cohorts for **(A)** Okuda stage I patients and **(B)** Okuda stage II patients. The historical cohort survival plots are based on the assumption that the historical survival distributions follow an exponential distribution $e^{-Œ^{a}*t}$, where $Œ^{a}$=ln(2)/median(days) *(65,69–71)*.

(range: 360–1012 days) compared with an historical median of 244 days. The advantage was even more pronounced in those with Okuda stage II (23 patients), with a median survival after microspheres of 302 days (range: 166–621 days) vs an historical median survival of 64 days. Toxicity and quality of life were good, with only one patient judged to have died of causes related to microsphere therapy. The quality-of-life report of this patient group compared hepatic artery infusion with cisplatin vs microspheres, revealing a small advantage to microsphere therapy. Toxicity and survival in a group of 14 patients with unresectable HCC by Kennedy et al. *(72)* and 16 patients by Soulen et al. *(73)* were very similar to those reported by Carr et al., with elevated enzymes, nausea, and fatigue being the most frequent common toxicity grade 2 or 3 findings. The dose delivered was different in all three studies; Kennedy et al. *(72)* delivered a median dose of 149 Gy (range: 128–174 Gy) to the whole liver with a 9-month survival of 75%, Soulen et al. *(73)* delivered a mean of 128 Gy (range: 97–182 Gy), and Carr et al. delivered a mean of 133 Gy *(65)*. Resin microspheres used by Lau et al. *(61)* in 71 patients with unresectable HCC demonstrated significant activity, with two patients found to have a pathological complete response after repeated treatments. Because the calculation of dose delivered is different regarding resin spheres and glass spheres, it is not possible to compare dose in Gy; however, the doses (cumulative) reported by Lau et al. *(61)* exceeded 500 Gy in the tumor. Previously, Lau et al. *(62)* suggested a dose–response (>120 Gy) in an 18-patient cohort of inoperable HCC patients.

Estimating dose delivered in the tumor vs normal liver is problematic in microsphere therapy *(74–78)*, but it is clear from the literature that in the doses used and reported in either glass or resin spheres, the toxicity profile is fairly low, and responses by imaging and tumor markers are consistently good and in agreement between various researchers. With the widespread availability of this treatment method in Europe, North America, and Asia, increasing numbers of centers are beginning treatment protocols using microspheres alone or in combination with chemotherapy.

REFERENCES

1. Zeman E. Biologic basis of radiation oncology. In: *Clinical Radiation Oncology* (Gunderson L, Tepper J, eds.), Churchill Livingstone, Philadelphia, 2000, pp. 1–41.
2. Sailer SL. Three dimensional conformal radiotherapy. In: *Clinical Radiation Oncology* (Gunderson L, Tepper J, eds.), Churchill Livingstone, Philadelphia, 2000, pp. 236–255.
3. Hall E. *Radiobiology for the Radiologist*, Lippincott Williams & Wilkins, Philadelphia, 2000, pp. 5–16, 80–87.
4. Kennedy AS, Raleigh JA, Varia MA, et al. Proliferation and hypoxia in human squamous cell carcinoma of the cervix: first report of combined immunohistochemical assays. *Int J Radiat Oncol Biol Phys* 1997;37:897–905.

5. Withers HR. Gastrointestinal cancer: radiation oncology. In: *Gastrointestinal Oncology: Principles and Practice* (Kelsen DP, Daly JM, Levin B, Kern SE, Tepper JE, eds.), Lippincott Williams & Wilkins, Philadelphia, 2002, pp. 83–96.
6. Lawrence TS, Robertson JM, Anscher MS, Jirtle RL, Ensminger WD, Fajardo LF. Hepatic toxicity resulting from cancer treatment. *Int J Radiat Oncol Biol Phys* 1995;31:1237–1248.
7. Ingold J, Reed G, Kaplan H. Radiation hepatitis. *Am J Roentgenol* 1965;93:200–208.
8. Ogata K, Hizawa K, Yoshida M. Hepatic injury following irradiation: a morphologic study. *Tukushima J Exp Med* 1963;9:240–251.
9. Austin-Seymour MM, Chen GT, Castro JR. Dose volume histogram analysis of liver radiation tolerance. *J Radiat Oncol Biol Phys* 1986;12:31–35.
10. Dawson LA, Ten Haken RK, Lawrence TS. Partial irradiation of the liver. *Semin Radiat Oncol* 2001;11:240–246.
11. Lawrence TS, Ten Haken RK, Kessler ML, et al. The use of 3-D dose volume analysis to predict radiation hepatitis. *Int J Radiat Oncol Biol Phys* 1992;23:781–788.
12. Fajardo LF, Berthrong M, Anderson RE. *Radiation Pathology*. Oxford University Press, New York, 2001.
13. Lawrence TS, Tesser RJ, Ten Haken RK. An application of dose volume histograms to the treatment of intrahepatic malignancies with radiation therapy. *Int J Radiat Oncol Biol Phys* 1990;19:1041–1047.
14. Lawrence TS, Davis MA, Maybaum J, et al. The potential superiority of bromodeoxyuridine to iododeoxyuridine as a radiation sensitizer in the treatment of colorectal cancer. *Cancer Res* 1992;52:3698–3704.
15. Lawrence TS, Kessler ML, Robertson JM. 3-D conformal radiation therapy in upper gastrointestinal cancer. The University of Michigan experience. *Front Radiat Ther Oncol* 1996;29:221–228.
16. Lawrence TS, Kessler ML, Robertson JM. Conformal high-dose radiation plus intraarterial floxuridine for hepatic cancer. *Oncology* 1993;7:51–57.
17. Lawrence TS, Dworzanin LM, Walker-Andrews SC, et al. Treatment of cancers involving the liver and porta hepatis with external beam irradiation and intraarterial hepatic fluorodeoxyuridine. *Int J Radiat Oncol Biol Phys* 1991;20:555–561.
18. Lawrence TS, Davis MA, Stetson PL, Maybaum J, Ensminger WD. Kinetics of bromodeoxyuridine elimination from human colon cancer cells in vitro and in vivo. *Cancer Res* 1994;54:2964–2968.
19. Dawson LA, McGinn CJ, Normolle D, et al. Escalated focal liver radiation and concurrent hepatic artery fluorodeoxyuridine for unresectable intrahepatic malignancies. *J Clin Oncol* 2000;18:2210–2218.
20. Dawson LA, Brock KK, Kazanjian S, et al. The reproducibility of organ position using active breathing control (ABC) during liver radiotherapy. *Int J Radiat Oncol Biol Phys* 2001;51:1410–1421.
21. McGinn CJ, Lawrence TS. Clinical results of the combination of radiation and fluoropyrimidines in the treatment of intrahepatic cancer. *Semin Radiat Oncol* 1997;7:313–323.
22. McGinn CJ, Ten Haken RK, Ensminger WD, Walker S, Wang S, Lawrence TS. Treatment of intrahepatic cancers with radiation doses based on a normal tissue complication probability model. *J Clin Oncol* 1998;16:2246–2252.
23. Ten Haken RK, Balter JM, Marsh LH, Robertson JM, Lawrence TS. Potential benefits of eliminating planning target volume expansions for patient breathing in the treatment of liver tumors. *Int J Radiat Oncol Biol Phys* 1997;38:613–617.
24. Ten Haken RK, Lawrence TS, McShan DL, Tesser RJ, Fraass BA, Lichter AS. Technical considerations in the use of 3-D beam arrangements in the abdomen. *Radiother Oncol* 1991;22:19–28.

25. Ten Haken RK, Martel MK, Kessler ML, et al. Use of Veff and iso-NTCP in the implementation of dose escalation protocols. *Int J Radiat Oncol Biol Phys* 1993;27:689–695.
26. Order SE, Pajak T, Leibel S, et al. A randomized prospective trial comparing full dose chemotherapy to I131 antiferritin: an RTOG study. *Int J Radiat Oncol Biol Phys* 1991;1:953–963.
27. Abrams RA, Pajak T, Haulk TL, et al. Survival results among patients with alpha-fetoprotein-positive, unresectable hepatocellular carcinoma: analysis of three sequential treatments of the RTOG and Johns Hopkins Oncology Center. *Cancer J* 1998;4:178–184.
28. Seong J, Keum KC, Han KH, et al. Combined transcatheter arterial chemoembolization and local radiotherapy of unresectable hepatocellular carcinoma. *Int J Radiat Oncol Biol Phys* 1999;43:393–397.
29. Seong J, Park HC, Han KH, et al. Local radiotherapy for unresectable hepatocellular carcinoma patients who failed with transcatheter arterial chemoembolization. *Int J Radiat Oncol Biol Phys* 2000;47:1331–1335.
30. Seong J, Park HC, Han KH, et al. Clinical results and prognostic factors in radiotherapy for unresectable hepatocellular carcinoma: a retrospective study of 158 patients. *Int J Radiat Oncol Biol Phys* 2003;55:329–336.
31. Park HC, Seong J, Han KH, et al. Dose-response relationship in local radiotherapy for hepatocellular carcinoma. *Int J Radiat Oncol Biol Phys* 2002;54:150–155.
32. Aoki K, Okazaki N, Okada S, et al. Radiotherapy for hepatocellular carcinoma: clinicopathological study of seven autopsy cases. *Hepatogastroenterology* 1994;41:427–431.
33. Guo WJ, Yu EX. Evaluation of combined therapy with chemoembolization and irradiation for large hepatocellular carcinoma. *Br J Cancer* 2000;73:1091–1097.
34. Suit H. The Gray Lecture 2001: coming technical advances in radiation oncology. *Int J Radiat Oncol Biol Phys* 2002;53:798–809.
35. Tokuuye K, Matsui R, Sakie Y. Proton therapy for hepatocellular carcinoma. In: *Proton Therapy Oncology Group XXXV Proceedings* 2001, pp. 57,58.
36. Matsuzaki Y, Osuga T, Saito Y, et al. A new, effective, and safe therapeutic option using proton irradiation for hepatocellular carcinoma. *Gastroenterology* 1994;106:1032–1041.
37. Herfarth KK, Debus J, Lohr F. Stereotactic single-dose radiation therapy of liver tumors: results of a phase I/II trial. *J Clin Oncol* 2001;19:164–170.
38. Ho S, Lau WY, Leung TW, Johnson PJ. Internal radiation therapy for patients with primary or metastatic hepatic cancer: a review. *Cancer* 1998;83:1894–1907.
39. Raoul JI, Guyader D, Bretagne JF. Randomized controlled trial for hepatocellular carcinoma with portal vein thrombosis: intra-arterial injection of 131I-labeled-iodized oil versus medical support. *J Nuclear Med* 1994;35(11):1782–1787.
40. Raoul JI, Guyader D, Bretagne JF, et al. Prospective randomized trial of chemoembolization versus intra-arterial injection of 131I-labeled-iodized oil in the treatment of hepatocellular carcinoma. *Hepatology* 1997;26:1156–1161.
41. Lau WY, Leung TW, Ho SK, et al. Adjuvant intra-arterial iodine-131-labelled lipiodol for resectable hepatocellular carcinoma: a prospective randomized trial. *Lancet* 1999;353: 943,944.
42. Dancey JE, Shepherd FA, Paul K, et al. Treatment of nonresectable hepatocellular carcinoma with intrahepatic 90Y-microspheres. *J Nucl Med* 2000;41:1673–1681.
43. Leung TW, Lau WY, Ho SK, et al. Radiation pneumonitis after selective internal radiation treatment with intraarterial 90yttrium-microspheres for inoperable hepatic tumors. *Int J Radiat Oncol Biol Phys* 1995;33:919–924.
44. Kennedy AS, Murthy R, Sarfaraz M, et al. Outpatient hepatic artery brachytherapy for primary and secondary hepatic malignancies. *Radiology* 2001;221P:468.
45. Van Echo DA, Kennedy AS, Coldwell D. TheraSphere (TS) at 143 Gy median dose for mixed hepatic cancers; feasibility and toxicities. *Am Soc Clin Oncol* 2001;260a:1038.

46. Coldwell D, Kennedy AS, Van Echo DA, et al. Feasibility of treatment of hepatic tumors utilizing embolization with yttrium-90 glass microspheres. *J Vasc Interv Radiol* 2001;12:S113.
47. Ariel IM. Treatment of inoperable primary pancreatic and liver cancer by the intra-arterial administration of radioactive isotopes (Y90 radiating microspheres). *Ann Surg* 1965;162: 267–278.
48. Ariel IM, Pack GT. Treatment of inoperable cancer of the liver by intra-arterial radioactive isotopes and chemotherapy. *Cancer* 1967;20:793–804.
49. Simon N, Warner RRP, Baron MG, Rudavsky AZ. Intra-arterial irradiation of carcinoid tumors of the liver. *Am J Roentgenol Radium Ther Nucl Med* 1968;102:552–561.
50. Murthy R, Line BR, Kennedy AS. Clinical utility of Brehmstralung scan (BRM-Scan) after TheraSphere (TS). *J Vasc Interv Radiol* 2002;13:S2.
51. Murthy R, Kennedy AS, Tucker G. Outpatient trans arterial hepatic 'low dose rate' (TAH-LDR) brachytherapy for unresectable hepatocellular carcinoma. *Proc Am Assoc Cancer Res* 2002;43:485.
52. Murthy R, Kennedy AS, Coldwell D. Technical aspects of TheraSphere (TS) infusion. *J Vasc Interv Radiol* 2002;13:S2.
53. Kennedy AS, Van Echo DA, Murthy R. Hepatic artery brachytherapy for neuroendocrine carcinoma. *Regulatory Peptides* 2002;108:32.
54. Gray BN, Anderson JE, Burton MA, et al. Regression of liver metastases following treatment with yttrium-90 microspheres. *Aust N Z J Surg* 1992;62:105–110.
55. Gray BN, Burton MA, Kelleher DK, Anderson J, Klemp P. Selective internal radiation (SIR) therapy for treatment of liver metastases: measurement of response rate. *J Surg Oncol* 1989;42:192–196.
56. Andrews JC, Walker SC, Ackermann RJ, Cotton LA, Ensminger WD, Shapiro B. Hepatic radioembolization with yttrium-90 containing glass microspheres: preliminary results and clinical follow-up. *J Nucl Med* 1994;35:1637–1644.
57. Blanchard RJ, Morrow IM, Sutherland JB. Treatment of liver tumors with yttrium-90 microspheres alone. *Can Assoc Radiol J* 1989;40:206–210.
58. Blanchard RJW. Treatment of Liver tumours with yttrium-90 microspheres. *Can J Surg* 1983;26:442,443.
59. Salem R, Thurston KG, Carr B. Yttrium-90 microspheres: radiation therapy for unresectable liver cancer. *J Vasc Interv Radiol* 2002;13:S223–S229.
60. Kennedy AS, Salem R. Comparison of two 90Yttrium microsphere agents for hepatic artery brachytherapy. In: *Proceedings of the 14th International Congress on Anti-Cancer Treatment* ICACT, Paris, France: 2003, pp. 156.
61. Lau WY, Ho S, Leung TW, et al. Selective internal radiation therapy for nonresectable hepatocellular carcinoma with intraarterial infusion of 90yttrium microspheres. *Int J Radiat Oncol Biol Phys* 1998;40:583–592.
62. Lau WY, Leung WT, Ho S, et al. Treatment of inoperable hepatocellular carcinoma with intrahepatic arterial yttrium-90 microspheres: a phase I and II study. *Br J Cancer* 1994;70: 994–999.
63. Houle S, Yip TK, Shepherd FA, et al. Hepatocellular carcinoma: pilot trial of treatment with Y-90 microspheres. *Radiology* 1989;172:857–860.
64. Carr B, Salem R, Sheetz M. Hepatic arterial yttrium labeled glass microspheres (TheraSphere) as treatment for unresectable HCC in 36 patients. *Proc Am Soc Clin Oncol* 2002, p. 139a.
65. Carr B, Torok F, Sheetz M. A novel and safe therapy for advanced-stage hepatocellular carcinoma (HCC): hepatic arterial 90Yttrium-labeled glass microspheres (TheraSphere). *Int J Cancer* 2002;(Suppl 13):459.
66. Willmott N, Daly JM. *Microspheres and Regional Cancer Therapy*. CRC Press, Boca Raton, FL, 1994, pp. 245.

67. Carr B. Hepatic arterial 90Yttrium glass microspheres (TheraSphere) for unresectable hepatocellular carcinoma: Interim safety and survival data on 65 patients. *Liver Transplant* 2004;10:S107–S110.
68. Steel J, Baum A, Carr B. Quality of life in patients diagnosed with primary hepatocellular carcinoma: hepatic arterial infusion of cisplatin versus 90-yttrium microspheres (Therasphere). *Psycho-Oncology* 2004;13:73–79.
69. Okuda K, Ohtsuki T, Obata H, et al. Natural history of hepatocellular carcinoma and prognosis in relation to treatment: study of 850 patients. *Cancer* 1985;56:918–928.
70. Pawarode A, Tangkijvanich P, Voravud N, et al. Outcomes of primary hepatocellular carcinoma treatment: an 8-year experience with 368 patients in Thailand. *J Gastroenterol Hepatol* 2000;15:860–864.
71. Sithinamsuwan P, Piratvisuth T, Tanomkiat W, et al. Review of 336 patients with hepatocellular carcinoma at Songklanagarind Hospital. *World J Gastroenterol* 2000;6:339–343.
72. Kennedy AS, Murthy R, Kwok Y. Hepatic artery brachytherapy for unresectable hepatocellular carcinoma: an outpatient treatment approach. *Proceedings of the 12th International Congress on Anti-Cancer Treatment* 2002;1:198,199.
73. Soulen M, Geschwind JF, Salem R. Y90 microsphere radioembolization of hepatoma: initial report of the U.S. multicenter trial. *Proc Soc Cardiovasc Intervent Radiol* 2002:175–176.
74. Burton MA, Gray BN, Jones C, Coletti A. Intraoperative dosimetry of 90Y in liver tissue. *Int J Radiat Appl Instrum B* 1989;16:495–498.
75. Burton MA, Gray BN, Kelleher DK, Klemp PF. Selective internal radiation therapy: validation of intraoperative dosimetry. *Radiology* 1990;175:253–255.
76. Ho S, Lau WY, Leung TW, et al. Partition model for estimating radiation doses from yttrium-90 microspheres in treating hepatic tumours. *Eur J Nucl Med* 1996;23:947–952.
77. Ho S, Lau WY, Leung TW, et al. Tumour-to-normal uptake ratio of 90Y microspheres in hepatic cancer assessed with 99Tcm macroaggregated albumin. *Br J Radiol* 1997;70: 823–828.
78. Sarfaraz M, Kennedy AS, Cao ZJ, Li A, Yu C. Radiation dose distribution in patients treated with Y-90 microspheres for non-resectable hepatic tumors. *Int J Radiat Biol Oncol Phys* 2001;51:32–33.

14 Putting It All Together

Practical Guidelines and Considerations for Physicians

Brian I. Carr, MD, *J. Wallis Marsh,* MD, *and David A. Geller,* MD

CONTENTS

From: *Current Clinical Oncology: Hepatocellular Cancer: Diagnosis and Treatment*
Edited by: B. I. Carr © Humana Press Inc., Totowa, NJ

A Patient With Any Tumor, Not for Transplant, With Child's B or C Cirrhosis, Encephalopathy, or Bilirubin Levels More Than 3.0 mg/dL
Clinical Evaluation and Work-up for Liver Transplant

1. INTRODUCTION

In the previous chapters, there was a systematic description of hepatocellular carcinoma (HCC) as a disease, its causes, clinical presentations, its various diagnostic tools, and treatment options that are available. This chapter offers some practical guidelines for the physician seeing a patient for the first time and some considerations of common management choices (Fig. 1).

2. SCREENING FOR HEPATOCELLULAR CARCINOMA

Much has been written on the subject of screening for HCC, including the usefulness of α-fetoprotein (AFP) as a marker and the best, simplest, and cheapest radiological method of treatment. There have been several papers showing that the cost–benefit of screening has not been proven, as judged by the cost for screening large populations that are known to be at risk compared with the small numbers of tumors that are detected at a treatable stage, as well as the false-positive outcomes. Without prejudice to the outcome of this ongoing debate, a patient in the United States who has chronic hepatitis B virus (HBV), chronic hepatitis C virus (HCV), or is known to be cirrhotic from any cause is at risk for subsequent development of HCC. Thus, cirrhosis is a premalignant condition. Considering that we know the cause of so few cancers of adult humans, it seems to us that the physician has an obligation to follow-up on patients with these diseases who are known to be at risk, in the hope of early diagnosis and, therefore, finding the HCC at a treatable stage. Therefore, it is our practice to perform twice-yearly computed tomography (CT) scans and AFP measurements, although the latter are elevated in only 50% of HCCs and there is no clear linearity between tumor size and AFP measurement. Given that the published figures for development of HCC in a patient with cirrhosis are between 2 and 5% per annum, it may be expected that routine annual or semiannual screening of patients with cirrhosis is likely to detect a reasonable number of HCCs at a treatable stage. All this needs to be weighed against the cost of managing patients at an advanced stage at diagnosis.

3. THE ROLE OF BIOPSY

Fine-needle aspiration biopsy is well-established, routine, and can detect cancer. It normally cannot supply the architecture for a confident diagnosis of

HCC Identified

Resection candidate

Resection
Noncirrhotic
Child's A
Single lesion
No metastasis

Transplant candidate

Transplant evaluation
1 lesion ≤ 5 cm
3 lesions ≤ 3 cm
Child's A/B/C
No gross vascular invasion
No metastasis

Yes
↓
Living donor transplant
Suitable donor

UNOS List (Cadaver)
MELD score (? > 3 mo)

No
↓
OLTX

Yes
↓
Neoadjuvant therapy
RFA/TACE/^{90}Yttrium

Not a surgical resect

Not a transplant Candidate
Co-morbid factors
≥ 4 lesions
Gross vascular invasi
LN (+) or Metastasis

PEI or Lap. RFA
Single lesion
< 5 cm
Child's A/B

Clinical Trials
← →

TACE/^{90}Yttrium/ New agents
Multi-focal
> 5 cm
Child's A/B/C
Bilirubin < 1.5

Palliative care/ Hormonal therapies
Child's C
Bilirubin ≥ 2
Metastases

Fig. 1. Treatment Decision Algorhythm.

HCC. Usually, only core-needle biopsy can do that. Recent practice in some areas, particularly in Europe, has been to avoid biopsy when there is presence of cirrhosis, a vascular liver lesion, and a rising AFP level. It is our practice to always perform a biopsy before treatment, whenever practical. We believe that this is important for two reasons. First, it gives us complete confidence that we have the correct diagnosis and the correct tumor histological type. Second, as we enter the age of molecular proteomics and molecular diagnostics, there are an increasing number of tests that allow us prognostic group stratifications that require tissue for either special stains, *in situ* hybridization, or gene expression. It has been argued that percutaneous needle biopsy is associated with a risk of spread by needle tracking. Although this has been reported, in our experience of the last 1300 needle biopsies for confirmation for the presence of HCC, we have seen this only in seven cases, and all of them have been in the track of the needle, typically the chest wall, and thus easily treated. As with everything in medicine, there is a risk-and-reward calculation that must be made. We believe that the benefit or reward of obtaining a correct tissue diagnosis and tissue for prognostication hugely outweighs the very low risk of needle tracking, an even rarer risk of tumor bleed, or other rarer complications associated with the presence of ascites.

4. WHAT IF THE FIRST BIOPSY COMES BACK NEGATIVE FOR CANCER OR IS INCONCLUSIVE?

There are several choices in this situation. They include a repeat biopsy, laparoscopic biopsy, or repeat CT scan and then biopsy in 3–4 months, especially if any one of the tumors appears to be growing. Sometimes there can be multiple nodules smaller than 1 cm and two or more biopsies have been negative. This can be a difficult situation, and repeat CT scan follow-up clearly is indicated in this situation.

5. METASTATIC DISEASE INVOLVING THE LUNGS, BONES, OR BRAIN

A symptomatic approach is required for all cancers, including brain radiation for brain metastases and spinal radiation for lytic or blastic metastases, that put any spinal vertebra or the pelvis at risk. The literature does not support any chemotherapeutic agent or combination of agents as being effective in this situation. We try to enroll all our patients in phase II or I studies for extrahepatic metastases. However, we often find patients whose disease is almost entirely confined to the liver, other than some periportal lymphadenopathy. In this situation, we focus on the 99% of the disease that is in the liver and we simply watch the lymph node disease. Quite often, this never seems to change. If the tumor does enlarge, however, it normally can be treated with external beam ionizing radiation.

6. WHAT IS THE BEST TREATMENT FOR ONE TO TWO HEPATIC LESIONS, EACH 3 CM OR SMALLER?

The choices here depend on the location of the tumor, specifically, its proximity to major vessels or bile ducts, but usually the treatment methods are PEI, radiofrequency ablation (RFA), or transarterial chemo-embolization (TACE). If the lesions are accessible, then either percutaneous ethanol injection (PEI) or RFA, depending on the operator skill and interest, would seem to be equivalent, and for small lesions at least, resection seems to be equal to PEI. The choice of treatment is also impacted by the severity of cirrhosis. Additionally, given the favorable curative new Model for Endstage Liver Disease (MELD) criteria, liver transplantation is a reasonable treatment option in this situation, especially in the presence of cirrhosis. We have a multidisciplinary weekly liver tumor conference, where all new and difficult cases are reviewed, before a treatment decision is made.

7. WHAT ARE THE TREATMENT OPTIONS FOR ONE TO TWO LESIONS OF ANY SIZE, WITH OR WITHOUT CIRRHOSIS AND WITH NORMAL LIVER FUNCTION TEST RESULTS?

A single lesion of any size in a noncirrhotic liver, or one with Child's A cirrhosis, and a small contralateral lesion has several treatment methods. Depending on the exact location and proximity to major blood vessels, resection of the single lesion and possibly either resection or RFA of the contralateral lesion may be a reasonable choice. If the main lesion cannot be resected, then TACE or hepatic ^{90}Yttrium microspheres are our preference. If cirrhosis is present, liver transplantation should be considered, given the favorable MELD score and the chance for cure.

8. WHO SHOULD OR CAN RECEIVE A LIVER TRANSPLANTATION?

The current guidelines include HCC as a single lesion less than 5 cm maximum in diameter or three HCC lesions, each 3 cm or smaller without gross vascular invasion of a main portal vein or portal vein branch or hepatic vein branch, and without metastases, regardless of the degree of cirrhosis. These patients have the highest possibility of complete cure because the liver transplantation treats both the cirrhosis as well as the HCC, unlike the above treatments. The United Network for Organ Sharing (UNOS) (cadaveric) and MELD scoring systems are updated regularly.

MELD was instituted on February 27, 2002, with a 6- to 40-point scale based on serum total bilirubin, international normalized ration (INR), and creatinine levels, with more severe disease having a higher score (http://www.unos.org/resources/meldpeldcalculator.asp). For patients with radiographic evidence of stage I HCC (one tumor up to 2 cm), 24 MELD points were assigned, and for those with stage II HCC (one tumor up to 5 cm, or up to three lesions all smaller than 3 cm, without gross vascular invasion or extrahepatic spread), 29 points were assigned. After 1 year, it became evident that this was too high a priority, and the points were decreased to 20 for stage I HCC and to 24 for stage II. Recently, the stage I HCC priority has been criticized, and a proposal to eliminate the stage I priority has been adopted.

9. WHAT ARE THE TREATMENT OPTIONS FOR ONE LESION MORE THAN 5 CM OR THREE LESIONS WITH ONE OR MORE BEING LARGER THAN 3 CM?

We approach this with TACE or hepatic ^{90}Yttrium in an attempt to downstage the size or the lesion in question. As soon as the patient has been restaged and can fit within the MELD score criteria for transplantation, then the patient undergoes a liver transplantation evaluation and is listed, if appropriate. Alternatively, the patient can undergo transplantation as a primary treatment (depending on the philosophy of the individual transplantation center), but the patient will not receive any additional MELD listing points.

10. A PATIENT WITH MULTIPLE LESIONS, ANY MORE THAN 5 CM AND WITHOUT METASTASES, WHO HAS A BLOOD GROUP-MATCHED FAMILY MEMBER WILLING TO ACT AS A LIVING-RELATED DONOR

Live donor transplantation has been used frequently in the past for patients with HCC because of the shortage of organs and rapidity of HCC growth. However, with the recent advent of the allowance of extra MELD listing points for patients with HCC (single lesion ,â§5 cm or three lesions none {GT}3 cm), the incidence of live donor transplantations for this group of patients has decreased. For those patients with single lesions larger than 5 cm or with more than three lesions, live donor transplantation is an option but is individualized within each transplantation program. Because the risk of recurrence in this group of patients is much higher, many programs will not offer live donor transplantations to this group. However, as we have recently found, patients with multiple lesions may have either multiple *de novo* tumors or intrahepatic metastases; these groups can be distinguished using currently available genotyping techniques. Patients with multiple small *de novo* could be considered for live donor transplantation, whereas the recurrence rate for patients with intrahepatic metastases is probably prohibitive. If the patient has a single, peripheral lesion larger than 5 cm without metastasis or hepatic or portal vein involvement, then the patient could be considered for live donor transplantation.

11. MULTIFOCAL HCC WITH TUMORS CONFINED TO THE LIVER WITH OR WITHOUT PORTAL VEIN THROMBOSIS AND BILIRUBIN LEVELS LESS THAN 2.0 mg/dL

These patients are treated with hepatic artery chemotherapy or chemoembolization (TACE) or ^{90}Yttrium glass microspheres into the hepatic artery. Patients seem to prefer the latter, because of the minimal side effects and the small total number of treatments that are usually required.

12. A PATIENT WITH ANY TUMOR, NOT FOR TRANSPLANT, WITH CHILD'S B OR C CIRRHOSIS, ENCEPHALOPATHY, OR BILIRUBIN LEVELS MORE THAN 3.0 MG/DL

These patients are normally referred for palliative or supportive care, or possibly phase II studies with noncytotoxic drugs, such as hormones or growth factor modulators.

13. CLINICAL EVALUATION AND WORK-UP FOR LIVER TRANSPLANT

The patients are evaluated by a multidisciplinary team at most transplantation centers that consists of transplantation surgeons, hepatologists, anesthesiologists, nurses, and social workers. The evaluation includes a thorough history and physical examination as well as an evaluation of the patient's cardiac and pulmonary functions. All patients undergo an endoscopy to assess for esophageal varices. Further, age-appropriate screening for other carcinomas should be performed (e.g., colonoscopy, mammography, pap smear, etc.). Blood work for tissue typing, tumor markers, viral disease (e.g., HBV, HCV, human immunodeficiency virus, cytomegalovirus, Epstein–Barr virus, etc.) and autoimmune markers are performed. All patients with HCC being considered for transplantation must have a current CT and MRI of the abdomen and pelvis as well as a CT of the chest. After the medical testing and fiscal clearance is obtained, the patient is presented at the transplant evaluation conference for listing.

Index

H

I

U

V,W, Y